Study Guide for Black & Hawks

Medical-Surgical Nursing

Clinical Management for Positive Outcomes

Seventh Edition

Susan Grinslade, PhD(c), RN
Assistant Professor
University of Texas Health Science Center
School of Nursing
San Antonio, Texas

Laurie J. Singel, MSN, RN, BC
Assistant Professor, Clinical
University of Texas Health Science Center
School of Nursing
San Antonio, Texas

Pamela L. Keys, MSN, RN
Instructor, Clinical
University of Texas Health Science Center
School of Nursing
San Antonio, Texas

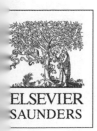

ELSEVIER
SAUNDERS

ELSEVIER
SAUNDERS
11830 Westline Industrial Drive
St. Louis, Missouri 63146

Study Guide for Medical-Surgical Nursing:
Clinical Management for Positive Outcomes, Seventh Edition

Copyright © 2005 by Elsevier Inc.

Previous editions copyrighted 2001, 1997, 1993

International Standard Book Number 1-4160-0258-8

Executive Publisher: Barbara Nelson Cullen
Senior Developmental Editor: Victoria Bruno
Publishing Services Manager: Gayle May

Printed in the United States of America

Last digit is the print number: 9 8 7 6 5 4 3 2

Preface

This Study Guide has been developed as a tool to assist you in evaluating your understanding of the information presented in the textbook *Medical-Surgical Nursing: Clinical Management for Positive Outcomes*, Seventh Edition. In mastering this information, you will obtain the knowledge and necessary skills that will be important to you in your nursing practice.

Learning will be enhanced by reading the textbook before class and by reviewing the study questions to guide your reading. The objectives that introduce each Study Guide chapter will also help guide you to the important content in the textbook chapter.

The introductory chapters provide a solid foundation with the sections "Understanding Terminology," "Theories and Trends," and "Reviewing Your Knowledge." The assessment chapters include anatomy and physiology labeling exercises with high-quality diagrams. Understanding the concepts covered in these sections will be basic to developing nursing care.

The clinical chapters will take you through the steps of nursing care. The section "Understanding Pathophysiology" covers the causes and mechanisms of disorders. The assessment of disorders and their clinical manifestations is covered in "Applying Your Knowledge," with short scenarios in selected chapters. "Best Practices" proceeds to implementing nursing care with diagnoses, interventions, and client education. "Keeping Drug Skills Sharp" covers pharmacological issues such as safety, dosage, indications for use, and contraindications.

Concept map exercises are included in selected chapters in the Study Guide. You can use these exercises to learn care of clients with specific disorders. The exercises are based on the concept maps that appear in your textbook.

Use the Study Guide as a review and then concentrate on content areas that are more difficult. If you are certain of the answer to a question, move on to the next one. You may find that what is most efficient for your time and learning is to only write in answers for questions that require you to use the textbook or for which you are not sure of the answer. Answers to all of the questions are included in the back of the Study Guide.

In nursing, a strong knowledge base is important, and understanding the basic concepts and principles is necessary in order to be prepared for patient care experiences. We hope that this Study Guide will assist you as you learn medical-surgical nursing care and that you will enjoy your experiences in clinical practice.

Contents

Chapter 1

Health Promotion

OBJECTIVES

1.1 Examine concepts of health, health promotion, and disease prevention.

1.2 Explore the nurse's role in implementing interventions to promote health.

1.3 Analyze specific risks and benefits of nutrition, exercise, social relationships, and the mind-body connection and health.

UNDERSTANDING TERMINOLOGY

1. State the WHO 1947 definition of health.

2. An integrated method of functioning which is oriented toward maximizing the potential of which the individual is capable within the environment where he or she is functioning is

_____.

3. True or False

_____ Disease is a failure of a person's adaptive mechanisms to adequately counteract stimuli and stresses, resulting in functional or structural disturbances.

4. Which of the following best describe the concept of illness?
   1. a state of being with social and psychological as well as biomedical components
   2. the presence of disease or infirmity
   3. a biological dysfunction which interferes with well-being
   4. a condition of being ill and unable to function optimally

5. Define *health promotion*.

6. Which of the following are true statements regarding risk factors?
   1. Risk factors, when present, indicate a disease or illness will occur.
   2. Family history is a behavioral risk factor.
   3. Risk factors, when present, are associated with an increased probability of disease.
   4. Pollution is a nonmodifiable risk factor.

7. List the three categories of risk factors and give an example of each.
   a.

   b.

   c.

8. Compare and contrast a modifiable and non-modifiable risk factor.

Modifiable Risk Factor	Non-modifiable Risk Factor

9. A judgment of one's ability to execute a specific behavior is _____ _____.

10. Another word to describe *self-efficacy* is _____.

11. Explain allostatic load.

12. Differentiate between recessive disease and a dominant disorder.

13. A cancer-causing substance is known as a _____.

THEORIES AND TRENDS

14. Dunn believes that health professionals focus on disease rather than wellness because _____
_____.

15. List the 10 leading health indicators that reflect the major public health concerns of Americans.

    a.

    b.

    c.

    d.

    e.

    f.

    g.

    h.

    i.

    j.

16. True or False

    _____ The belief that individuals want to avoid personal threats or illness is a basic premise of
    the Health Belief Model.

17. Match the Stages of Change from Prochaska and DiClimente's Transtheoretical Model to the appropriate description.

	Stages of Change		**Description**
_____	a.	Precontemplation	1. taking steps to avoid relapse
_____	b.	Contemplation	2. thinking about making a change in the near future
_____	c.	Preparation	3. making overt change
_____	d.	Action	4. planning actively and starting a behavior change
_____	e.	Maintenance	5. thinking seriously about making a change

8. Explain the principle behind gene therapy.

19. Which of the following is not a benefit of mind-body therapy?
    1. alter the immune system
    2. increase the pain experience
    3. reduce stress
    4. decrease anxiety

REVIEWING YOUR KNOWLEDGE

20. Explain why it is important to have a broad definition of health.

21. Within the nurse-client relationship, which of the following reflect the nurse's role with regard to the client's health? (Select all that apply)
    1. Display respect for the client's health choices and decisions.
    2. Assist the client to change his or her view of health.
    3. Support the client's participation in actualizing his or her health.
    4. Assist the client in understanding the priority of his or her values and perceptions.

22. High-level wellness requires what three actions?
    a.

    b.

    c.

23. What is the primary document that guides the United States' efforts to prevent disease and promote health?

24. True or False

    _____ Based on the epidemiology of how diseases originate and spread, interventions can be taken to reduce risk.

    _____ A benefit of beta-carotene that reduces the risk of cancer is that beta-carotene regulates cellular differentiation.

    _____ A client's definition of health remains static throughout his or her lifetime.

    _____ Wellness is the absence of clinical manifestations.

    _____ A person can have a disease without feeling ill.

    _____ According to the ANA, a nurse who is socially and politically active is not practicing nursing.

    _____ Unhealthy lifestyles account for more cancer than environmental chemical contamination.

_____ Children who drink milk are still subject to developing rickets if they have no exposure to sunlight.

_____ The manner in which an individual copes with everyday stressors can contribute to deficient levels of pituitary growth hormone.

_____ Health requires that individuals engage in meaningful relationships.

_____ Social support is believed to buffer individuals from the negative effects of stress.

_____ Planning and setting goals facilitates coping with stress.

25. The risk for disease or illness can be assessed through a _____
_____.

26. Which of the following are examples of the ways that fat appears to be a cancer promoter? (Select all that apply)
    1. causes the body to secrete fewer hormones
    2. increases the secretion of estrogen
    3. increases secretion of bile into the intestines
    4. alters cell membranes and changes them to be less resistant to carcinogens

27. Foods thought to reduce the risk of cancer are _____
    and _____.

28. Explain the benefits of alcohol to health.

29. An abnormal response to the allostatic load is _____.

30. What two diseases are associated with increased exposure to air pollution?
    a.

    b.

31. Match the following diseases with the appropriate vitamin deficiency.

Disease	Vitamin Deficiency
_____ a. Scurvy	1. Niacin
_____ b. Beriberi	2. Vitamin C
_____ c. Pellagra	3. Thiamine

32. Which of the following are true statements about the recommendation for exercise? (Select all that apply)
    1. One hour of exercise is recommended daily.
    2. To be beneficial exercise must be completed at one time each day.
    3. Exercise tones and strengthens the musculoskeletal system.
    4. Exercise reverses pathophysiologic changes.
    5. Exercise increases the production of endorphins.
    6. Exercise increases production of LDLs.

33. Describe the benefits of social support in chronic illness.

34. Which type of support group is an example of a Twelve-Step program?

35. Which of the following is a characteristic of a support group?
    1. facilitates repression of painful experiences
    2. fosters social isolation
    3. fosters dependence
    4. fosters self-esteem

APPLYING YOUR KNOWLEDGE

36. A client asks a nurse what foods he can eat to increase his consumption of antioxidants. The nurse's best answer would be:
    1. red meat
    2. milk
    3. carrots
    4. lima beans

37. The nurse is counseling a client with high cholesterol and advises the client to reduce saturated fat in his diet to less than _____.

BEST PRACTICES

38. Which of the following is the best example of primary intervention?
    1. screening for diabetes
    2. referral to rehabilitation after injury
    3. performing self-breast examination
    4. immunization against hepatitis A

39. Which of the following is the best example of secondary intervention?
    1. assessing a client's home for risk of falls
    2. teaching a client to apply sunscreen before sun exposure
    3. monitoring a client's blood pressure after starting antihypertensives
    4. immunizing a client with the flu vaccine

40. Which of the following is the best example of tertiary intervention?
    1. dental hygiene
    2. physical therapy after a back injury
    3. immunizing a client with the pneumonia vaccine
    4. wearing seat belts

41. Describe ways that nurses can empower clients.

42. Describe the four interventions to increase self-efficacy.
    a.
    b.
    c.
    d.

43. A nurse is assisting a client to make a behavior change related to diet. Which of the following nursing actions is most likely to increase the client's self-efficacy?
    1. providing the client with a handout on the Food Pyramid
    2. giving the client several opportunities to select healthy foods from a food menu
    3. admonishing the client when she makes an unhealthy food choice
    4. telling the client she will never succeed unless she is willing to give up all sweets

44. When health promotion teaching to change a client's health behavior is ineffective, the nurse's best action is to:
    1. recognize that the client is noncompliant.
    2. provide the client with additional information.
    3. assess the client's perception of his or her ability to change.
    4. reinforce previous teaching, using different teaching strategies.

45. Describe nursing interventions that can be implemented to prevent disease and disability associated with aging.

46. The most effective intervention to relieve stress is _____
    _____.

Health Promotion in Middle-Aged Adults

OBJECTIVES

2.1 Utilize *Healthy People 2010* and evidence-based guidelines for nutrition, activity, and prevention recommendations to promote the health of young and middle-aged adults.

2.2 Develop and implement nursing interventions which assist young and middle-aged adults decrease health risks.

2.3 Utilize effective strategies to assist young and middle-aged adults modify lifestyles and promote health.

UNDERSTANDING TERMINOLOGY

1. Match the negative health effects of stress to the type of response. Items may be used more than once.

Negative Effect	Type of Response
_____ a. depression	1. behavioral
_____ b. decreased ability to think	2. emotional
_____ c. headaches	3. physical
_____ d. chest discomfort	
_____ e. disrupted sleep	
_____ f. impatience	
_____ g. fatigue	

2. The three components of stress management intervention are:

a.

b.

c.

THEORIES AND TRENDS

3. Explain why a 3-day dietary log is most helpful in recognizing problematic eating behaviors.

4. Which of the following principles are used to guide the development of a realistic plan for addressing problem eating patterns/behaviors? (Select all that apply)
   1. decreasing the amount of certain types of foods
   2. substituting certain foods
   3. totally eliminating certain foods
   4. increasing certain foods

5. Current activity recommendations for adults state that they should accumulate _____ hour(s) of moderate activity every day.

6. Why is physical activity an effective intervention for stress management?

7. The goal of cognitive reappraisal is to change _____ or _____ of events as stressors.

8. List the risk factors for hepatitis B which indicate that a client should receive the hepatitis B vaccination series:
   a.

   b.

   c.

   d.

   e.

   f.

REVIEWING YOUR KNOWLEDGE

9. Which of the following are true statements about healthy activity? (Select all that apply)
   1. Sixty percent of adults get no leisure-time physical activity.
   2. Women are more inactive than men.
   3. Physical activity improves mood.
   4. Physical activity decreases the risk for heart disease.

10. List the four components of an exercise prescription:
    a.

    b.

    c.

    d.

11. Research has determined that people who successfully incorporate physical activity in their daily lives share three characteristics. List these characteristics:
    a.

    b.

    c.

12. True or False

    _____ To implement a successful healthy eating and physical activity prescription, a plan is needed to recognize and overcome probable barriers.

    _____ Tobacco is the single greatest cause of premature death in the United States.

    _____ Healthy eating is an effective intervention to resist stress.

13. The first step in helping a client manage stress is _____.

14. The nurse recognizes the goal of stress resistance is to _____ _____ the body's response to stress.

15. Explain how each of the following interventions is helpful for cognitive reappraisal:
    a. thought stopping

    b. refuting irrational ideas

c. guided imagery

d. effective coping

16. Young adults die prematurely for a number of reasons. Select the greatest causes of premature death in young adults. (Select all that apply)
    1. diabetes
    2. motor-vehicle accidents
    3. suicide
    4. heart disease
    5. stroke
    6. homicide

17. CAGE is a mnemonic that guides assessment of problem drinking. Which of the following assessment questions would the nurse use to assess the "A" component?
    1. Have you ever been told to avoid drinking?
    2. How much alcohol do you consume per day?
    3. What activities are associated with your drinking?
    4. Have people annoyed you by criticizing your drinking?

18. Which of the following is a characteristic of women at risk for violence?
    1. high self-esteem
    2. experience hopefulness
    3. married at age 25 or older
    4. living in households with high stress

19. Which of the following characteristics of a woman's partner increase her risk for abuse?
    1. been abused as a child
    2. social drinker
    3. shares relationship decision-making
    4. verbally supportive

APPLYING YOUR KNOWLEDGE

20. Identify the four nursing actions that can be implemented to assist in meeting *Healthy People 2010* goals for young and middle-aged adults.
    a.

    b.

c.

d.

21. Which of the following clients would be classified as obese?
    1. BMI of 15
    2. BMI of 21
    3. BMI of 27
    4. BMI of 32

22. An obese client states "I don't understand why I keep gaining weight; I eat much less than my sister." The nurse's best response would be?
    1. "Is your sister overweight also?"
    2. "Your sister probably does more exercise than you do."
    3. "Sometimes we think that we don't eat much but we really do."
    4. "It is not just the quantity of foods you eat but also the quality which contributes to weight gain."

23. The nurse is conducting a nutrition class about decreasing cancer risk through healthful eating. Which of the following clients' diets would the nurse recognize as potentially decreasing cancer risk?
    1. red meats, refined/processed grains, dairy products, and fruits
    2. fish and poultry, complex and concentrated carbohydrates, and vegetables.
    3. fish, whole grains, fruits, and vegetables
    4. fish, poultry, and red meats, refined/processed grains, fruits, and vegetables.

24. A nurse is counseling a client experiencing stress. The goal is to help the client: (Select all that apply)
    1. recognize stressors.
    2. cope effectively with stress.
    3. learn decision-making skills.
    4. learn positive thinking skills.
    5. recognize irrational thinking.

25. A nurse assesses a client for behavioral manifestation of stress. A positive finding would be:
    1. sore neck and shoulder muscles.
    2. increased blood pressure.
    3. anger.
    4. increased alcohol use.

26. When the nurse is planning a personalized eating and exercise prescription with the client, it is most important to consider:
    1. history.
    2. alternatives to exercise.
    3. perceived and actual barriers.
    4. penalties for non-compliance.

27 . Key factors when assessing a client for stress are: (Select all that apply)
   1. taking a history of manifestations.
   2. determining stressful situations.
   3. examining current coping behaviors.
   4. developing ineffective coping.
   5. developing a plan for coping.

28. When evaluating effectiveness of a stress management intervention, the nurse would know the intervention was effective when the client:
   1. overeats.
   2. has disrupted sleep.
   3. complains of a sore neck.
   4. practices relaxation techniques.

29. Which of the following foods would a client choose to promote coping with stress?
   1. red beans and rice
   2. noodle casserole
   3. chicken with mixed vegetables
   4. multigrain cereal and coffee

30. Which of the following describe physical and mental relaxation techniques? (Select all that apply)
   1. Progressive relaxation promotes how to relax all muscle groups.
   2. Breathing techniques are part of relaxation.
   3. Meditation increases blood pressure.
   4. Tai Chi is an active form of relaxation.

31. A nurse is teaching a defensive driving course for young adults. Discuss the prevention counseling that should be included and the rationale for each.

32. A nurse uses the Alcohol Use Disorders Identification Test (AUDIT) to assess a client for problem drinking. A client who scores _____ is considered a problem drinker.
   1. 2 or more
   2. 4 or more
   3. 6 or more
   4. 8 or more

33. A client is experiencing health consequences due to exposure to environmental tobacco smoke. Which of the following is the best example of a nurse acting in an advocacy role?
   1. telling family members of the client to stop smoking
   2. supporting social efforts to limit smoking in public places
   3. advising the client to switch jobs
   4. advising the client to wear a mask when exposed to environmental smoke

34. The highest priority nursing intervention for a client currently in a violent relationship is _____ _____.

~~B~~EST PRACTICES

5. According to the Institute of Medicine report on a healthy diet, the nurse would recommend total level of calories based on which of the following? (Select all that apply)
   1. age
   2. gender
   3. height
   4. weight
   5. body mass index (BMI)
   6. body fat %
   7. activity level

6. What is the underlying purpose of using PACE (Patient-centered Assessment and Counseling for Exercise and Nutrition) when counseling clients concerning physical activity?

7. Provide a rationale for the recommendation or non-recommendation for each of the following for stress management.
   a. eating simple carbohydrates

   b. overeating

   c. eating fruits

   d. adequate sleep and rest

8. A client comes to the clinic and presents with hypertension and diabetes. A health history reveals a 10-year, 2-pack-per-day smoking history. Using the stepped process for intervention, outline the five nursing actions to take with this client.
   a.

   b.

   c.

   d.

   e.

39. State the rationale for screening every female client for a history of or current abuse:

40. The two activities that are essential to protecting young adults from infectious diseases are:
    a.

    b.

41. State the frequency and rationale for the following recommended screenings for a 32-year-old woman.

Screening	Frequency	Rationale
a. height and weight		
b. Papanicolaou test		
c. assessment of problem drinking		

42. When a woman reaches the age of 50, what preventive screening measures are added on an annual basis?
    a.

    b.

Chapter 3

Health Promotion in Older Adults

OBJECTIVES

3.1 Examine sociodemographic and other factors related to the person over the age of 65 that influence health care services and quality.

3.2 Discuss physiologic and psychosocial factors which influence aging and functional status of older adults.

3.3 Describe support resources and ethical/legal issues which influence people over the age of 65.

UNDERSTANDING TERMINOLOGY

1. Differentiate between ADLs and IADLs.

2. Define *ageism*.

3. Define substance use disorders.

4. True or False

   _____ Competence is a legal term used to describe one's ability to make decisions for oneself.

   _____ Capacity is one's ability to make decisions, understand consequences, and manage one's affairs.

   _____ A durable power of attorney for health care is a legal document which grants another person the authority to make health care decisions if the grantor is unable to do so.

THEORIES AND TRENDS

5. What is the rationale behind the assessment of self-care abilities?

6. Describe the effects of ageism in our society.

7. List the six factors which contribute to poor relocation adjustment:
   a.

   b.

   c.

   d.

   e.

   f.

REVIEWING YOUR KNOWLEDGE

8. Nurses may need to advocate for quality health care and equitable distribution of health care resources for older women. Identify the factors which contribute to this need. (Select all that apply
   1. Only 43% of older women live with spouses.
   2. Traditionally these women assume dependent roles.
   3. Many elderly women are widows.
   4. The life expectancy for women is greater than for men.

9. According to the U.S. 2000 Census, what percentage of older adults lives in poverty?
   1. 7%
   2. 10.2%
   3. 12.4%
   4. 20%

10. Which of the following groups of older adults are least likely to have a high school education?
    1. white non-Hispanics and Hispanics
    2. African Americans and Native Americans
    3. Hispanics and African Americans
    4. Native Americans and white non-Hispanics

11. Quality of life (QOL) is a subjective perception of health capacities. List five factors known to affect perceived quality of life:
    a.

    b.

    c.

    d.

    e.

2. List five positive effects of physical activity on health in older adults.
    a.

    b.

    c.

    d.

    e.

3. A nurse is conducting a home visit of an older client and notes that the client's weight has been decreasing gradually over the last few months. What factors would the nurse consider which might contribute to this? State a rationale for each.

Factor	Rationale
a.	
b.	
c.	
d.	
e.	

14. True or False

_____ Older adults often fail to seek help for treatable conditions by accepting changes as inevitable.

_____ The combined effect of disease and disability effects on one's ability to perform tasks of everyday living is a person's functional ability.

_____ The presence of chronic illnesses in an older adult results in limitations of activities of daily living.

_____ All adults are presumed competent.

_____ Capacity is absolute.

_____ Advance directives encourage individuals to be partners in guiding medical treatment and to claim their rights in treatment decisions.

_____ In general, a living will affirms a person's right and desire to refuse life-prolonging interventions.

15. A thorough assessment of an older person's functional ability can be used: (Select all that apply)
    1. to detect problem areas.
    2. serve as a basis for recommendations that foster independence.
    3. to measure activities of daily living.
    4. to determine need for personal care.
    5. to plan long-term care.

16. Describe changes in sleep patterns experienced by older adults.

17. Explain why it is important for the nurse to assess the older adult for sensory impairments.

18. What percentage of nursing home admissions is related to falls?

19. List the three substances most often abused by older adults.
    a.

    b.

    c.

20. Two types of advance directives are _____ and
_____.

APPLYING YOUR KNOWLEDGE

1. Explain why family support is important to the older adult.

2. Which of the following is an appropriate goal for a health promotion program for older adults?
   1. maintain levels of independence
   2. increase productivity
   3. maintain mortality
   4. increase morbidity

3. The nurse is providing care to an older adult. During the assessment of self-care process, the nurse would emphasize the client's _____ rather than his or her _____.

4. A nurse is teaching the importance of physical activity to a group of seniors at a senior nutrition site. A senior asks why they should exercise, stating, "I'm too old and fat." The nurse's best response would be that exercise will:
   1. "help lower your blood pressure."
   2. "decrease osteoporosis."
   3. "decrease body fat and build lean muscle."
   4. "increase sense of well-being."

5. The experience of stress by an older adult may alter physical and emotional health. Which of the following factors are known to influence one's ability to cope with stress? (Select all that apply)
   1. personality
   2. past coping ability
   3. confidence in overcoming obstacles
   4. spirituality
   5. socioeconomic status

6. Which of the following is an effective teaching strategy when providing health education to an older client?
   1. Provide the most important information last.
   2. Speak in a louder than normal voice.
   3. Use large, easy to read typeface.
   4. Use blue and green paper for handouts.

7. The nurse is caring for an older client in the hospital. Nursing assessment for this client should be guided by an understanding that:
   1. acute illnesses are not effected by underlying chronic disease.
   2. diseases often have an atypical presentation.
   3. clinical manifestations are consistent with expected disease presentations.
   4. age and the number of pathologic conditions are indirectly correlated.

8. Explain why nurses should be concerned with polypharmacy in the older adults.

29. List two advantages of advance directives.
    a.

    b.

30. Research has determined that _____ impairments are early indicators of active illness in the older adult.

31. Discuss the advantage of an integrated system of care.

Chapter 4

Health Assessment

OBJECTIVES

4.1 Describe the purpose of, procedure for, and the nurse's role in conducting and documenting a comprehensive health assessment including the health history and physical examination.

4.2 Differentiate between different physical examination techniques and screening physical examinations.

4.3 Analyze different diagnostic procedures and tests and the related nursing responsibilities.

UNDERSTANDING TERMINOLOGY

1. The _____ is the client's subjective statement of the reason he or she is seeking health care.

2. Match each associated factor to explore during a symptom analysis (manifestation) with the appropriate description.

Associated Factor
_____ a. timing
_____ b. quality
_____ c. quantity
_____ d. location
_____ e. precipitating factor
_____ f. aggravating or relieving factor
_____ g. associated factors

Description
1. determines if anything causes the manifestation to be worse or better.
2. identifies where the manifestation occurs in the body and whether or not it is stationary or moves. May not be assessed if the answer is apparent.
3. determines if anything else has occurred in conjunction with the manifestation.
4. determines when the manifestation first occurred and what might have caused it.
5. asks for a description of the size, amount, number or extent of the manifestation in terms of intensity. Determines how the manifestation has affected other aspects of the client's life.
6. determines when the manifestation started, how long it has been present, and how often it occurs.
7. asks the client to describe the manifestation in terms of sharpness, dullness, etc.

3. Match each term associated with the mental status assessment with the appropriate definition.

Term	Definition
_____ a. flat affect	1. recall information within hours
_____ b. immediate memory	2. ability to perceive the self realistically and accurately
_____ c. mood	3. ability to focus or concentrate on a task or activity over time
_____ d. recent memory	4. observable, outward demeanor that depicts the current emotional state
_____ e. general fund of knowledge	5. recall information within minutes
_____ f. affect	6. actions and decisions made in daily living
_____ g. blunted affect	7. subjective description of a personal emotion that is pervasive and sustained
_____ h. remote memory	8. lack of any facial expression or emotional response accompanied by a monotonous voice
_____ i. attention span	9. inability to discriminate reality from misperceptions
_____ j. perceptual distortion	10. reduced in intensity but still appropriate to the situation
_____ k. insight	11. within hours, months, or years
_____ l. judgment	12. identification of common places, events, and people

4. Define each term related to vital sign measurement.
   a. hyperthermic

   b. hypothermic

   c. tachycardia

   d. bradycardia

   e. tidal volume

   f. hypotension

   g. hypertension

   h. pulse pressure

   i. auscultatory gap

5. Match each term with the appropriate definition.

	Term		Definition
_____	a. specificity	1.	ability of a test to correctly identify a disease
_____	b. sensitivity	2.	results of a test indicate the client has a disease when in fact the client does not have the disease
_____	c. false-positive	3.	results of a test indicate the client is free of a disease when in fact the client has the disease
_____	d. false-negative	4.	ability of a test to correctly identify a person who is disease free.

6. Compare and contrast genetic and somatic risk.

7. _____ is a radiographic technique that uses a contrast agent to assess blood vessels and the flow of blood through them.

8. Define *endoscopy*.

9. Match each term with the appropriate definition or description.

	Term		Definition or Description
_____	a. cytology	1.	special needle cuts a specimen from tissues not in view
_____	b. Pap test	2.	thin slice of tissue is cut and examined for a rapid microscopic diagnosis
_____	c. biopsy	3.	study of the anatomy, physiology, pathology, and chemistry of a cell
_____	d. needle aspiration biopsy	4.	entire lesion and a margin of surrounding normal tissue is removed
_____	e. excisional biopsy	5.	removal of tissue for diagnostic study
_____	f. frozen section	6.	aspirated cells are removed through a trocar or needle
_____	g. core needle biopsy	7.	test used to study vaginal or cervical cells

THEORIES AND TRENDS

10. Describe the advantages of using a computerized health history assessment.

11. Explain why Gordon's functional health patterns are a helpful way to organize health history information.

REVIEWING YOUR KNOWLEDGE

12. Which of the following describes nursing skill necessary to perform a health assessment? (Select all that apply.)
    1. It identifies physical and psychosocial needs.
    2. Advanced assessment techniques are required.
    3. It requires observation and decision-making skills.
    4. Proficiency requires practice.
    5. It requires ability to discriminate.
    6. It is comprised of several parts.

13. True or False

    _____ The health assessment begins with the physical examination.

    _____ One of the primary uses of a PET scan is to measure blood flow.

    _____ Health history formats are standardized across health care settings.

    _____ When a client enters the health care system, the nurse becomes the client's exclusive social network.

    _____ Inadequate financial resources can increase risk for accidental injury or trauma.

    _____ If a client has a modifiable risk factor present, he or she should always be provided with information about changing behavior and referred to a community resource.

    _____ Screening procedures are performed to determine potential or actual health problems.

    _____ The purpose of the physical examination is to differentiate normal from abnormal physical findings.

    _____ A balance scale is preferred for assessing a client's weight because of its accuracy.

    _____ The physical examination provides an excellent opportunity for the nurse to provide health teaching.

    _____ The SI System is a comprehensive modern form of the metric system that provides a common international language for measurement.

_____ Serial port sampling causes greater client discomfort due to multiple venipunctures.

_____ One of the benefits of fluoroscopy is that joint actions, organs, and entire body systems can be observed directly.

4. Compare and contrast the long versus the short health history format.

Long Format	Short Format

5. Identify the five essential components of a health history.
   a.

   b.

   c.

   d.

   e.

6. When gathering data about past health history, the nurse would not gather information about:
   1. usual childhood illnesses.
   2. family members' causes of death.
   3. hospitalizations.
   4. obstetric visits.
   5. allergies.

7. Which of the following variables affect a client's ability to respond to specific questions during a mental status exam? (Select all that apply)
   1. level of education
   2. cultural background
   3. degree of exposure to knowledge and information
   4. familiarity with the language and vocabulary
   5. perceived acceptance by the doctor

18. The cultural assessment is very broad in nature because it seeks information about:
    1. individual values.
    2. what the larger group's tenets mean to the individual.
    3. individual beliefs.
    4. individual behaviors.

19. Match each type of risk factor with the appropriate description.

	Type of Risk Factor	Descriptor
_____	a. genetic / biologic	1. living in an area subject to floods
_____	b. behavioral	2. family history
_____	c. environmental	3. diet high in fat

20. A foundation of _____ and _____ is key to developing skill in physical assessment

21. List and describe each of the four primary techniques used in physical assessment.
    a.

    b.

    c.

    d.

22. The physical examination begins with a _____.

23. The Romberg Test is used to assess the client's _____.

24. _____ is a systemic disease caused by bacteria and the toxins in the blood.

25. Which of the following are true statements about wound cultures? (Select all that apply)
    1. Cultures are performed to identify the presence of microorganisms in wounds.
    2. Specimens are collected using aseptic technique.
    3. Cultures are collected after antibiotic therapy is initiated.
    4. Additional precautions may be needed when collecting cultures from draining wounds.

26. The site for specimen collection using a microcapillary collection method is usually the
_____.

27. An early-morning urine specimen gives more definitive results because:
    1. the urine is not concentrated.
    2. clients are less likely to have difficulty providing a specimen when the bladder is full.
    3. the urine is not influenced by diet.
    4. it is an acceptable time for a random sample collection.

28. List the three purposes of x-ray examinations:
    a.

    b.

    c.

29. An advantage of an MRI over a CT scan is that the client is _____
_____.

APPLYING YOUR KNOWLEDGE

30. It is important for the nurse to observe the client closely:
    1. throughout the health history.
    2. at the beginning of the interview.
    3. during psychological assessment.
    4. when assessing risk factors.

31. To ensure an accurate health history the nurse should:
    1. obtain information from a secondary source.
    2. assume meaning if the client is reluctant to be forthcoming.
    3. be cognizant that the nurse's perceptions are always accurate.
    4. continually validate information gathered with the client.

32. During the family health history, the nurse assesses:
    1. immunization status.
    2. problems related to heart disease.
    3. quality, quantity, and duration of symptoms.
    4. frequency of social interactions.

33. During the general appearance component of the psychosocial assessment, the nurse assesses:
    1. grimacing.
    2. crying.
    3. orientation to time.
    4. manner of dress.

34. A client's motivation is influenced by:
    1. external resources.
    2. spiritual beliefs.
    3. personal needs and desires.
    4. genetic predisposition.

35. A client's socioeconomic status is influenced by:
    1. employment status.
    2. health habits.
    3. sleep patterns.
    4. leisure activities.

36. A nurse is assessing a client about the date a specific screening procedure was performed. Which question by the nurse is the best way to elicit this data?
    1. "You should have had a mammogram last month, did you?"
    2. "Why haven't you been to the dentist in over two years?"
    3. "When was your last eye examination and what were the results?"
    4. "With your history, you do go for a Pap smear every year, don't you?"

37. Match the following descriptions of physical examinations to their types.

	Description	**Type of Physical Examination**
_____	a. updates baseline data and assesses changes in health status	1. complete
_____	b. focuses on a specific body system	2. periodic head-to-toe
_____	c. superficial check of major body systems	3. regional
_____	d. comprehensive and includes ancillary procedures	4. screening

38. Match the components of the general appearance and behavior assessments with the appropriate description or indicator.

	Components of General Appearance	**Description or Indicator**
_____	a. level of cooperation	1. assessments are specific to the client
_____	b. body and breath odor	2. healthy or frail
_____	c. dress	3. obvious sign of pain or breathing difficulty
_____	d. gait	4. distribution of weight and height
_____	e. body build	5. erect, with hips and shoulders aligned over knees and ankles
_____	f. state of health	6. smooth and coordinated with arms swinging
_____	g. mental status	7. purposeful and controlled without tremors, tics, fasciculations, or spasticity
_____	h. hygiene and grooming	8. appropriate to time of year, temperature, age, and socioeconomic status
_____	i. movements	9. pleasant image
_____	j. posture	10. deficient hygiene
_____	k. distress or discomfort	11. level of consciousness
_____	l. age, sex, and race	12. interest and willingness to discuss information

39. A nurse assesses a client's vital signs as 101° F, 52 pulse, 16 respirations, 92/70 blood pressure. The client's vital signs are best described as:
    1. hypothermic, bradycardic, hypotensive, pulse pressure of 20.
    2. hyperthermic, tachycardic, hypotensive, pulse pressure of 22.
    3. hyperthermic, tachycardic, hypertensive, pulse pressure of 32.
    4. hyperthermic, bradycardic, hypotensive, pulse pressure of 22.

BEST PRACTICES

40. Which of the following are true statements regarding the processing of physical assessment data? (Select all that apply)
    1. Compare findings from one side of the body to the other.
    2. The human body is exactly symmetrical which makes detection of abnormalities easier.
    3. Normal parameters are the benchmark for comparing findings.
    4. Examine suspected problem areas revealed during the health history carefully.

41. An example of an interdependent nursing intervention related to diagnostic tests is:
    1. writing orders.
    2. interpreting test results for immediate action.
    3. directing laboratory and radiology technicians.
    4. ordering follow-up procedures.

42. A nurse is collecting a urine specimen from a client with an indwelling catheter. In order to collect the specimen, the nurse would:
    1. clamp the tubing below the collection port for 60 minutes.
    2. separate the drainage tube from the catheter.
    3. use a GU syringe to collect specimen from the catheter.
    4. cleanse and collect the specimen from the collection port.

43. An abnormal result in a client's urinalysis is:
    1. specific gravity 1.120.
    2. opacity clear.
    3. color yellow.
    4. glucose negative.

44. A client is scheduled for a CT scan using contract media. In preparing the client for the procedure, the nurse's most important action would be to:
    1. adjust food and fluid intake based on client history.
    2. explain the procedure and ensure that the client has given consent.
    3. assess the client for a history of claustrophobia.
    4. assess the client for an allergy to iodine.

45. Which statement made by a client scheduled for a CT scan with sedation indicates that the nurse needs to provide further teaching?
    1. "I shouldn't drink alcohol but I can have coffee on the day of the exam."
    2. "I shouldn't eat for 2 hours before the scan."

46. A client returns from an angiography procedure using a femoral approach. Which assessment finding would alert the nurse to potential complications?
    1. blood pressure 132/86, pulse 84
    2. voided 350 cc clear yellow urine
    3. capillary refill greater than 3 seconds
    4. a 1 inch diameter spot of dark blood on the femoral dressing

47. True or False

    _____ Prior to the client having an ultrasound of the uterus, the nurse should instruct her to void and empty her bladder.

    _____ Because emotional reactions to life situations and problems vary, the psychosocial history may be less reliable than objective assessment data.

48. A nurse is collecting blood for multiple blood studies. Explain why the nurse would collect blood in a red top tube before collecting blood in a lavender top tube.

Chapter 5

Complementary and Alternative Therapies

OBJECTIVES

5.1 Differentiate between complementary and alternative medicine.

5.2 Describe the five major domains of CAM therapies.

5.3 Discuss the nurse's role in assessing client use of CAM therapies and associated education.

UNDERSTANDING TERMINOLOGY

1. Define *complementary and alternative medicine*.

2. Define *integrative medicine*.

3. Explain what a placebo effect is.

4. Explain what a redox agent is.

5. Describe therapeutic touch.

THEORIES AND TRENDS

6. Differentiate between complementary and alternative medicine as described by NCCAM.

7. List the five major domains of CAM therapies:
    a.

    b.

    c.

    d.

    e.

8. True or False

    _____ About 30% of all modern medicines come from plant sources.

    _____ About 80% of the population in the United States has used CAM at some point.

    _____ The most rapidly growing area of CAM is the use of dietary supplements.

    _____ A new ruling by the FDA will allow food companies to make health claims on labels if most of the scientific evidence supports a benefit.

REVIEWING YOUR KNOWLEDGE

9. True or False

    _____ Dietary supplement and herb manufacturers are held to the same strict standards as are manufacturers of pharmaceuticals.

10. State the main problem with the DSHEA ruling of 1994.

11. What two dietary supplements have been demonstrated to have a positive effect on age-related macular degeneration?
    a.

    b.

12. An example of a CAM alternative medical system is:
    1. homeopathic medicine.
    2. shamanism.
    3. dietary supplements.
    4. massage.
    5. magnetic therapy.

13. An example of CAM mind-body interventions is:
    1. acupuncture.
    2. hypnosis.
    3. alternative diets.
    4. chiropractic medicine.
    5. Reiki.

APPLYING YOUR KNOWLEDGE

14. Explain what actions the nurse initiates to assess information about a client's use of CAM.

Chapter 6

Overview of Health Care Delivery

OBJECTIVES

6.1 Discuss the major government influences on the health care delivery system.

6.2 Describe the various social, political, and economic factors which have influenced health care services and delivery.

6.3 Examine major strategies to contain rising health care costs.

THEORIES AND TRENDS

1. Discuss why American industries are concerned about rising health care costs.

2. Explain how public values about health care are changing.

REVIEWING YOUR KNOWLEDGE

3. The government department that oversees federal government health care efforts is the
    _____.

4. List five major sources of government health care expenditures and identify if they are federal, joint (federal and state), or state:
    a.

    b.

c.

d.

e.

5. List the two major sources of federal funding for biomedical research and training.
   a.

   b.

6. The federal government funds public health programs through the _____
   _____.

7. The organization that represents hospitals' efforts to influence legislation, regulation, judicial decisions, and health policy is the _____.

8. Explain why private sector, employers, and insured clients pay more for health care.

9. What two groups of individuals of the non-elderly population are affected the most by being uninsured or underinsured?
   a.

   b.

10. Discuss the socioeconomic effect of the introduction of commercial insurance such as Blue Cross/Blue Shield.

11. The purpose of the Hill-Burton Act of 1946 was to:

12. Explain how the constructions of health care facilities under the Hill-Burton Act contribute to the access of health care by indigent clients.

13. The social program that provided the impetus for the passage of Medicare was the _____
_____.

14. Complete the following table to compare and contrast Medicare and Medicaid.

	Medicare	**Medicaid**
a. Type of program		
b. Source of funding		
c. Services provided		

15. The purpose of the Balanced Budget Act of 1997 was to:

16. The three major purposes of the Health Insurance Portability and Accountability Act of 1996 were to:

a.

b.

c.

APPLYING YOUR KNOWLEDGE

17. What happens if hospitals do not comply with regulations promulgated by the federal government related to health care delivery?

18. List five strategies that have been used to decrease rising health care costs:

a.

b.

c.

d.

e.

19. List the six major strategies used during the period of regulation and cost containment to curtail rising health care costs:

a.

b.

c.

d.

e.

f.

BEST PRACTICES

20. What was the major objective of *Nursing's Agenda for Health Care Reform*?

Chapter 7

Ambulatory Health Care

OBJECTIVES

7.1 Examine the characteristics of ambulatory care settings within the health care delivery system.

7.2 Discuss the nursing role in ambulatory care settings including types of interventions, challenges, and legal issues.

7.3 Describe future trends and challenges to nursing practice in ambulatory care settings.

UNDERSTANDING TERMINOLOGY

. Differentiate between primary health care and primary care.

. Define *telehealth nursing practice*.

THEORIES AND TRENDS

. The ambulatory setting is a major site for health care delivery because:
   1. the number of hours and days clients stay in hospital has increased.
   2. new technology for surgery and procedures is available.
   3. private insurance will not reimburse for in-hospital care.
   4. the acuity of clients in ambulatory settings is decreasing.

4. List six challenges to ambulatory care nurses based on demographic and socioeconomic trends:
   a.

   b.

   c.

   d.

   e.

   f.

REVIEWING YOUR KNOWLEDGE

5. True or False

   _____ Autonomy is a characteristic of nursing practice in ambulatory care settings.

   _____ Ambulatory nursing care is episodic and lasts 24 to 48 hours.

   _____ Clinical services provided in the ambulatory care setting have traditionally been provided based on the medical model of care.

   _____ The major role of nurses in hospital outpatient departments is client and family education and case management.

   _____ Working with a multidisciplinary team in the ambulatory care setting is challenging because nurses may be asked to provide care beyond their scope of practice.

   _____ Nursing competence is based on knowledge, skill, and ability to effectively carry out a given role.

   _____ Nursing certification in ambulatory care nursing is a means of demonstrating competence.

6. Describe why nursing assessment is a challenge in the ambulatory care setting.

7. The three classifications of ambulatory care settings are _____ _____, and _____.

8. Describe the three means of classifying ambulatory clients.

9. Explain the nurse's role in telephone triage.

10. The two types of telephone surveillance (or monitoring) that are in common practice are
_____ and _____.

11. Explain what should be included in the documentation of a telehealth encounter in the client's medical record.

12. Explain the purpose of accreditation of ambulatory care settings:

13. List the three organizations which provide accreditation for ambulatory care settings:
    a.

    b.

    c.

APPLYING YOUR KNOWLEDGE

14. Characteristics of clients seen for care in ambulatory care settings include: (Select all that apply)
    1. Men make more visits than women.
    2. Older adults make more visits than children.
    3. African Americans are more likely to use hospital outpatient departments.
    4. Difficulty breathing is a common reason for visits.

15. Explain the rationale for the nurse to have an understanding of cultural competence in the ambulatory care setting.

16. The benefits of the Interstate Compact for nursing licensure include: (Select all that apply)
    1. reduced barriers to interstate practice.
    2. improved tracking for disciplinary purposes.
    3. cost-effectiveness.
    4. unduplicated counts of nurses in practice.
    5. decreased consumer access to nurses in their state.

BEST PRACTICES

17. An example of a primary prevention health promotion activity is:
    1. blood glucose screening.
    2. immunizations.
    3. cardiac rehabilitation.
    4. nutrition education.

18. An example of secondary prevention activity is:
    1. blood glucose screening.
    2. immunizations.
    3. cardiac rehabilitation.
    4. nutrition education.

19. An example of tertiary prevention activity is:
    1. blood glucose screening.
    2. immunizations.
    3. cardiac rehabilitation.
    4. nutrition education.

Acute Health Care

OBJECTIVES

8.1   Examine the historical trends in the evolution of hospital/acute care nursing.

8.2   Describe hospitals including setting, types, mode of admission, and other factors which contribute to the provision of quality of care.

8.3   Analyze the nursing role when working in an acute care setting including legal and ethical responsibilities.

UNDERSTANDING TERMINOLOGY

1. Match each type of hospital admission to the appropriate description.

Type of Admission	Description
_____ a. emergency	1. client is seen in physician's office and it is determined that the client needs nursing care and specialized monitoring
_____ b. direct	2. client has elected to undergo a special diagnostic or surgical procedure
_____ c. scheduled	3. Client is seen in an outpatient department and it is determined that client needs surgery, nursing care, or monitoring and cannot manage the disease at home

2. Describe a physician hospitalist.

3. Explain the term "swing bed."

4. Match each type of care provided by nurses in acute care settings with the appropriate description.

	Type of Care	Description
_____	a. interdependent	1. processes that support actual bedside nursing
_____	b. direct	2. provision of treatment or administration of medications
_____	c. indirect	3. assess, care for, educate, and comfort clients

5. Explain what is meant by "one-level-of-care."

6. Define *culturally competent care.*

7. Define *risk management.*

THEORIES AND TRENDS

8. True or False

_____ The expected outcome of using a nursing classification system for staffing is a reduction in costs, improvement in care, and an increase in client satisfaction.

9. Explain the purpose of hospital surveys by regulating agencies.

10. A future trend that will influence the delivery of care in hospitals is:
    1. technology will decrease the acuity of clients.
    2. health care will be directed at individuals.
    3. bioterrorism concerns.
    4. fewer health care workers will be immigrants.

REVIEWING YOUR KNOWLEDGE

11. The new prospective payment system implemented in 1983 to stem the rise in health care costs was _____.

12. In the 1990s, hospitals changed from a _____-driven, fee-for-service system to a _____-driven, capitated, and managed care system.

13. True or False

_____ As a consequence of cost containment efforts, hospitals merged in the 1990s to become "health-care systems."

_____ A hospital is described as an institution whose function is to provide diagnostic and therapeutic client services for a variety of medical conditions.

_____ Voluntary/not-for-profit hospitals are only concerned about meeting expenses on an on-going basis.

_____ The requirement for nursing care is the primary reason clients are hospitalized.

_____ Postacute care is designed to fill the gap between home-care and long-term care.

_____ A certified lactation specialist is a formal nurse educator who teaches clients in the hospital and provides follow-up care in the community.

_____ Research of clinical practices contributes to efforts to contain costs.

_____ Most hospitals use one type of nursing care delivery.

_____ Today's client is submissive to suggestions for care.

_____ It is appropriate for incident reports to be used for punitive activity.

_____ Lawsuits rely upon information revealed in an incident report.

4. List the three types of hospitals:
   a.

   b.

   c.

5. List the three goals of case management:
   a.

   b.

   c.

6. Explain the purpose of work-redesign.

7. The purpose of skill-mix between RNs and other non-licensed personnel is achieved when

_____.

18. _____ staff are used to make staffing adjustments caused by fluctuation of census data and acuity levels.

19. The use of _____ has helped hospitals to make the most effective use of available nursing staff.

20. Identify the federal legislation associated with each impact or purpose.

Impact or Purpose	Federal Legislation
a. requires places of employment to be free from recognized hazards	
b. laid the foundation for equal employment	
c. take affirmative action to recruit, hire, and advance handicapped people	
d. promote employment of older people	
e. eliminate workplace discrimination against Americans with disabilities	

21. List the five categories of highest risk in a hospital setting:
    a.

    b.

    c.

    d.

    e.

APPLYING YOUR KNOWLEDGE

2. Nursing at the beginning of the 20th century is best characterized as: (Select all that apply)
   1. Nurses worked in hospitals on a fee-for-service basis.
   2. Most nurses worked in private duty.
   3. Hospitalized clients were poor and generally had communicable diseases.
   4. It was desirable for affluent clients to be admitted to hospitals.

3. Following the Great Depression, the demand for hospital-based nurses increased due to:
   1. the increased demand for nurses to work in private duty.
   2. hospitals providing room and board instead of salary.
   3. the availability of hospital insurance through Blue Cross.
   4. a decrease in the number of nursing graduates.

4. Compare and contrast informal versus formal education provided to clients or groups.

5. Functional nursing requires that:
   1. care provided under this model is done solely by RNs.
   2. all caregivers are licensed.
   3. the RN provides basic, bedside care to the client.
   4. the RN coordinates care for an entire team or unit.

6. A major advantage of team nursing is:
   1. it is economical.
   2. the RN knows clients well.
   3. care is less fragmented.
   4. the team is comprised of multiple RNs.

BEST PRACTICES

7. List six characteristics that describe a *magnet hospital*:
   a.

   b.

   c.

   d.

   e.

   f.

28. True or False

_____ Research has conclusively demonstrated that the use of unlicensed assistive personnel improves client outcomes.

_____ Evidence-based practice uses research findings and client characteristics to guide clinical practice.

_____ If something is not documented in the medical record, it is assumed that it was not done

29. List nine factors that should be considered when developing a plan for quality client care:
a.

b.

c.

d.

e.

f.

g.

h.

i.

30. The one indicator of quality of care that hospitals should always consider is _____ _____.

Critical Care

OBJECTIVES

9.1   Discuss the historical development of Critical Care Nursing.

9.2   Explore reasons for caring for certain clients in the ICU.

9.3   Analyze the role of the critical care nurse.

THEORIES AND TRENDS

. Which of the following factors contributed to the further development of critical care environments during the 20ᵗʰ century? (Select all that apply)
1.   "shock wards" used during World War II
2.   an oversupply of nurses after the second world war
3.   the polio epidemic
4.   the development of mechanical ventilators

REVIEWING YOUR KNOWLEDGE

. True or False

_____   The critical care unit is where care is provided to clients who are unstable or potentially
unstable.

_____   John Hopkins Hospital established the first "critical care" environment in the 1890s.

_____   ICUs often use a password system which allows the nurse to share information about
the client via the telephone.

_____   Research has demonstrated that despite their beliefs nurses and physicians caring for clients in the ICU underestimate family needs for information, proximity, and assurance.

_____   The physician is primarily responsible for coordinating the care of a client in the ICU.

Explain why clients with each type of disorder require nursing care in an ICU.
a.   respiratory disorders
b.   circulatory disorders
c.   neurological changes
d.   life-threatening infections
e.   metabolic problems
f.   major surgical procedures
g.   postoperative with history of cardiac or pulmonary disease

4. The delirium that is often experienced by a critically ill client is called
   _____.

5. List three settings where critical care nursing is practiced.
   a.

   b.

   c.

6. Which nursing role is considered to be the backbone of critical care nursing?

7. Describe the following advanced practice roles in the ICU as to educational requirements and job descriptions.
   a. Critical care clinical nurse specialist

   b. Acute care nurse practitioner

8. Identify the two professional organizations that provide the ICU nurse with practice guidelines, educational programs, and professional publications among other benefits.
   a.

   b.

APPLYING YOUR KNOWLEDGE

9. A possible consequence of inadequate sleep quantity and quality for the ICU client is:
   1. a decrease in oxygen consumption.
   2. a decrease in carbon dioxide production.
   3. a positive nitrogen balance.
   4. impaired immunity and delayed healing.

10. Explain environmental controls the nurse can initiate to decrease stress experienced by a client in the ICU and the expected outcome of these interventions.

1. List four complementary and alternative therapies the nurse can implement to assist in providing a healing environment for the client in the ICU:

   a.

   b.

   c.

   d.

BEST PRACTICES

2. Explain why it is important for the ICU nurse to manage stress experienced by the client's family.

3. Explain the benefit of using "Visitor Assistants" for family members of clients in the ICU.

4. Explain why it is important for the ICU nurse to act in an advocacy role for the client and family.

5. Explain why it is imperative that the ICU nurse engage in continuing education.

Chapter 10

Home Health Care

OBJECTIVES

10.1 Examine trends contributing to the growth of home health services.

10.2 Describe the philosophy of community-based care including the delineation of core values and principles.

10.3 Discuss the Omaha System and Nightingale Tracker including their application and use in home health care practice.

UNDERSTANDING TERMINOLOGY

. Define *home health care nursing*.

THEORIES AND TRENDS

. All of the following have contributed to the growth of home health services, except:
   1. shrinking health care costs.
   2. aging of the population.
   3. federal legislation.
   4. the increase in managed care.

. List the four purposes of legislative and regulatory changes made in 1997 that reduced Medicare-Medicaid reimbursement to home health agencies:

   a.

   b.

   c.

   d.

REVIEWING YOUR KNOWLEDGE

4. Explain the primary role of the nurse case manager employed by home health agencies.

5. The Boy Scout motto that applies to home health care is _____
_____. Explain why this is critical for the nurse.

6. Invaluable resources that a nurse takes with her to a home visit that contribute to her ability to provide high-quality care are _____,
_____, and _____.

7. The most important thing for a nurse to do during the initial visit with the home health client is to establish _____.

8. List and explain the four levels of the Problem Classification Scheme in the Omaha System:
   a.

   b.

   c.

   d.

9. Describe the Problem Rating Scale for Outcomes of the Omaha System.

10. True or False

_____ Community health nursing provides an umbrella under which all types of home health care are practiced.

_____ Ideally the shift of health care services from the hospital to the community decreases fragmentation of care, increases collaboration among health care team members, and increases accountability.

_____ It is common practice for the home health nurse to be the individual to verify financial data and source of payment with the client during the initial intake.

_____ A hospice team is comprised of representatives of multiple health care disciplines whose goal is to support end-of-life decisions made by clients and their families.

_____ The client and nurse establish goals of care in home health nursing.

_____ The Problem Rating Scale for Outcomes in the Omaha System provides the nurse with an opportunity to compare client status at different points in time to determine nursing effectiveness.

APPLYING YOUR KNOWLEDGE

11. Nursing activities that a nurse would implement during the initial client visit include: (Select all that apply)
    1. gathering subjective data.
    2. assessing the physical environment.
    3. objective data about the client only.
    4. interpretation of data and problem identification.

12. Explain the Intervention Scheme of the Omaha System.

13. Explain the purpose and use of the Nightingale Tracker.

BEST PRACTICES

14. Explain the importance of communication and collaboration among home health care staff.

15. Discuss the basic core values central to the community-oriented philosophy of care practiced in home health agencies.

16. Describe basic principles that nurses who practice in home health care can incorporate to maximize outcomes of care.

Chapter 11

Long-Term Care

OBJECTIVES

11.1 Describe the historical development of long-term care facilities.

11.2 Describe the federal legislation which has impacted the development and regulation of long-term care facilities.

11.3 Describe the nursing activities related to care of residents in long-term care facilities.

THEORIES AND TRENDS

. Early long-term care facilities were characterized by: (Select all that apply)
   1. adequate supplies to care for clients.
   2. sound nutritional food.
   3. residents being forced to sleep on floors.
   4. overcrowding.
   5. residents being forced to work for keep.
   6. open drunkenness and sexual relations.

. True or False

_____ Long-term care facilities historically had their origin in the tradition in European countries to segregate the aged and disabled from the rest of society.

_____ Historically, the development of community institutions to care for individuals with long-term care needs was developed so that clients did not remain in hospital beds for extended periods of time.

REVIEWING YOUR KNOWLEDGE

The federal legislation which provided funds for the construction of nursing homes was the _____.

The federal legislation passed in 1987 which provided strict regulations and produced profound reform in nursing home care was the _____.

5. List the two specific nursing staffing requirements specified by federal regulations for long-term care facilities:

    a.

    b.

6. Residents of long-term care facilities must have an assessment completed within _____ days of admission. They must be reassessed at least _____ or whenever there is a _____.

7. The tool used to document the assessment and used as a basis for care planning is the _____.

8. List seven skills that are essential for an effective manager in a long-term care facility:

    a.

    b.

    c.

    d.

    e.

    f.

    g.

9. True or False

    _____ The passage of the Social Security Act provided a means for older adults to purchase care through an informal system of care.

    _____ Medicare and Medicaid were developed to ensure a minimum level of health care for the aged and poor.

    _____ Lobbying efforts by the American Medical Association and owners of long-term care facilities ensured provisions for reimbursement for nursing home care in Medicare and Medicaid.

    _____ Long-term care facilities which do not meet required conditions and regulations may have Medicare and Medicaid reimbursement terminated.

    _____ Nurses and nursing organizations played an active role in the development of regulations and guidelines for long-term care facilities.

    _____ The role of nurses may vary in LTCF from performing selected roles such as medication administration to providing total care.

    _____ It is not uncommon for residents and their families to experience negative reactions when the resident transitions to living in a LTCF.

_____ Nurses working in long-term care facilities function in a variety of management roles which require them to be familiar with regulations, reimbursement programs, legal aspects of nursing practice, and employee-employer relations.

APPLYING YOUR KNOWLEDGE

10. A condition that long-term care facilities must meet to receive reimbursement through Medicare and/or Medicaid is that residents must:
    1. be totally dependent.
    2. have a comprehensive health assessment within the first 3 weeks of care.
    3. have personal funds managed by facility personnel.
    4. have nursing care consistent with level of care and needs.

11. Characteristics of residents of long-term care facilities include: (Select all that apply)
    1. the risk of being in an LTCF decreases with age.
    2. women residents outnumber men.
    3. the majority of residents are African American.
    4. most residents have some impairment of self-care.
    5. a medical diagnosis is a key criteria for admission.
    6. change in caregiver status often precipitates admission.

12. Describe problems with the MDS as an assessment tool which may impact nursing care planning.

BEST PRACTICES

13. Regulations specify components of the care plan used in a long-term care facility. List six characteristics of the care plan:
    a.

    b.

    c.

    d.

    e.

    f.

14. Explain the importance of effective communication and documentation for nursing caregivers of long-term care facility residents.

15. List six activities a nurse can implement to ensure safety in telephone orders from physicians for long-term care facility residents:

    a.

    b.

    c.

    d.

    e.

    f.

Chapter 12

Rehabilitation

OBJECTIVES

12.1 Examine the concepts, definitions, and goals of rehabilitation nursing.

12.2 Describe the concepts central to understanding functional ability.

12.3 Describe the principles and processes of rehabilitation nursing and the nurse's role.

THEORIES AND TRENDS

1. List two factors that have contributed to an increased number of clients requiring rehabilitation services:

   a.

   b.

REVIEWING YOUR KNOWLEDGE

2. Rehabilitation nursing is defined as the diagnosis and treatment of human responses of individuals to actual or potential health problems relative to _____.

3. Using WHO International Classification of Functioning, Disability, and Health as a guide, match each term with the appropriate definition.

Term	Definition
_____ a. body structure	1. external physical, social, and attitudinal conditions that can influence an individual's capacity to perform functions
_____ b. activities	2. problems that deviate significantly from the expected norm
_____ c. personal factors	3. physiological and psychological components of body systems
_____ d. participation	4. organs, limbs, and their components
_____ e. impairments	5. involvement in life situations
_____ f. body functions	6. execution of a task or action by an individual
_____ g. environmental factors	7. non-health conditions of an individual's life

4. List the five different types of rehabilitation service settings:
   a.

   b.

   c.

   d.

   e.

5. Describe factors that are used to determine the most appropriate setting for a client's rehabilitation.

6. True or False

   _____   Ongoing evaluation of progress toward rehabilitation goals is achieved through team conferences.

   _____   Anticipatory guidance is an effective intervention to help clients transition successfully from one level of care to another.

   _____   Encouragement from a nurse for the client to achieve independence is viewed as poor quality of care.

   _____   Before discharge, clients and families are usually very competent in their ability to manage all aspects of client care at home.

APPLYING YOUR KNOWLEDGE

7. Medicare requires that a client must be able to participate actively in at least _____ hours of therapy a day and need at least _____ therapeutic modalities in addition to rehabilitation _____ and _____.

8. Explain each of the following key principles related to the focus of rehabilitation and the nurse's role for each.
   a. client-centered

   b. goal-oriented

c. focus on functional ability

d. use of a team approach

e. client finding acceptable quality of life

f. wellness focus

g. adapting to change

h. coping and adjusting

i. understanding role of culture

j. client and family education

9. A factor that can interfere with an effective rehabilitation process is:
   1. the attitude of the client.
   2. the support of family members.
   3. adequate financial resources.
   4. available community resources.

10. True or False

   _____ The most important reason for nurses to understand the rehabilitation component of the continuum of care is that it enables them to make appropriate referrals and to prepare clients for the rehabilitation experience.

BEST PRACTICES

11. Explain why it is important for the nurse to make sure the client and family members understand the differences between acute care and rehabilitation settings.

Chapter 13

Clients with Fluid Imbalances

OBJECTIVES

13.1 Identify common terminology related to fluid and electrolyte imbalances.

13.2 Define the etiology and pathophysiology of fluid imbalances.

13.3 Describe how to assess a client's fluid status.

13.4 Identify high-risk clients who may develop fluid imbalances.

13.5 Describe nursing interventions used to help treat clients with fluid imbalances.

13.6 Identify systemic complications associated with fluid imbalances.

ANATOMY & PHYSIOLOGY REVIEW

1. Label the structures of the cell.

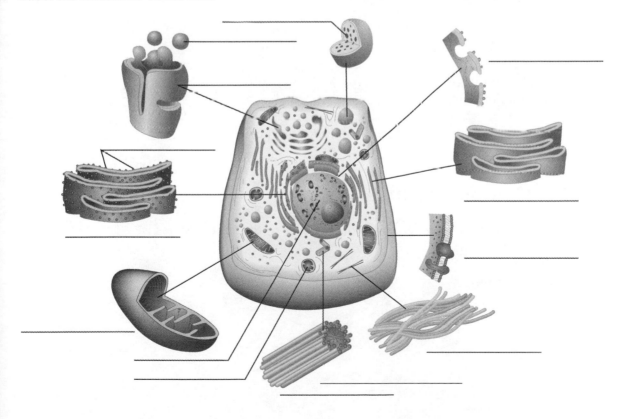

UNDERSTANDING PATHOPHYSIOLOGY

2. A patient suffering with extracellular fluid volume deficit (ECFVD) can also be said to be
   _____.

3. Thirst is inhibited by _____.

4. List the two types of fluid shifts:
   a.

   b.

5. What hormone is responsible for increasing water and sodium reabsorption?
   1. ADH and aldosterone
   2. estrogen
   3. thyroxin
   4. calcium

6. Identify the three types of extracellular fluid (ECF) volume deficits.
   a.

   b.

   c.

7. Decreased urine output is a classic sign of _____.

8. Clinical signs that a client is dehydrated include: (Select all that apply)
   1. dry mucous membranes.
   2. sunken eyes.
   3. decreased skin turgor.
   4. elevated alkaline level.

9. Oral rehydration is inhibited by cola drinks because they contain _____
   and _____.

APPLYING YOUR KNOWLEDGE

10. The most common fluid and electrolyte disturbance in the United States is:
    1. hypokalemia.
    2. dehydration.
    3. sodium retention.
    4. obesity.

11. Physiological regulators of fluid balance include: (Select all that apply)
    1. thirst.
    2. hormones.
    3. the lymphatic system.
    4. the kidneys.

12. Clients with a high risk of developing fluid imbalances include clients with: (Select all that apply)
    1. dysphagia.
    2. dementia.
    3. diabetes insipidus.
    4. renal failure.

13. Dehydration can be caused by: (Select all that apply)
    1. unmonitored use of potent diuretics.
    2. severe vomiting.
    3. diarrhea.
    4. excessive exercise.

14. Older clients are at risk for excessive fluid loss for several reasons, including: (Select all that apply)
    1. decreased renal concentration of urine.
    2. altered ADH response.
    3. increased body fat.
    4. diminished thirst.

15. A client with inadequate fluid volume would have which of the following clinical signs? (Select all that apply)
    1. decreased blood pressure
    2. weak pulse
    3. decrease in central venous pressure
    4. elevated respirations

6. The nurse should notify the team leader if a client has not had at least
   _____ of urine output for 8 consecutive hours.

7. Complications of too-rapid IV fluid infusion can result in _____
   and _____.

8. In evaluating renal function in clients, which lab test critical in maintaining adequate renal output?
    1. creatinine
    2. CBC
    3. ADH level
    4. lipase

BEST PRACTICES

19. Which conditions predispose clients to fluid loss? (Select all that apply)
    1. fever
    2. hyperglycemia
    3. gastrointestinal suctioning
    4. ileostomy
    5. burns
    6. hyperventilation

20. A 78-year-old female is starting to experience cerebral anoxia due to fluid loss. What sign would indicate this and need to be reported to the physician? (Select all that apply)
    1. restlessness
    2. apprehension
    3. headache
    4. confusion

21. The goals of treatment for fluid volume deficit are to: (Select all that apply)
    1. restore normal fluid volumes by using fluids similar in composition to those lost.
    2. replace ongoing losses.
    3. correct the underlying problems (such as vomiting or diarrhea).
    4. ensure replacement of magnesium to the system.

22. Which of the following assessment criteria are critical when managing patients with fluid volume deficits? (Select all that apply.)
    1. urine output
    2. body weight
    3. sodium and potassium lab value
    4. osmolality
    e. BUN

23. When weighing a client, it is important to: (Select all that apply)
    1. rely on what the client tells you his or her weight is.
    2. weigh the client daily.
    3. use the same scale for each weight.
    4. weigh the client at the same time each day.
    5. have the patient void prior to weighing.

24. Respiratory assessment that would indicate fluid volume excess are: (Select all that apply)
    1. diminished lung sounds
    2. crackles, ronchi
    3. coughing
    4. dyspnea

25. What intravenous fluid would be used to provide intracellular fluid hydration?

26. What intravenous fluid would be used to provide extracellular fluid deficit?

KEEPING DRUG SKILLS SHARP

27. Mild diuretics and digitalis promote _____ and improve _____ .

28. Clients taking diuretics and digitalis need to be monitored for: (Select all that apply)
    1. plasma electrolytes.
    2. digitalis toxicity.
    3. hypokalemia.
    4. hypernatremia.

29. True or False

    _____ Unmonitored use of potent diuretics can cause hyperkalemia.

    _____ Lemon and garlic are safe low-sodium salt substitutes.

    _____ Clients taking ACE inhibitors can use potassium salt substitutes sparingly.

    _____ Digitalis toxicity is common in the elderly.

30. The therapeutic effect will be greater for a client receiving albumin if the infusion is regulated to run:
    1. rapidly, and fluids are encouraged.
    2. slowly, and fluid intake is restricted.
    3. rapidly, and fluid intake is withheld.
    4. slowly, and fluids are encouraged liberally.

31. The nurse will administer albumin to a client to assist in:
    1. clotting of blood.
    2. formation of red blood cells.
    3. activation of white blood cells.
    4. development of oncotic pressure.

Chapter 14

Clients with Electrolyte Imbalances

OBJECTIVES

14.1   Define terms related to electrolyte imbalances.

14.2   Describe etiologies of potassium, calcium, and magnesium imbalances.

14.3   Identify people who are at risk for developing specific electrolyte imbalances.

14.4   Describe teaching guidelines for clients with electrolyte imbalances.

UNDERSTANDING PATHOPHYSIOLOGY

. Anyone with decreased intake, decreased availability, or increased loss of electrolytes is at risk for
_____.

. Nursing diagnoses that may apply to clients with electrolyte imbalances include:
   a.

   b.

   c.

   d.

. Define *hyponatremia*.

. Define *hypernatremia*.

. Factors that can alter oxygen and carbon dioxide exchange include: (Select all that apply.)
   1. tachypnea.
   2. dyspnea.
   3. shortness of breath.
   4. fluid in the alveoli.

6. Hypernatremia is usually associated with _____ or
_____.

7. List three conditions in which sodium retention occurs:
   a.

   b.

   c.

8. The most ominous result of hypocalcemia is _____ .

9. *Hypokalemia* is defined as a plasma K+ level less than _____.

10. Clinical manifestations of hypokalemia include: (Select all that apply.)
    1. abnormal findings on EKG.
    2. GI abnormalities.
    3. muscle weakness.
    4. leg cramps.

11. Dysrhythmias with hypokalemia are due to _____
_____.

12. The underlying cause of hyperkalemia is often associated with _____
_____ kidney function.

13. Define *Trousseau's sign*.

14. Define *Chvostek's sign*.

15. The three most common causes of hypercalcemia are: (Select all that apply)
    1. metastatic malignancy.
    2. hyperparathyroidism.
    3. thiazide diuretics.
    4. corticosteroid induced.

APPLYING SKILLS

16. Athletes and outdoor laborers are at risk for _____ due
to _____.

17. Hyponatremia causes which of the following gastrointestinal (GI) manifestations in clients? (Select all that apply)
    1. hyperactive bowel sounds
    2. abdominal cramping
    3. diarrhea
    4. nausea

18. A plasma sodium level less than 135 meq/L confirms a diagnosis of _____ _____.

19. What EKG changes would a nurse expect to find in the client with hypokalemia? (Select all that apply)
    1. depressed and prolonged ST segment
    2. depressed and inverted T waves
    3. prominent U waves
    4. wide QRS complexes

BEST PRACTICES

20. Which clinical manifestations should be expected when clients lose vascular volume secondary to sodium and water loss? (Select all that apply)
    1. decreased systolic and diastolic blood pressure
    2. orthostatic hypotension
    3. weak thready pulse
    4. heart murmurs

21. Clients with sodium levels of 125meq/L or less should receive _____ _____.

22. Hypertonic saline must be given very slowly by IVPB infusion in a large vein in order to decrease the risk of: (Select all that apply)
    1. hypernatremia.
    2. pulmonary overload.
    3. phlebitis.
    4. renal shutdown.

23. Oral potassium (chloride and gluconate) is extremely irritating to gastric mucosa and must be administered with: (Select all that apply)
    1. juice.
    2. meals.
    3. milk.
    4. a glass of water.

KEEPING DRUGS SKILLS SHARP

24. A diuretic often given intravenously to prevent pulmonary fluid overload is:
    1. tetracycline.
    2. Lasix.
    3. mannitol.
    4. HCTZ.

25. Declomycin (demeclocycline hydrochloride), an agent that antagonizes the antidiuretic hormone (ADH), is the preferred drug for treating:
    1. hypernatremia.
    2. hyponatremia.
    3. hypokalemia.
    4. hyperkalemia.

26. To prevent rapid elevation of plasma sodium and exacerbation of vasospasm in people with subarachnoid hemorrhage, the solution of choice is:
    1. $D_5$1/2 NS.
    2. NS.
    3. D_5W.
    4. Ringer's lactate.

27. Older clients, because of their low percentage of total body water, are at risk for
    _____ after even mild attacks of diarrhea.

28. Medications that commonly cause hypokalemia include: (Select all that apply)
    1. thiazide diuretics.
    2. osmotic diuretics.
    3. steroids.
    4. digitalis preparations.

29. Clients who have acute hypocalcemia and develop tetany will be treated with: (Select all that apply)
    1. IV calcium chloride.
    2. IV calcium gluconate.
    3. Lasix.
    4. vitamin D.

Acid-Base Balance

OBJECTIVES

15.1 Discuss general concepts of regulation of acid base balance.

15.2 Define acid base compensation.

15.3 Describe the process of arterial blood gas analysis.

15.4 Discuss acid base imbalances.

15.5 Identify clinical manifestations of acid base disturbances.

15.6 Identify complex acid base disorders.

UNDERSTANDING PATHOPHYSIOLOGY

1. A normal serum pH is _____.

2. An acidic solution has a pH of less than _____.

3. An alkaline solution has a pH of greater than _____.

4. Acids that cannot be converted to gases must be eliminated in _____
_____.

5. True or False

_____ The kidneys regulate serum pH by secreting H into the urine and by regenerating HCO_3.

6. The organ that regulates the electrolyte balance in the body is the:
   1. liver.
   2. kidneys.
   3. heart.
   4. parathyroid.

7. Acid base compensation acts to restore the normal ratio of _____
and normalize _____.

8. _____ refers to any pathologic process that causes a
relative excess of acid.

9. _____ refers to excess acid in the blood.

10. _____ indicates a primary condition resulting in excess base in the body.

11. _____ refers more narrowly to elevation of serum pH.

12. Aldosterone is primarily secreted by the adrenal cortex in direct response to:
    1. decreased water intake.
    2. loss of sodium and water.
    3. decreased serum osmolality.
    4. increased potassium level.

APPLYING SKILLS

13. Which of the following pH values are considered in range of being potentially fatal? (Select all that apply)
    1. pH below 6.8
    2. pH above 7.8
    3. pH equal to the alkaline ratio
    4. pH above the acid ratio

14. Hyperkalemia refers to _____ potassium level.

15. Hypokalemia refers to _____ potassium level.

16. Hyponatremia refers to _____ sodium level.

17. Hypernatremia refers to _____ sodium level.

18. Match each blood gas value with its corresponding condition.

	Blood Gas Value	**Condition**
_____	a. pH 7.53; $PaCO_2$ 33 mm Hg; HCO_3 25 mEq/L	1. respiratory alkalosis
_____	b. pH 7.4; $PaCO_2$ 26 mm Hg; HCO_3 16 mEq/L	2. respiratory acidosis
_____	c. pH 7.31; $PaCO_2$ 58 mm Hg; HCO_3 25 mEq/L	3. metabolic acidosis
_____	d. pH 7.64; $PaCO_2$ 48 mm Hg; HCO_3 47 mEq/L	4. metabolic alkalosis

19. Match each condition with its corresponding acid base disturbance.

	Condition	**Acid Base Disturbance**
_____	a. sedative or narcotic overdose	1. Respiratory acidosis
_____	b. mechanical overventilation	2. Respiratory alkalosis
_____	c. diabetic ketosis	3. metabolic acidosis
_____	d. respiratory failure	4. metabolic alkalosis
_____	e. renal failure	
_____	f. prolonged vomiting	

20. High-risk clients for whom it is essential that nurses be alert for signs of acid base imbalance include: (Select all that apply)
    1. pulmonary and cardiovascular and renal system patients.
    2. clients receiving total parenteral nutrition or enteral tube feedings.
    3. clients receiving mechanical ventilation.
    4. clients with diabetes mellitus.
    5. clients with vomiting, diarrhea.
    6. older clients.

BEST PRACTICES

21. _____ must be used to treat hypoxemia.

22. What test is performed to ensure adequate circulation in the hand prior to a radial artery puncture for an arterial blood gas?
    1. Allen's
    2. Open hand draw
    3. Arterial compliant test
    4. CBC

KEEPS DRUG SKILLS SHARP

23. A client who is receiving furosemide (Lasix) and digoxin (Lanoxin) should be observed for symptoms of electrolyte depletion caused by:
    1. hyperkalemia.
    2. hyponatremia.
    3. hypocalcemia.
    4. azotemia.

24. Clients receiving digitalis preparations should be evaluated for a loss of
    1. sodium.
    2. calcium.
    3. potassium.
    4. phosphate.

16

Clients Having Surgery

OBJECTIVES

16.1   Describe perioperative nursing.

16.2   Discuss perioperative nursing assessments, interventions, and responsibility.

16.3   Discuss intraoperative nursing assessments, interventions, and responsibility.

16.4   Discuss PACU nursing assessments, interventions, and responsibility.

16.5   Discuss postoperative nursing assessment, interventions, and responsibility.

UNDERSTANDING PATHOPHYSIOLOGY

1. The use of tricyclic antidepressants presurgically can cause increased risk for
    _____ postsurgically.

2. Explain the additional surgical risks a client who smokes faces versus a client who does not
    smoke.

3. Clients with diabetes are at increased risk for _____
    and _____.

4. The stage of general anesthesia at which surgery is performed is:
    1. I.
    2. II.
    3. III.
    4. IV.

5. List the seven potential causes of postoperative hypotension:

   a.

   b.

   c.

   d.

   e.

   f.

   g.

6. Older adults with _____ or _____ impairments may take longer to regain orientation postoperatively.

7. Clinical manifestations of postoperative hypoxia include: (Select all that apply)
   1. orientation.
   2. restlessness.
   3. pink, moist skin.
   4. pulse oximetry below 90%.
   5. warm skin.

8. The postoperative client at greatest risk for thrombus and devastating emboli is the client who had _____ surgery.

9. The three clinical manifestations which may alert the nurse to thrombus are:

   a.

   b.

   c.

10. Explain why obese clients have a delayed return of consciousness after anesthetic procedures.

11. True or False

    _____ Postoperatively, temporary deficits in memory and recall are considered normal.

    _____ For clients to heal surgical wounds effectively they must be in a state of negative nitrogen balance.

    _____ Caudal anesthesia is commonly used with obstetric clients.

APPLYING SKILLS

12. Explain each component of the ABCDE mnemonic used to gather information from the preoperative client.

    A

    B

    C

    D

    E

13. Which assessment findings should be reported to surgeon and anesthesia immediately?
    1. recent upper respiratory infection
    2. failure of the client to stop smoking until two days ago
    3. diminished breath sounds in both bases with expiratory wheezing
    4. clear breath sounds

14. Identify the two laboratory studies performed before surgery to diagnose respiratory conditions and explain why they are performed.

15. List the three common preoperative tests ordered to assess renal function:
    a.

    b.

    c.

16. List the laboratory tests used to determine nutritional status in the preoperative client:
    a.

    b.

    c.

    d.

17. Of the following clients scheduled for surgery, which is at greatest risk for a poor surgical outcome?
    1. 19-year-old athlete
    2. 30-year-old obese housewife
    3. 45-year-old height and weight proportionate office manager
    4. 50-year-old running coach

18. A Penrose drain works by:
    1. wicking
    2. gravity
    3. low-suction
    4. aspiration

19. Explain the role of each of the following members of the surgical team.
    a. surgeon:

    b. anesthesiologist/nurse anesthetist:

    c. circulating nurse:

    d. scrub personnel:

20. When using a unipolar electrosurgical unit (ESU), the OR nurse would: (Select all that apply)
    1. inspect the plug and wires for intactness.
    2. place a ground pad under the thigh.
    3. place a ground pad under the shoulder.
    4. place a ground pad over a previous surgical scar.
    5. ensure that skin is intact before placing a ground pad.

21. List the three phases of the postoperative period:
    a.

    b.

    c.

22. Which of the following is part of breathing assessment in the PACU?
    1. pulse oximeter
    2. wound status
    3. respiratory assistance devices
    4. breath sounds

23. The minimum temperature a client must have to be discharged from the PACU is
    _____.

24. The three characteristics to include in assessment of postoperative drainage are:
    a.

    b.

    c.

BEST PRACTICES

25. The priority teaching implemented preoperatively to prevent hypoventilation with an obese client is _____.

26. Which of the following methods for getting out of bed should the nurse teach a client having abdominal surgery to minimize pain and discomfort?
    1. Raise the HOB to 90 degrees and swing legs to the side of the bed.
    2. From a flat supine position, sit-up in bed and swing legs to the side of the bed.
    3. Turn onto side, use arms to push self into an upright position.
    4. Raise HOB to 45 degrees and swing legs to the side of the bed.

27. Which of the following should the nurse teach the client about postoperative pain control?
    1. Pain medication will be provided and the client should ask for medication when the pain is becoming unbearable.
    2. Pain medication will be provided sparingly due to a high risk for addiction.
    3. Pain medication will be given when the client is participating in postoperative ambulation exercises.
    4. Pain medication will be available and the client should ask for medication when he or she begins to feel uncomfortable.

28. When providing preoperative teaching for the older client, the nurse should consider factors such as: (Select all that apply)
    1. decreased sensory ability.
    2. difficulty hearing high-pitched sounds.
    3. glare from lights may bother the eyes.
    4. increased susceptibility to hypothermia.

29. Informed consent can be provided by:
    1. 10-year-old girl with written permission from an absent parent.
    2. 17-year-old high school senior.
    3. 16-year-old married boy.
    4. 18-year-old college freshman.

30. Explain safety measures the nurse provides for the client after preoperative medications are given.

31. A postoperative client who had spinal anesthesia complains of a headache. An appropriate nursing intervention would be to:
    1. place the client in Trendelenburg position.
    2. provide a warm compress.
    3. keep the client flat.
    4. restrict fluid intake.

32. Identify four factors the nurse considers when positioning a client on the operating table.
    a.

    b.

    c.

    d.

33. The circulating nurse notices a break in surgical asepsis by the surgical assistant when he touched his mask with a gloved hand. Which action should the nurse take?
    1. Record the break in technique on the OR record.
    2. Ask the assistant to leave the OR.
    3. Change the assistant's mask.
    4. Change the assistant's glove.

34. Which of the following actions are initiated to promote a smooth transport from the OR to the PACU? (Select all that apply)
    1. Move the client rapidly from the OR table to the stretcher.
    2. Maintain the client's modesty.
    3. Avoid kinking the IV tubing.
    4. Provide warm blankets.
    5. Keep the side rails up on the stretcher.

35. The client is positioned in PACU to ensure _____ and the preferred position is _____.

36. A major complication in the PACU is airway obstruction. The primary nursing intervention to prevent this is:
    1. suctioning.
    2. use of an oral airway.
    3. use of a nasal airway.
    4. positioning of the head.

37. The nursing intervention for a client experiencing laryngospasm after endotrachial extubation is
    _____.

38. If shock is suspected, an appropriate nursing intervention for the PACU nurse to initiate would be to:
    1. place the client is a flat supine position.
    2. increase the rate of IV fluids.
    3. decrease the oxygen flow rate.
    4. raise the head of the bed.

39. If a nurse were in doubt about how to describe a postoperative wound, the most appropriate action would be to _____.

40. Explain the nursing actions to be initiated if a client eviscerates a postoperative wound.

41. Explain the postoperative instructions that should be reviewed with a client and caregiver before discharge.

42. True or False

_____ Alterations in skin integrity not due to the surgical procedure are preventable by the surgical nurse and operative team.

_____ The nurse encourages family members of surgical clients to go home while the client is in surgery.

_____ A client experiences a cardiac arrest in the OR and it is the circulating nurse's responsibility to call a "Code Blue."

KEEPING DRUG SKILLS SHARP

43. Preoperative medications are given in order to: (Select all that apply)
    1. lower blood pressure.
    2. allay anxiety.
    3. increase oxygen availability.
    4. decrease pharyngeal secretions.
    5. reduce anesthesia side effects.
    6. promote urinary retention.

44. Match each preoperative medication with the correct desired effect (may be used more than once).

	Medication	**Desired Effect**
_____	a. diazepam (Valium)	1. antiemetic effect
_____	b. atropine sulfate	2. inhibit gastric acid production
_____	c. cimetidine	3. control secretions
_____	d. droperidol (Inapsine)	4. decrease anxiety

45. It is important to monitor a client for malignant hyperthermia and shivering if he or she received:
    1. enflurane (Ethrane).
    2. fentanyl citrate-droperidol (Innovar).
    3. nitrous oxide.
    4. fluothane (Halothane).

46. List the eight methods for administering regional anesthesia:
    a.

    b.

    c.

    d.

    e.

    f.

    g.

    h.

47. A highly toxic topical anesthetic agent is:
    1. procaine.
    2. tetracaine.
    3. lidocaine.
    4. cocaine.

48. What is the action of the medication Dantrolene?
    1. vasoconstriction
    2. vasodilation
    3. muscle relaxation
    4. diuresis

Chapter 17

Perspectives in Genetics

OBJECTIVES

17.1 Describe the basic concepts of genes and chromosomes.

17.2 Discuss the primary categories of genetic conditions.

17.3 Identify characteristics of Alzheimer's disease, diabetes mellitus, and cancer, and how genetic factors are related to them.

17.4 Discuss genetic diseases and family assessment.

17.5 Identify the role of genetic testing in clinical practice.

UNDERSTANDING PATHOPHYSIOLOGY

1. _____ are a basic unit of heredity.

2. Humans have _____ pairs of chromosomes.

3. Chromosome pairs 1-22 are called _____.

4. Females have _____ chromosomes and males have
   _____ chromosomes.

5. DNA is made up of two long, twisted strands. Each strand is composed of smaller chemical units
   called _____.

6. Transcription and translation is concerned with the _____
   or the nucleic acid for these processes.

7. Alzheimer's disease is the most common cause of _____
   in late life.

8. Mature onset of diabetes of the young (MODY), a subset of NIDDM, can be inherited as an
   _____ trait.

9. Most cancers result from an accumulation of _____
   that occur over time in somatic body cells.

APPLYING SKILLS

10. Select the three primary categories of genetic conditions.
    1. chromosomal
    2. single gene (Mendeliam)
    3. multifactorial (complex trait)
    4. direct trait line

11. Babies with Down syndrome have which chromosome disorder?
    1. Trisomy 21
    2. Trisomy 29
    3. United ALS
    4. CFR-88

12. True or False

    _____ Cystic Fibrosis (CF) is a common autosomal recessive genetic disorder in the Caucasian population.

    _____ Parents of children with cystic fibrosis are heterozygous carriers for the CF gene.

BEST PRACTICES

13. During prenatal counseling, it is critical to explain to families with histories of X-linked conditions that: (Select all that apply)
    1. the mother of a boy affected with an X-linked condition may be a carrier of the condition.
    2. the son may be affected as a result of a new mutation that occurred during periconceptual period.
    3. a male child inherits his X chromosome only from his mother.
    4. a male child inherits his Y chromosome only from his father.

14. Alzheimer's disease is most accurately described as: (Select all that apply)
    1. adult onset, slowly progressive dementia.
    2. personality changes.
    3. memory loss and deterioration of cognitive functions.
    4. deposition of amyloid neuritic plaques and tangles in the cerebral cortex.

15. Disorders for which carrier testing is recommended include: (Select all that apply)
    1. Tay-Sachs disease.
    2. sickle cell.
    3. cystic fibrosis.
    4. thalassemia.
    5. fragile X syndrome.

16. State the primary goal of prenatal genetic testing.

Chapter 18

Perspectives in Oncology

OBJECTIVES

18.1 Discuss critical terminology related to cancer.

18.2 Discuss basic concepts related to cancer.

18.3 Review factors predisposing individuals to cancer.

18.4 Discuss the incidence and prevalence of cancer today.

18.5 Discuss the impact of cancer on individuals.

18.6 Describe the classifications of cancer.

18.7 Compare and contrast characteristics of normal cells and cancer cells.

UNDERSTANDING TERMINOLOGY

1. The word *tumor* simply refers to a _____.

2. A neoplasm is an abnormal _____ that serves no useful purpose and may harm the host organism.

3. *Metastasis* refers to _____ _____ _____.

4. The term *oncology* refers to the:
   1. medical specialty that deals with the diagnosis, treatment, and study of cancer.
   2. study of regional lymph nodes and dissection of tumors.
   3. study of veins and graphs of nodes.
   4. medical study of epidemiology.

5. A person with expertise in treating cancer with chemotherapy or biotherapy and in handling general medical problems is referred to as a _____.

6. _____ is the study of distribution and determinants of diseases and health.

7. Match each term with the appropriate definition.

    _____ a. incidence rates for cancer   1. total number of people with cancer alive today

    _____ b. prevalence of cancer   2. reflects the number of new cases of cancer occurring in a specified population during a year

    _____ c. mortality rates   3. number of deaths caused by cancer that occur in the specified population in a given year

8. Match each term with the appropriate definition or description.

    _____ a. fibromas   1. common benign neoplasm that arises in adipose tissue

    _____ b. lipomas   2. may grow anywhere in the body, but frequently make their home in the uterus

    _____ c. leiomyomas   3. expands in size as it grows, but does not infiltrate or metastasize

    _____ d. benign tumor   4. represent a serious threat to the life and well being of the host

    _____ e. malignant neoplasms   5. benign neoplasm of smooth muscle origin, most common benign tumor in women

    _____ f. carcinoma in situ   6. neoplasm of epithelial tissue that remains confined to the site of origin

    _____ g. malignant fibrosarcomas   7. tumors are similar to benign fibromas, tend to grow in the same sites, and may originate as benign fibromas, later becoming malignant

    _____ h. bronchogenic carcinomas   8. tumors account for 90% of all cases of lung cancer

THEORIES AND TRENDS

9. The process through which normal cells are transformed into malignant or cancer cells is called _____.

10. Briefly describe the three stages of a metastatic cascade.
    Stage 1

    Stage 2

    Stage 3

11. The _____ usually defends against bacterial or viral invaders and plays a key role in controlling the growth of cancer cells.

12. True or False

_____ Cancer is a genetic disease.

REVIEWING YOUR KNOWLEDGE

13. _____ causes more cancer in the U.S. than do all other known causes combined.

14. True or False

_____ Certain viruses are strongly associated with cancer.

15. Some host characteristics that influence cancer susceptibility include: (Select all that apply)
    1. age.
    2. sex.
    3. genetic predisposition.
    4. ethnicity or race.

16. A specific tumor marker for prostate cancer can be detected by an elevated result on which blood test?
    1. PSA (prostate specific antigen)
    2. Alpha feta protein
    3. EAS
    4. RNA factor

17. Cancer can be associated with: (Select all that apply)
    1. radiation.
    2. chemicals.
    3. viruses.
    4. other physical agents.

Clients with Cancer

OBJECTIVES

19.1   Discuss the nurse's role in cancer prevention.

19.2   Discuss the nurse's role in cancer diagnosis.

19.3   Discuss the role of surgery in cancer diagnosis and treatment.

19.4   Discuss radiation therapy as a treatment for neoplastic disorders, its potential side effects, and nursing care.

19.5   Discuss chemotherapy as a treatment modality for neoplastic disorders, its side effects, and nursing care.

UNDERSTANDING PATHOPHYSIOLOGY

1. Risk factors associated with many cancers include: (Select all that apply)
    1. smoking.
    2. dietary habits.
    3. alcohol consumption.
    4. ingestion of proteins.

2. The American Cancer Society recommends that women perform monthly breast self-examination beginning at age _____.

3. True or False

    _____   Lung cancer is the leading cause of cancer among Americans.

    _____   Colorectal cancer has the highest incidence of all cancers in men.

    _____   African American men have the highest incidence of prostate cancer in the world.

    _____   Cancer staging is the process of determining the extent of disease as the basis for treatment decisions.

    _____   Women are at greater risk of head and neck cancer than men.

4. The main objective of chemotherapy is to _____
    _____.

5. Clinical manifestations of an immediate hypersensitivity reaction include: (Select all that apply)
   1. dyspnea.
   2. chest tightness.
   3. pruritus.
   4. urticaria.
   5. tachycardia, dizziness.

APPLYING SKILLS

6. Tests and procedures used in early detection of cancers include: (Select all that apply)
   1. mammograms.
   2. Pap smears.
   3. endoscopy.
   4. radiologic imaging studies.

7. True or False

   _____ The Pap smear detects cancer in a pre-malignant stage.

8. Side effects of radiation therapy include: (Select all that apply)
   1. skin reactions.
   2. fatigue.
   3. diarrhea.
   4. nausea and vomiting.
   5. esophagitis and dysphagia.

9. _____ is the cardinal sign of an infection in a client with cancer.

BEST PRACTICES

10. True or False

    _____ The American Cancer Society recommends that cervical cancer screening begin 3 years after the onset of vaginal intercourse, but no later than the age of 21.

    _____ The U.S. Nuclear Regulatory Commission requires that radiation exposure of people be kept as low as reasonably achievable.

11. The first actions taken by the nurse when a hypersensitivity reaction occurs after drug administration include: (Select all that apply)
    1. immediately stopping drug administration.
    2. maintaining IV access with 0.9% normal saline.
    3. maintaining airway.
    4. taking the client's temperature.

12. The three key principles that the nurse should follow to protect him- or herself and others from excessive radiation exposure are _____, _____, and _____.

13. The physician may prescribe _____ to elevate or maintain the erythrocyte level and decrease the need for transfusions.

14. Decisions made at the time of first diagnosis of cancer are crucial because _____.

15. Cytological specimens are best obtained _____.

16. Surgery is not always the first phase of treatment for cancer clients. Many treatment protocols begin with _____ or _____.

17. Vascular access devices (VAD) are used during initial treatment of cancer clients who require: (Select all that apply)
    1. continuous chemotherapy.
    2. multiple access.
    3. parenteral fluids.
    4. antibiotics.
    5. frequent blood testing.

KEEPING DRUG SKILLS SHARP

18. Combination chemotherapeutic agents are used to: (Select all that apply)
    1. destroy more malignant cells.
    2. produce fewer side effects.
    3. strike cancer cells at different points in the cell cycle.
    4. individualize complex regimens.

19. When administering chemotherapeutic agents, the following steps are critical: (Select all that apply)
    1. verification of the drug
    2. verification of the dose of drug
    3. verification of schedule of drug
    4. verification by two nurses against written orders

20. The most common complications of vascular access devices for use with chemotherapy are _____ and _____.

21. Medication administration during chemotherapy has greatly improved with advent of: (Select all that apply)
    1. serotonin receptor antagonists.
    2. Zofran.
    3. Kytril.
    4. Anzemet.

22. Radiation therapy is frequently employed to kill residual cancer cells left behind after
    _____.

23. Chemotherapy doses are usually based on: (Select all that apply)
    1. body surface area in square meters (m²).
    2. client's height and weight.
    3. client's last hemoglobin.
    4. previous chemotherapy orders.

24. _____ is the term used for when some of the drug escapes from the vein.

25. True or False

    _____ Corticosteroids used in many treatment protocols can leave a client vulnerable to cancer-associated infections because they suppress immune functions.

Clients with Wounds

OBJECTIVES

20.1   Describe the processes involved in normal wound healing.

20.2   Identify the types of wound healing intention.

20.3   Discuss the impact of inflammation on normal wound healing.

20.4   Identify rationales for different types of wound dressings.

20.5   Describe nursing care and medical management for various types of wounds.

UNDERSTANDING PATHOPHYSIOLOGY

. The first component necessary for proper wound healing to occur is: (Select all that apply)
   1. vascular response.
   2. nutrition.
   3. antibiotic therapy.
   4. oxygen.

. Compare and contrast the activities that occur in each of the four phases of wound healing.

Phase	Activity
Vascular	
Inflammation	
Proliferative	
Maturation	

3. Capillary dilation increases blood flow to the site of injury and: (Select all that apply)
   1. delivers more carbon dioxide to the area.
   2. delivers more nutrients to the area.
   3. carries phagocytes away from the area.
   4. dilutes toxins secreted by invading organisms.

4. Increased numbers of _____ indicate a bacterial invasion as the bone marrow releases immature cells to combat the infection.

5. Chronic wounds that do not heal are said to have an imbalance of
   _____.

6. True or False

   _____ Wound remodeling can take over a year to complete.

   _____ Scar tissue is stronger than original tissue because it is thicker.

   _____ Eosinophils secrete antihistamine and basophils secrete histamine.

   _____ Kinins decrease vascular permeability to control excessive bleeding at the site of injury.

   _____ Neutrophils can squeeze through the lining of a capillary wall through a process called diapedesis.

   _____ "No inflammation, no healing."

   _____ Platelets release growth factors to stimulate healing

   _____ Inflammation does not occur when dead cells are present.

   _____ Neutrophils can handle up to 100,000 bacteria invading a wound.

   _____ Angiogenesis is a process which assists platelets to stop bleeding.

   _____ An obese client with a large wound should have carbohydrate calorie restrictions but sufficient protein intake.

   _____ Autolytic debridement can be used with infected wounds less than 5 cm.

   _____ Hyperalimentation is sometimes used to facilitate wound healing.

   _____ The key to prevention of pressure ulcers is turning and repositioning.

   _____ Clean sandwich baggies can be used as alternative gloves by clients doing dressing changes in their homes.

   _____ To obtain appropriate wound culture specimens, remove the exudate and then swab the wound bed.

7. Identify each type of wound healing as primary, secondary, or tertiary intention.

A _____

B _____

C _____

8. Identify the pathological effects of each factor on wound healing.

Factor	Effect
Diabetes mellitus	
Lack of Vitamin C	
Neuropathy	
Foreign bodies	
Protein malnutrition	
Smoking	

9. Why is inflammatory exudate from a wound considered helpful?

10. Nutritional impairment can delay wound healing. The lab value indicative of the nutritional status of the client is the _____.

APPLYING SKILLS

11. Purulent exudate from a wound is a manifestation of _____
_____.

12. A nurse must check for an edematous area on a client's leg to monitor for increased swelling. Identify the appropriate action to ensure accurate measurements.

13. Prior to beginning a dressing change, the nurse should assess the client's
_____.

14. True or False

_____ Exudate from a wound can help in the healing process.

_____ A blister is an example of a serous exudate.

_____ Low-grade fever should be treated with antipyretics.

_____ When assessing edema, the nurse should use the uninvolved side as a baseline.

_____ Surgical incisions normally appear pink and swollen.

_____ Proper wound healing includes an internal scar known as a "healing ridge."

_____ Eschar helps to protect wound during the healing process.

15. Compare and/or contrast the types of wound appearance and the clinical significance of these assessment findings.

Wound Appearance	Clinical Significance
Edges approximated	
Open wound, edges apart	
Healing ridge under skin	
Serous exudate	
Purulent exudate	
Eschar	
Granuloma	

BEST PRACTICES

16. State the rationale for applying ice only for the first 24 to 72 hours to the site of an injury, then following it with heat.

7. When teaching a client how to care for a surgical incision, the nurse should emphasize all of the following except:
   1. clinical manifestations of infection.
   2. how to care for and empty drain reservoir.
   3. use of water to cleanse a suture line.
   4. when to return for suture removal.

18. Define the methods for debridement:

Method	Procedure
Sharp debridement	
Mechanical	
Enzymatic	
Autolytic	

19. A _____ solution is recommended as safe for wound care.

20. Identify the action the nurse would perform to enhance the effect of enzymatic ointment on dry, thick eschar over a wound.

KEEPING DRUG SKILLS SHARP

21. A client who is taking steroids is at risk for developing infections. Identify the mechanism for the increased risk.

22. True or False

_____ Diabetic clients with wounds should maintain blood glucose levels below 200 mg/dl to promote proper wound healing.

_____ Glucocorticoids help reduce inflammation and speed wound healing.

_____ Carbon monoxide is a vasoconstrictive agent that slows blood supply to wound site and delays healing.

_____ Vitamin C in high doses is harmful to a wound due to its acidic content.

_____ NSAIDs can be used to reduce inflammation in wounds.

CONCEPT MAP EXERCISES

The following questions are based on the concept map *Understanding Inflammation and Its Treatment* in your textbook.

23. How does the "RICE" treatment affect the inflammatory process?

24. How do NSAIDs reduce inflammation?

25. Steroids are given to block the release of _____ from mast cells.

Chapter 21

Perspectives on Infectious Disorders

OBJECTIVES

21.1 Discuss the impact of infectious disease on human history.

21.2 Describe the process of an infection and methods to prevent and/or contain it.

21.3 Identify sources of nosocomial infections in hospitalized clients and methods to prevent them.

21.4 Discuss the impact of immunization programs on the prevention and containment of infectious diseases.

21.5 Describe methods used to prevent and contain infectious diseases in long-term care facilities and community settings.

UNDERSTANDING PATHOPHYSIOLOGY

. Factors that resulted in the dramatic decrease of infectious diseases during the period from 1950 to 1980 include: (Select all that apply)
   1. social, public health and medical control efforts.
   2. environmental sanitation.
   3. international vaccination programs.
   4. restraint in prescribing antibiotics.
   5. development of new anti-infectives.

. Factors that have resulted in a steady increase in infectious diseases since the 1980s include: (Select all that apply)
   1. new infectious agents.
   2. decreasing vaccination rates.
   3. increasing populations of chronically ill, malnourished, and immunocompromised clients.
   4. restraint in prescribing antibiotics.

. List the common reservoirs for infection:
   a.
   b.
   c.
   d.
   e.
   f.

4. Explain why the identification of a "carrier" is of critical importance in controlling infection.

5. Portals of entry for a pathogen into a new host include: (Select all that apply)
   1. ingestion.
   2. exhalation.
   3. contact with mucous membranes.
   4. the percutaneous route.
   5. the transplacental route.

6. How can ethnicity be considered a factor which might increase the susceptibility of a client to disease?

7. First-line defences against infection include all of the following except:
   1. gag and cough reflexes.
   2. inflammatory response.
   3. peristalsis in GI tract.
   4. flushing action by tears, saliva.

8. Invasion of an organism that allows replication without clinical manifestation or detectable immune response is referred to as _____.

9. The period of time during which a pathogen is replicating but before it is shed from the host is called the _____.

10. The _____ is the period of time from invasion of the disease to appearance of clinical manifestations.

11. Common nosocomial infections that health care workers are at particular risk for contracting include: (Select all that apply)
    1. HIV.
    2. hepatitis B.
    3. pneumonia.
    4. tuberculosis.

12. True or False

    _____ The entire population needs to be immune to prevent disease epidemic.

    _____ Herd immunity decreases the likelihood of disease transmission.

13. Common portals of exit for infectious diseases include: (Select all that apply)
    1. bodily secretions.
    2. body fluids.
    3. exhaled air.
    4. excretions (urine and feces).
    5. open lesions.
    6. exudates from wounds.

APPLYING SKILLS

14. Describe for each category of clients how their risk for developing nosocomial respiratory infections occurs.

Category	Etiology
Postoperative	
Diminished consciousness	
Impaired gag reflex	
Intubation	
Tracheostomy	
Old age	
Chronic lung disease	
Cardiac disease	
Renal insufficiency	
Malignancies	

BEST PRACTICES

15. Explain why it is important for the nurse to recognize subclinical infectious states when caring for clients.

16. State the rationale for discontinuing the practice of pre-operative shaving of the surgical site.

17. A _____ dressing placed over an insertion site may contribute to the development of an infection because it allows for growth of normal skin flora.

18. _____ and the use of _____ hand rubs are the most effective ways to prevent the spread of infection.

19. List the common protective barriers used by health care workers to prevent transmission of infection.
    a.
    b.
    c.
    d.

20. List three transmission-based client care precautions for clients with known infections to contain transmission:
    a.
    b.
    c.

KEEPING DRUG SKILLS SHARP

21. The mechanisms that allow bacteria to develop resistance to antiobiotics include all of the following except:
    1. producing an enzyme that will inactivate or destroy the antibiotic.
    2. altering the target site to evade action of the antibiotic.
    3. overprescribing of penicillin.
    4. preventing antibiotic access to the target site on bacterium.

22. Measures to reduce the incidence of antimicrobial resistance include: (Select all that apply)
    1. Obtaining appropriate specimens for culture before starting antibiotics.
    2. Checking sensitivity reports to ensure antibiotic is appropriate.
    3. Thorough hand washing.
    4. Strict aseptic techniques.
    5. Use of barrier precautions.

23. True or False

_____ Tetanus boosters are due every 10 years after the primary series.

_____ Women of childbearing age should avoid immunizations for Rubella.

_____ A child who has had a varicella infection does not need the immunization.

_____ Influenza vaccine is recommended for people older than 65, nursing home residents, and people with chronic cardiac or pulmonary disorders.

_____ Pertussis vaccine is given only after age 60 to prevent complications.

_____ People born before 1957 have natural immunity to Measles, Mumps, and Rubella.

_____ Older people need vaccinations because of a decline in their immune system function.

_____ OSHA requires all employers to provide Hepatitis B vaccination to at-risk employees at the employer's expense.

Chapter 22

Clients with Pain

OBJECTIVES

22.1 Discuss the phenomenon of pain and how various factors affect its perception by the client and health care providers.

22.2 Discuss the types of pain and pain syndromes experienced by clients.

22.3 Describe nursing and medical/surgical management of the client with pain.

22.4 Compare and contrast analgesics and methods of administration.

22.5 Identify non-pharmaceutical interventions for the client with pain.

UNDERSTANDING PATHOPHYSIOLOGY

1. Explain how pain can be beneficial to the client.

2. Explain how unrelieved pain can result in pulmonary complications in the postoperative client.

3. Compare and contrast the characteristics of acute pain and chronic pain.

Type	Characteristics
Acute Pain	
Chronic Pain	

Copyright © 2005 by Elsevier Inc. All rights reserved.

113

4. Identify examples of each type of chronic pain.
   a. nonmalignant:

   b. intermittent:

   c. malignant:

5. Identify the three classifications for sources of pain in the body and give examples of each.
   a.

   b.

   c.

6. True or False

   _____ Cutaneous pain tends to be diffuse, poorly localized, and vague.

   _____ Somatic pain is poorly localized and may cause nausea.

   _____ Skeletal muscle is sensitive to stretching and ischemia which will cause pain.

   _____ Each dermatome is served by only one spinal nerve and dorsal root.

   _____ Pain in the GI tract is the result of inflammation, ulcers, or muscle spasms.

7. _____ causes pain in the client with HIV due to lesions causing blockage of the lymphatic drainage, thereby increasing pressure and pain.

8. List the factors that affect how pain is perceived.
   a.

   b.

   c.

   d.

   e.

   f.

9. Differentiate between pain threshold and pain tolerance.

10. Factors that affect the duration of action of pain medications include: (Select all that apply)
    1. pain intensity.
    2. route of administration.
    3. dose size.
    4. the client's ability to absorb, biotransform, and eliminate medication.

11. The _____ provides pain relief by delivering electrical bursts through the skin which mask the pain signals to the brain.

APPLYING YOUR KNOWLEDGE

12. Margo McCaffery's definition of pain is "whatever the experiencing person says it is and existing whenever the person says it does." Explain how this definition affects a nurse's assessment of a client in pain.

13. Clients can undergo behavioral changes when experiencing pain for prolonged periods of time. Common characteristics of clients experiencing chronic pain syndrome include: (Select all that apply)
    1. depression.
    2. increased/decreased appetite and weight.
    3. social withdrawal.
    4. poor sleep and chronic fatigue.
    5. decreased concentration.
    6. drastically increased activity level.

14. Clients may exhibit which of the following behaviors in an attempt to adapt to pain? (Select all that apply)
    1. guarding the painful area
    2. showing a blank expression
    3. exhibiting decreased activity
    4. reporting pain frequently
    5. increased physical activity
    6. exhibiting sleepiness
    7. reporting pain only if asked
    8. showing painful expressions

15. List the five new JCAHO standards for pain management:
    a.

    b.

    c.

    d.

    e.

16. Identify the single most important indicator of pain intensity.

17. The _____ scale is more appropriate for assessing pain in children than numerical or visual descriptor scales.

18. Critical factors to determine when assessing pain in clients include: (Select all that apply)
    1. location.
    2. quality.
    3. duration.
    4. distress.

BEST PRACTICES

19. State the nurse's role as part of the healthcare team in addressing pain relief needs for the client.

20. List two responsibilities of the nurse to correct misinformation about pain.
    a.
    b.

21. True or False

    _____ The health care team can determine a person's pain tolerance level.

    _____ Past experience with pain can alter a client's perception of pain.

    _____ Many health care providers believe that the amount of pain can be based on a medical condition.

    _____ Pain perception does not depend exclusively on the degree of physical damage.

22. Identify three nursing interventions to assist the client in pain in addition to providing pain medication.
    a.
    b.
    c.

23. The nurse should not identify complete pain relief as a realistic outcome for a client with _____ _____ pain.

24. Identify an independent action can the nurse implement to relieve pain.

KEEPING DRUG SKILLS SHARP

25. List the three steps of the "pain ladder" developed by The World Health Organization.
    a.
    b.
    c.

26. True or False: According to the American Pain Society, the following statements should be implemented as standards for pain management:

_____   Nurses should individualize route, dosage, and schedule of pain medications for each client.

_____   Analgesics should be given on a PRN basis according to orders.

_____   The use of meperidine [Demerol] should be avoided.

_____   The use of placebos is appropriate for children and older clients.

_____   The nurse must recognize and treat side effects of pain medications.

_____   Health care providers should expect physical dependence and prevent withdrawal manifestations.

_____   Nurses must use caution when changing to a new opioid or route.

_____   Clients who develop tolerance to a medication should have dosages reduced to prevent addiction.

27. _____ are only used with caution for HIV clients because of reports of cross-reaction with acetaminophen drugs used to treat the HIV infection.

28. The ceiling for maximum dosage of morphine that can be administered to clients with pain is
_____.

29. Describe the characteristics of the common anesthetic agents Lidocaine and Bupivacaine.

Agent	Characteristics
Lidocaine	
Bupivacaine	

30. Application of _____ 45 minutes to 1 hour prior to the site of venipuncture, injection, or heel sticks will reduce pain by providing local anesthesia.

31. A major contraindication for using celecoxib (Celebrex) is _____ allergy.

32. List three common medications used to treat constipation as a side-effect of meperidine.
   a.

   b.

   c.

33. Morphine is a powerful opioid that can cause respiratory depression. Identify the time frames for the nurse to assess respiratory status after administering morphine via the following routes:

    IV:

    IM:

    SC:

    Epidural:

34. For each type of adjuvant medication, identify the medication category and indication for use.

Medication	Category	Indication
Tegretol		
Dilantin		
Neurontin		
Decadron		
Lioresal		

35. List the two nontraditional routes of administration that have been developed for Fentanyl (long-acting morphine):

    a.

    b.

36. Explain the advantage of patient-controlled analgesia (PCA) over PRN administration of pain medication by the nurse.

37. Rectal doses are _____ oral preparations.
    1. less than
    2. equal to
    3. greater than

Perspectives in Palliative Care

OBJECTIVES

23.1   Discuss the development of hospice and its impact on end of life care.

23.2   Identify the five phases of the normal death and dying experience according to Kubler-Ross.

23.3   Identify clinical manifestations experienced by the client at the end of life.

23.4   Discuss nursing care and medical management for the client at the end of life.

23.5   Describe nursing interventions to assist clients and their families coping with end of life issues.

UNDERSTANDING PATHOPHYSIOLOGY

1. List the five phases of the normal death and dying experience as identified and defined by Elizabeth Kubler-Ross.
    a.

    b.

    c.

    d.

    e.

2. State the focus of palliative care.

3. The chronic diseases that are major causes of death in the United States include: (Select all that apply)
    1. heart disease.
    2. cancer.
    3. stroke.
    4. COPD.
    5. dementia.

119

4. Identify four factors that define quality of life.
   a.
   b.
   c.
   d.

5. Possible *reversible* causes for delirium are: (Select all that apply)
   1. medications, especially opioids, sedatives.
   2. hypoxia.
   3. dehydration.
   4. metabolic causes [hyponatremia].
   5. sepsis.
   6. polypharmacy.
   7. increased ICP from metastatic disease.

6. Provide examples of the common causes of fatigue in the hospice client.

Problem	Example
Disease/treatment-related	
Physiologic	
Psycho-emotional	
Spiritual	

APPLYING SKILLS

7. A client's _____ is determined by a thorough history and physical evaluation of the client's status and wants/desires.

8. The most effective instrument for assessing changes in cognitive status is the _____ _____.

9. Clinical manifestations that occur during the active dying process include: (Select all that apply)
   1. decrease in urinary output; urinary retention or incontinence.
   2. increase in anxiety.
   3. mottling of skin color with peripheral cyanosis.
   4. tachypnea or Cheyne-Stokes respirations.
   5. impaired swallowing, loss of gag reflex.
   6. delirium, altered cognition.
   7. acute confusion, anxiety.

10. The sense of _____ remains intact throughout the dying process.

11. A 72-year-old grandmother has been diagnosed with metastatic breast cancer and has been told her prognosis is less than 6 months. Her family is concerned with her increasing fatigue and wants to reduce her pain medication dosages to allow her to interact more with the family when they visit. Explain how can the nurse differentiate between effects of medications and true fatigue to help maintain the client's comfort level and improve the quality of family interactions.

12. A client has been battling liver cancer for over a year and has begun to show clinical manifestations of an active dying process. Identify the clinical presentations the hospice nurse would observe to indicate an active dying process rather than a stable chronic condition.

BEST PRACTICES

13. Nursing interventions to assist the client with dyspnea include: (Select all that apply)
    1. calming presence.
    2. breathing exercises.
    3. a fan blowing in room.
    4. relaxation therapy.
    5. offering cold fluids.
    6. incentive spirometer therapy.
    7. massage.
    8. pursed-lip breathing.

14. Nursing interventions to correct reversible causes of fatigue include all of the following except:
    1. administering prescribed transfusions or erythropoietin to correct anemia.
    2. counseling, education, relaxation and massage to address stress.
    3. limiting fluid intake.
    4. modifying activity and rest patterns.
    5. administering prescribed corticosteroids to lessen effects of tumor induced substances and increase appetite.
    6. administering prescribed psychostimulants to increase energy.

15. Identify nursing interventions to assist the client and his or her family cope with the last days of life.

    a.

    b.

    c.

    d.

16. List the four tasks of mourning for conclusion of bereavement.

    a.

    b.

    c.

    d.

KEEPING DRUG SKILLS SHARP

17. Common opioids used to provide pain relief include: (Select all that apply)
    1. morphine.
    2. amitriptyline.
    3. hydromorphone.
    4. Fentanyl.

18. The maximum amount of opioid that can be administered to a hospice client is

    _____.

19. Compare and contrast common adjuvant medications used in hospice care.

Medication	Action	Indication
NSAIDs		
Tricyclic antidepressants and anticonvulsants		
Anticholinergics		
Benzodiazepines		

20. True or False

_____ Therapeutic levels of analgesics must be maintained at all times for clients with persistent or chronic pain.

_____ Around-the-clock scheduling of medications is the most appropriate for hospice clients.

_____ Immediate-release oral morphine should be given every 5-6 hours as needed.

_____ Controlled-release medications may be given every 8, 12, or 24 hours.

_____ Short-acting medications should be given to cover a spike in client's pain.

_____ A client experiencing pain 2 hours after a rescue dose should wait until the next scheduled dose to prevent oversedation and respiratory depression.

_____ Morphine is used to relieve dyspnea (difficulty breathing).

21. _____ _____ is the drug of choice for hallucinations.

22. Medications used for sleep disturbances include all of the following except:
    1. zolpidem (Ambien).
    2. flurazepam (Dalmane).
    3. oxazepam (Serax).
    4. oxycontin (Oxycodone).
    5. temazepam (Restoril).

23. _____ are effective medications for treating smooth muscle spasms.

24. Clients with neuropathic pain described as "shooting," "burning," or "shock-like" can be treated with _____ medications.

25. If an intracranial tumor causes increased pressure, _____ would be effective in reducing the edema.

Clients with Sleep and Rest Disorders and Fatigue

OBJECTIVES

24.1 Describe the phenomenon of sleep and common sleep pattern disturbances.

24.2 Analyze common sleep disorders including risk factors, characteristics, therapeutic interventions, and nursing care.

24.3 Discuss the association of sleep pattern disturbances to underlying medical and psychological disorders and related nursing interventions.

24.4 Analyze chronic fatigue syndrome.

UNDERSTANDING PATHOPHYSIOLOGY

1. True or False

    _____ Sleep is a normal state of altered consciousness during which the body rests.

    _____ Poor sleep habits can contribute to transitory periods of insomnia.

    _____ Narcolepsy is characterized by excessive daytime sleepiness and is not associated with disturbed nocturnal sleep.

    _____ Nightmares are parasomnias associated with REM sleep.

    _____ Fatigue is a subjective state in which the client feels a sense of physical exhaustion but is mentally rested.

2. Characteristics of sleep and sleep pattern disturbances include: (Select all that apply)
    1. During a given year approximately 1/2 of the population has some problem.
    2. Sleep disturbances may be secondary to environmental stressors.
    3. Sleep disturbances have a reciprocal relationship to underlying illness and disorders.
    4. Sleep pattern disturbance is always transitory.

3. Which of the following statements about the physiology of sleep are true? (Select all that apply)
    1. The production of melatonin, a potent sleep inducer, is controlled by the pituitary.
    2. The retina provides information about darkness and light to the suprachiasmatic nucleus.
    3. Decreased concentrations of serotonin are associated with non-rapid eye movement sleep.
    4. Cytokines are linked to the sleep cycle.

4. All of the following are polysomnography parameters of sleep except:
   1. brain wave activity.
   2. eye movements.
   3. respiratory rate and depth.
   4. muscle tone.

5. Match each description of NREM and REM sleep to the appropriate type of sleep. (Descriptions may be used more than once)

   Descriptions   **Type of Sleep**

   _____ a. light stage of sleep from which when wakened, clients   1. NREM
             deny being asleep

   _____ b. ventilatory response to hypoxia and hypercapnia is   2. REM
             decreased

   _____ c. dreams are thought-like ruminations about recent
             events

   _____ d. dreams are vivid, story-like, emotional, and bizarre

   _____ e. burst of activity are called sleep spindles

6. Psychophysiologic insomnia is associated with increased physiologic response to
   _____.

7. Cataplexy is best described as:
   1. excessive daytime sleepiness.
   2. a circadian rhythm in the sleep cycle.
   3. the time it takes to fully awaken from a sleep cycle.
   4. a loss of muscle tone at times of unexpected emotion.

8. List the three primary contributing factors for obstructive sleep apnea syndrome in children:
   a.

   b.

   c.

9. List and briefly describe the three circadian rhythm sleep disorders:
   a.

   b.

   c.

10. Sleep disorders are often secondary to other medical or psychological problems. List the three primary neurotransmitter imbalances associated with sleep disorders and briefly discuss each:
    a.

    b.

    c.

11. Match each hormonal imbalance with the appropriate description of the sleep pattern disturbance associated with it.

	Hormonal Imbalance		**Description**
_____	a.	hyperthyroidism	1. less slow-wave sleep
_____	b.	hypothyroidism	2. nightmares and early morning headaches
_____	c.	diabetes mellitus	3. snoring and obstructive sleep apnea
_____	d.	premenstrual syndrome	4. fragmented, short, sleep periods
_____	e.	menopause	5. excessive sleepiness
_____	f.	postmenopausal	6. poor sleep quality and mood changes

12. An internal stimuli that contributes to sleep fragmentation is:
    1. nocturnal temperature.
    2. bruxism.
    3. the urge to void.
    4. room light.

13. State the factors that contribute to sleep deprivation in clients in a critical care unit.

14. Defining characteristics of chronic fatigue include: (Select all that apply)
    1. verbalization of a lack of energy.
    2. disruption of usual routines.
    3. emotional stability.
    4. increased libido.
    5. accident proneness.

APPLYING SKILLS

15. True or False

    _____ Chronobiology is the study of biologic changes as they occur in relation to time.

16. A nurse who is planning care would anticipate a sleep pattern disturbance during hospitalization in which of the following clients because of altered circadian rhythms?
    1. a 20-year-old male
    2. a 35-year-old female
    3. a 45-year-old female
    4. a 75-year-old male

17. What factors that influence sleep patterns in older adults should the nurse consider when planning care?

18. Clients who experience early-morning awakenings should be screened for _____ _____.

19. The primary diagnostic test for sleep disorders is _____.

20. What visible signs of sleep disorder should the nurse observe for during the physical assessment?

Case Study

A client is being evaluated for a possible sleep disorder. The client is a male, aged 49, height 5'10", weight 254 lbs. His chief complaint is that he feels tired in the morning when he wakes up, "Like I haven't been to sleep at all. But my wife says I had to have been sleeping because my snoring is keeping her awake." The client states that he had seen a physician about 6 months ago and was given a prescription for benzodiazepine for "anxiety." When questioned further, the client states that he doesn't think the medicine has helped; if anything, he feels worse. When asked if there were other things the client was concerned about, he stated that he was having trouble maintaining an erection during intercourse. The client's history and physical exam is unremarkable although the nurse notes that his neck is short and thick and that he drinks 1 or 2 beers 3–4 nights a week.

21. What factors are present which place this client at risk for obstructive sleep apnea syndrome?

22. What clinical manifestations does the client present which suggest obstructive sleep apnea syndrome?

23. What in the client's history should the nurse report to the physician immediately and why?

A diagnosis of Obstructive sleep apnea syndrome is made. The client is encouraged to lose weight, reduce or cease consumption of alcohol, and use CPAP during sleep.

24. What is the rationale for encouraging the client to decrease alcohol consumption?

25. What should the nurse teach the client about CPAP?

BEST PRACTICES

26. Based on an understanding of ultradian cycles, a nurse working the night shift would plan to awaken clients (if necessary) not any more frequently than every _____ minutes.

27. The nurse is caring for a client with psychophysiologic insomnia. Which of the following nursing interventions should the nurse implement to promote sleep?
    1. Introduce the client to relaxation exercises and have him or her initially practice them at bed-time.
    2. Allow the client to vary time of rising to accommodate periods of unrest.
    3. Allow the client to take short power naps during the day.
    4. Curtail the time the client is allowed in bed to the minimum necessary.

28. Appropriate interventions for a client with narcolepsy include: (Select all that apply)
    1. Emphasize good sleep hygiene.
    2. Allow variation in the sleep schedule.
    3. Provide naps at pre-set times in the awake cycle.
    4. Plan naps for periods associated with sleepiness.
    5. Develop a safety plan to cope with potential disruptions.

29. A client with SAD asks the nurse to explain why she needs to buy a special light and can't use the floor lamp. What explanation should the nurse provide?

30. Explain what precautions the nurse should take with clients who experience REM-associated erections and also have an indwelling catheter.

31. List the nursing interventions the nurse can implement to assist hospitalized clients with sleep onset difficulty:
    a.

    b.

    c.

    d.

32. A nurse is caring for a client with a nursing diagnosis of sleep pattern disturbance related to changes in sleep routine secondary to hospitalization. An appropriate nursing intervention would be to:
    1. have the client turn out the lights and television at least one hour before the usual sleep time.
    2. encourage the client to sleep with fewer covers.
    3. provide a low carbohydrate, high protein snack at bedtime.
    4. provide a back rub and dim lights and noise.

33. Explain why the client with chronic fatigue syndrome should be taught to balance periods of gentle activity with frequent rest periods.

34. When teaching a client with chronic fatigue syndrome about exercise, the nurse would advise the client to:
    1. engage in vigorous aerobic activity daily.
    2. maintain ongoing physical activity to alleviate symptoms.
    3. engage in a balanced plan of gentle activity.
    4. avoid active, aerobic physical activity.

KEEPING DRUG SKILLS SHARP

35. Based on an understanding of chronopharmacology, a nurse would anticipate that clients receiving continuous intravenous heparin would have a greater risk of bleeding in the
_____.

36. Explain why antidepressants are part of the treatment for narcolepsy.

37. Explain the rationale for prescribing clonazepam or baclofen to clients with periodic limb movement disorder.

38. Initial pharmacotherapy for clients with chronic fatigue syndrome who are experiencing pain would be:
    1. antihistamines.
    2. sedatives.
    3. antidepressants.
    4. anti-inflammatory agents.

Chapter 25

Clients with Psychosocial and Mental Health Concerns

OBJECTIVES

25.1 Explore the importance of psychosocial concepts to health.

25.2 Differentiate among major psychiatric disorders with can co-occur with medical illness, their outcome management, and nursing interventions.

25.3 Apply psychosocial concepts to care of clients with medical-surgical illnesses.

UNDERSTANDING PATHOPHYSIOLOGY

1. It is important for the nurse to understand the psychological and social aspects of a client's health because: (Select all that apply)
   1. physical health may be altered by underlying psychological processes.
   2. the stress of physical illness may alter a client's normal emotional response.
   3. social abilities may alter a client's ability to negotiate the health care delivery system.
   4. the manner in which clients respond psychologically to physical illness may vary.

2. List the four universal psychosocial concepts and related factors which influence response to stressors.
   a.

   b.

   c.

   d.

3. Anxiety is:
   1. a strong feeling of fear or dread with an unknown cause.
   2. a phenomenon occurring between a person and the environment which endangers well-being.
   3. a response to a stressor that is emotion-focused.
   4. an unconscious response to a stressor.

4. Compare and contrast emotion-focused and problem-focused coping behavior.

5. Match each type of self-esteem with the typical client response.

	Type of Self-Esteem	**Typical Response**
_____	a. High self-esteem	1. consistently pessimistic
_____	b. Low self-esteem	2. positive expectations

6. Identify the two causes of psychiatric disorders and briefly explain each.

7. A positive clinical manifestation of schizophrenia is:
   1. blunted affect.
   2. avoidance of social contact.
   3. auditory hallucination.
   4. lack of attention to hygiene.

8. Match each clinical manifestation associated with mood disorders with the appropriate type of disorder (may be used more than once).

	Clinical Manifestation	**Type of Disorder**
_____	a. Sad mood	1. Depressive Mood Disorder
_____	b. Increased libido	2. Mania
_____	c. Negative thinking	
_____	d. Change in sleep pattern	
_____	e. Rapid speech	
_____	f. Preoccupation with somatic complaints	
_____	g. Increased energy	
_____	h. Impulsive behavior	

9. A typical manifestation of a client with a depressive type mood disorder is:
   1. an overabundance of energy.
   2. an optimistic attitude.
   3. increased motivation.
   4. hopelessness.

10. Major depressive disorders are characterized by: (Select all that apply)
   1. occurrance of onset between 20-50 years of age.
   2. prevalence in adolescent and adult men.
   3. co-occurance with other psychiatric and medical illness.
   4. suicide.

11. True or False

   _____ Clients who experience the same event will have the same stress response.

_____ When verbal and nonverbal communication is incongruent, the verbal communication reflects the true meaning.

_____ Anxiety disorders are the most common psychiatric disorder in the United States.

_____ The key element in mood disorders is that the person cannot control the severity of the feeling.

APPLYING SKILLS

12. The ego defense mechanism most frequently used by clients with a serious illness is
_____.

13. Which of the following have a high risk for suicide?
    1. young adults and school age children
    2. a person just before a psychiatric hospitalization
    3. a person with a history of a previous attempt
    4. a person with a signed safety contract

14. True or False

    _____ Ego defense mechanisms operate at the conscious level to disguise a real threat and protect the person from feeling anxious.

BEST PRACTICES

15. A nurse is providing care to a client with anxiety about a recent diagnosis. A nursing intervention to help to decrease the client's anxiety would be to:
    1. refer all questions the client has to the physician.
    2. provide a brightly lit environment with noise for distraction.
    3. avoid looking directly at the client during communication.
    4. acknowledge the client's feelings and help the client to explore them.

16. List the four components of basic client and family teaching for a client with a psychiatric disorder:
    a.

    b.

    c.

    d.

17. When providing health teaching to a client with a pre-existing mental illness, the nurse should always include a _____ in the teaching.

18. An appropriate intervention for interacting with a client with an anxiety disorder would be to:
    1. establish a pattern of making eye contact, looking away, and reestablishing eye contact.
    2. speak in a loud firm voice.
    3. avoid using touch when talking.
    4. answer questions honestly.

19. True or False

    _____ Mood disorders can almost always be managed with a combination of medication and psychotherapy.

KEEPING DRUG SKILLS SHARP

20. Match each description with the type of side effect associated with antipsychotic agents used in the treatment of schizophrenia. The type of side effect may be used more than once.

Description	Type of Side Effect
_____ a. requires emergency hospitalisation	1. extrapyramidal symptoms
_____ b. drooling and acute muscle spasms of the tongue	2. tardive dyskinesia
_____ c. occurs in one-third of clients	3. neuroleptic malignant syndrome
d. extreme muscle rigidity, high fever, sweating, and fluctuations in consciousness	
e. involuntary movements of the tongue, face, hands, and legs	
f. treated with anticholinergic agents	

Clients with Substance Abuse Disorders

OBJECTIVES

26.1 Examine the theories of substance abuse.

26.2 Describe characteristics of substance abuse.

26.3 Describe common substances that are abused and associated effects.

26.4 Describe nursing care of clients who abuse substances.

26.5 Discuss the abuse of substances in health professionals.

UNDERSTANDING PATHOPHYSIOLOGY

1. A biologic theory of substance abuse would maintain that:
   1. Biochemical abnormalities predispose individuals to alcoholism.
   2. Native American experience tachycardia, a sensation of warmth, flushing, and generalized discomfort when they consume alcohol.
   3. Asian Americans have the highest rate of alcohol consumption.
   4. Acetaldehyde, a metabolic by-product, provides a sense of well-being when alcohol is consumed.

2. Compare and contrast the psychoanalytic, psychodynamic, behavioral, and family system theories that predispose individuals to substance abuse.

3. Match each substance abuse term with the appropriate definition.

	Term		Definition
_____	a.	Substance abuse	1. any factor that increases the likelihood of an event occurring
_____	b.	Substance dependence	2. return to a normal state of health
_____	c.	Addiction	3. discontinuation of a substance by a dependent person
_____	d.	Intoxication	4. continued use of a psychoactive substance despite accompanying problems
_____	e.	Tolerance	5. a compulsion, loss of control, and progressive pattern of drug use
_____	f.	Predisposition	6. a range of symptoms indicating that a person persists in using a substance
_____	g.	Withdrawal	7. an altered physiologic state resulting from the use of a psychoactive drug
_____	h.	Recovery	8. person needs to increase amounts of a drug to achieve the same effects

4. Which statements accurately characterize polysubstance abuse? (Select all that apply)
   1. Polysubstance abuse may be a coping strategy for clients with a chronic illness.
   2. Polysubstance abuse applies to multiple use of illegal substances only.
   3. Clients with polysubstance abuse require special care during withdrawal.
   4. Use of alcohol and nicotine is polysubstance abuse.

5. The immediate result of overconsumption of any psychoactive substance is _____ _____.

6. Factors which influence the withdrawal process in persons who sharply reduce or stop using psychoactive substances include: (Select all that apply)
   1. overall physical health.
   2. the reason for use.
   3. the type of drug used.
   4. the method of intake.

7. A client is withdrawing from alcohol. Which of the following clinical manifestations would the nurse expect to see 2 to 3 days after the last drink was ingested?
   1. below normal body temperature
   2. hypotension
   3. disorientation
   4. chest pain

8. The two body systems most directly affected by cocaine use are _____ and _____.

9. Which statements accurately characterize the physiologic effects of inhalants? (Select all that apply)
   1. Inhalants cause CNS excitement within minutes of use.
   2. Inhalants increase heart rate, respirations, and overall mental activity.
   3. Continuous use may result in bone marrow dysfunction.
   4. Sudden death is a potential outcome.

10. The human body produces a natural opioid called _____,
    which facilitates a feeling of well-being.

11. A manifestation associated with marijuana intoxication is:
    1. improved memory capacity.
    2. precise hand-eye coordination.
    3. decreased body temperature.
    4. lower heart rate.

12. Select correct descriptions of phencyclidine (PCP) and the body's response to it. (Select all that
    apply)
    1. increased production of dopamine
    2. papillary dilation
    3. diploplia
    4. excreted in the urine
    5. hypotensive
    6. psychosis-like state

13. The classic symptom associated with caffeine withdrawal is _____
    _____.

14. The most commonly used illegal drug in the United States is
    _____.

15. True or False

    _____ Alcoholism, as evidenced by research, has a genetic component.

    _____ According to the sociocultural framework of addiction, the societal environment con-
    tributes to drug use, treatment, and recovery.

    _____ Alcohol is a CNS stimulant that affects all levels of the brain.

    _____ Marijuana residues in the lungs are more carcinogenic than tobacco residue.

    _____ Nicotine use is the leading cause of preventable death in the United States.

    _____ The most common health consequences of abusing drugs and alcohol are disorders of
    the cardiovascular system.

    _____ Nurses have a higher prevalence of substance abuse than other health care professionals
    such as physicians.

    _____ Clients who abuse hallucinogens are at high risk for acts of violence.

    _____ The effects of hallucinogens on individuals are predictable.

APPLYING SKILLS

16. When conducting a drug and alcohol assessment, the nurse needs to consider that: (Select all that apply)
    1. one of the purposes is to determine the relationship between the abuse and other health problems.
    2. clients who abuse drugs or alcohol are forthcoming about their problem.
    3. the ability to conduct a comprehensive assessment may be influenced by the nurse's personal beliefs and feelings.
    4. all clients need to be assessed for drug and alcohol abuse.

17. Explain the rationale for the nurse to monitor the respiratory status of clients experiencing acute intoxication.

18. The purpose of the blood alcohol level test is to detect and estimate the level of alcohol in the _____. The legal limit in most states is _____%.

19. A nurse is caring for a client in the ER four hours after ingesting a hallucinogen. Assessment findings would reveal:
    1. pinpoint pupils.
    2. hypotension.
    3. eupnea.
    4. tachycardia.

20. A client who has abused a CNS depressant such as a sedative may require gastric lavage if the substance was taken within the last _____ to _____ hours.

21. Signs of chemical dependence in a professional colleague include: (Select all that apply)
    1. mood changes.
    2. pale complexion.
    3. impeccable appearance.
    4. wearing a sweater constantly.
    5. frequent breaks in the nurse's lounge.
    6. attention to detail in client assignments.

22. True or False

    _____ A nurse caring for a client who abuses cocaine and who was admitted from the ER eight hours ago should assess the client for cocaine intoxication.

BEST PRACTICES

23. Prior to being effective in establishing a therapeutic relationship and providing treatment to substance abusers, the nurse must first engage in _____.

24. The nursing intervention with the highest priority in a client experiencing an opioid overdose is to:
    1. monitor cardiac status.
    2. maintain airway.
    3. establish IV access.
    4. administer naloxone (Narcan).

25. The treatment for opiod addiction recommended by the National Institutes of Health is _____ _____.

26. When providing nursing care for clients who have taken an overdose of a sedative, hypnotic, or anxiolytic, the priority areas of care are:
    a.

    b.

    c.

27. A "therapeutic intervention" for a substance abuse client:
    1. is used with clients who agree with the family that drug and alcohol treatment is needed.
    2. requires involvement of family and friends to be effective.
    3. follows a loosely constructed script to allow for flexibility.
    4. is implemented with firm, abrasive communication to emphasize the seriousness of the problem.

28. Identify the primary, secondary, and tertiary treatment options for a substance-abusing client.
    a.

    b.

    c.

29. Interventions implemented to prevent relapse in a substance abuser include: (Select all that apply)
    1. build on the client's coping skills.
    2. keep environmental variables constant.
    3. discuss measures to handle craving.
    4. encourage support group participation.
    5. teach strategies for a healthy lifestyle.

30. True or False

    _____ A key component of education for the substance abusing client and family concerns the role the family plays in the addiction.

    _____ The major nursing intervention for a client experiencing withdrawal from alcohol is to promote a safe, calm, and comfortable environment.

    _____ In the client who abuses caffeine, nursing intervention begins with recognizing manifestations of excessive use and withdrawal.

KEEPING DRUG SKILLS SHARP

31. Explain the rationale for using benzodiazepines in clients withdrawing from alcohol.

32. Alcoholic Anonymous (AA) opposes the use of naltrexone hydrochloride (ReVia) for the treatment of alcoholism because: (Select all that apply)
    1. use of this drug is not consistent with a total abstinence model.
    2. its use is seen as a crutch.
    3. clinical evidence does not support the drug's effectiveness.
    4. clients who use the drug have a higher relapse rate.

33. List the three areas of focus for nursing care of the client who abuses amphetamines:
    a.

    b.

    c.

34. Which statements accurately characterize cocaine and cocaine use? (Select all that apply)
    1. Cocaine may be used intravenously, snorted, or chewed.
    2. Cocaine prevents dopamine reuptake.
    3. Cocaine is metabolized and excreted in the liver.
    4. Cocaine use can lead to cardiac failure.
    5. Upon withdrawal clients may experience euphoria.

Assessment of the Musculoskeletal System

OBJECTIVES

27.1 Describe significant health history information and subjective data needed for assessment of the musculoskeletal system.

27.2 Explain the critical elements used in performing a neurovascular assessment for musculoskeletal disorders.

27.3 Describe diagnostic procedures used to evaluate musculoskeletal disorders.

27.4 List important medications used to treat musculoskeletal disorders, as well as their potential adverse effects.

ANATOMY & PHYSIOLOGY REVIEW

1. Label the principal muscles of the body.

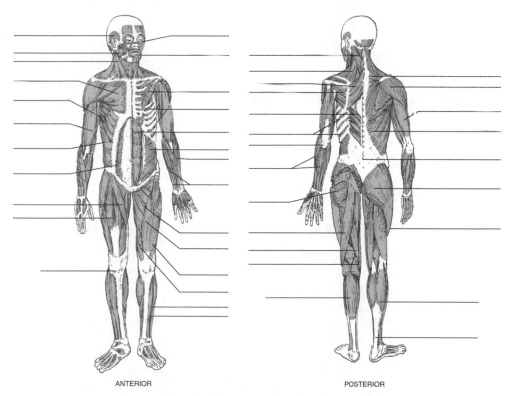

ANTERIOR   POSTERIOR

2. Label the principal bones of the adult human skeleton.

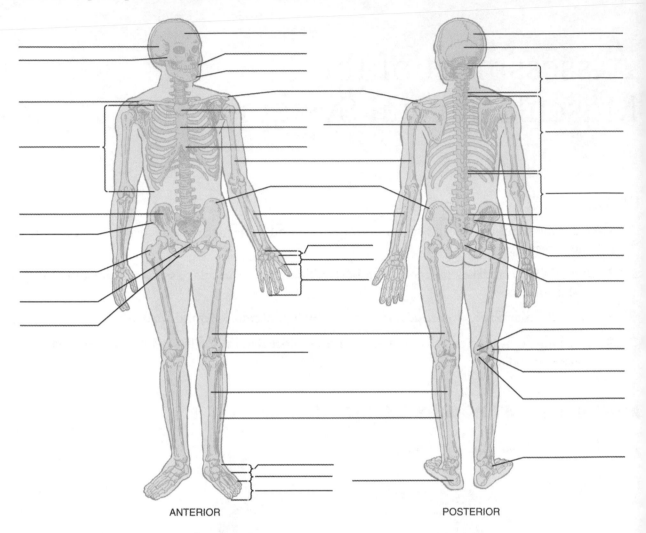

ANTERIOR   POSTERIOR

UNDERSTANDING PATHOPHYSIOLOGY

3. When a 38-year-old female with bone problems asks about nutrition and dietary intake, the nurse stresses which of these points regarding the patient's musculoskeletal health? (Select all that apply)
   1. Poor calcium intake can lead to bone decalcification and fractures.
   2. The patient should take a nutritional supplement.
   3. Adequate dietary intake of Vitamin A, D, and protein are critical to the patient's musculoskeletal health.
   4. The patient should take niacin twice daily.

4. Define these terms:
   a. Kyphosis

   b. Scoliosis

c. Lordosis

d. Genuvarum

e. Genuvalgum

5. Identify the each type of musculoskeletal deformity observable during assessment.

A _____   B _____   C _____

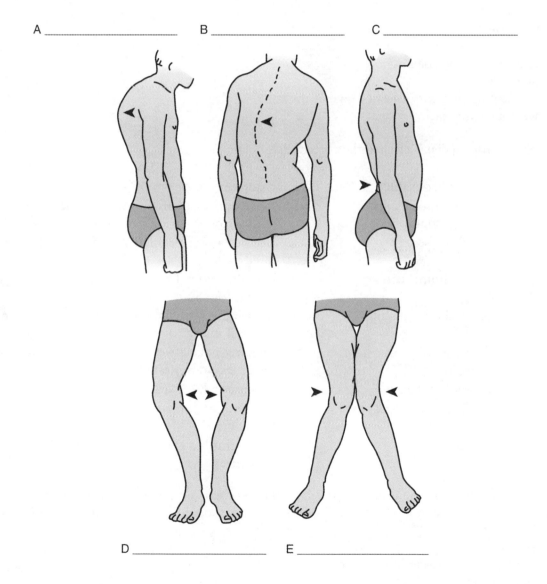

D _____   E _____

APPLYING SKILLS

6. The nurse is examining a 45-year-old male with painful, limited range of motion in his fingers and swelling in his right wrist, which he has had over the last 4 weeks. He explains that he plays golf 4 days a week and that the pain has gotten progressively worse. Which parts of the client's health history are important for the nurse to ascertain? (Select all that apply)
   1. chief complaint
   2. health history
   3. lifestyle data
   4. medications taken

7. When assessing musculoskeletal injuries, which of the following are important to note? (Select all that apply)
   1. pain, swelling
   2. tenderness
   3. joint stiffness
   4. cramps, muscle spasms
   5. deformity
   6. reduced movement or joint range of motion
   7. weight-height ratio

8. Match the appropriate letter to the correct diagnostic exam.

   _____ a. Arthrography
   _____ b. Sinography and myelography
   _____ c. Bone scan
   _____ d. Gallium scan
   _____ e. Indium imaging
   _____ f. Arthrocentesis
   _____ g. Arthroscopy
   _____ h. Electromyography
   _____ i. Biopsy

   1. Examination of sample of tissue
   2. Fiber optic arthroscope allows endoscopic examination of various joints
   3. Used to assess problems as muscle weakness, altered gait
   4. Use of Indium 111, connected to leukocytes, to detect bone infections
   5. Aspirating synovial fluid, blood, pus via a needle inserted into a joint cavity
   6. Images of skeleton obtained past radioisotope injected and migrated to bone
   7. Specific to bone disorders
   8. Injection of contrast agents and taking of x-ray films
   9. Radiographic examination of soft tissue joint structures

9. The nurse evaluated the laboratory results of her 67-year-old female client with arthritis. Which results, if elevated, would indicate bone and joint disease and cause the nurse to notify the physician?
   1. SGOT
   2. ESR (erythrocyte sedimentation rate)
   3. hemoglobin
   4. INR

10. Use the Neurovascular Check Sheet below to practice recording assessments in laboratory practice and in the clinical setting with your client who requires neurovascular assessment. Check for pain on passive stretch in the lower extremity by dorsiflexing the client's foot, or in the upper extremity by flexing the client's wrist. It is important to check for pain on passive stretch, one of the earliest indications of compartment syndrome. Compartment syndrome is a serious complication that could result in the loss of a limb. Any possible early signs of compartment syndrome must be reported to the physician.

EXTREMITY TO BE ASSESSED:				FREQUENCY OF ASSESSMENT:				
Date & Time	Color	Capillary Refill	Motion	Sensation	Pain on Passive Stretch	Is Extremity Elevated	Initial	

REPORT ANY SIGNIFICANT CHANGE TO PHYSICIAN

Color: Pink, Pale, Cyanotic, Black
Capillary Filling: Rapid, Sluggish
Motion: Present, Decreased, Absent
Extremity Elevated: Yes, unless ordered otherwise

Sensation: Present (with or without stimuli—specify)
  Decreased, Absent
Pain on Passive Stretch: Present, Absent

BEST PRACTICES

11. When performing a neurovascular assessment of clients with musculoskeletal injuries, which clinical signs and indications should be noted and documented? (Select all that apply)
    1. pain
    2. pallor
    3. temperature
    4. pulses
    5. capillary refill
    6. parenthesis
    7. mobility of affected joints

12. When the 62-year-old client who fell from a ladder and broke his leg 2 hours ago complains of increasing pain, the nurse is aware this could indicate:
    1. pain increasing on movement.
    2. joints needing replacement.
    3. peripheral warmth of lower extremities.
    4. edema and nerve compression.

13. Pallor, coolness, and cyanosis of an extremity due to an injury can indicate
    _____ in that the particular limb.

14. The nurse is examining an 18-year-old male with a fractured left ankle due to a football injury. Checking his pulses and capillary refill bilaterally will help determine the:
    1. function of knee joints above the injury.
    2. adequacy of blood supply to small peripheral vessels.
    3. rotation of muscle mass to extremity.
    4. joint range of motion extension.

15. Physicians order which non-invasive test for diagnostic evaluation of musculoskeletal injuries?
    1. DEXA scan.
    2. bone density.
    3. x-ray study (radiography).
    4. gallium scan.

16. Noninvasive diagnostic procedures used to evaluate musculoskeletal injuries include:
    a.

    b.

    c.

    d.

    e.

    f.

KEEPING DRUGS SKILL SHARP

17. With musculoskeletal injuries, pain from inflammation is usually relieved by the administration of which types of medications?
    1. steroids
    2. anticoagulants
    3. aspirin or nonsteroidal anti-inflammatory (NSAIDs)
    4. antihypertensives

18. A 67-year-old man has been admitted to the hospital with gastrointestinal (GI) bleeding, stomach pains, and pain to the right hip for the past 2 months. While obtaining admission history data, the nurse discovers the client is taking all of the medications below. Which medication could cause GI bleeding?
    1. NSAIDs
    2. diuretics
    3. cardiotonics
    4. hypotensive agents

Chapter 28

Management of Clients with Musculoskeletal Disorders

OBJECTIVES

28.1 Describe the clinical manifestations and diagnostic findings for osteoarthritis.

28.2 Explain the current treatment for osteoarthritis.

28.3 Describe nursing management for patients having total hip and knee replacements.

28.4 Identify primary musculoskeletal bone deformities of the foot.

28.5 Discuss risk factors for osteoporosis.

UNDERSTANDING PATHOPHYSIOLOGY

1. True or False

_____ Osteoarthritis is now recognized as a chronic, progressive process in which new tissue is produced in response to joint insults and cartilage deterioration.

_____ Osteoarthritis has no systemic involvement and inflammation is not typical.

2. Osteoarthritis accounts for substantial disability in the lower extremities as a result of its effects on _____.

3. Studies have show that overweight people have higher rates of osteoarthritis of the _____ than people of normal weight.

4. Match the following descriptions and definitions with the correct disorder (answers may be used more than once).

Descriptions/Definitions	Disorder
_____ a. most often treated with braces or corsets to straighten the spine	1. osteoporosis
_____ b. common in bones of spine hip and wrist	2. Paget's disease
_____ c. deformity caused by flexion contracture of PIP joint	3. osteomalacia
_____ d. loss of total bone mass substance	4. kyphosis
_____ e. pain when walking and change in gait pattern	5. osteomyelitis
_____ f. replacement of normal marrow with vascular connective tissue	6. bunions
_____ g. may occur as a result of local irritation of restrictive footwear	7. hammer toe
_____ h. bowed legs and cranial enlargement	
_____ i. occurs most frequently in femur, tibia, sacrum, and heels	
_____ j. results from vitamin D deficiency	
_____ k. generalized bone decalcification with bone deformity	
_____ l. idiopathic blood disorder/abnormal accelerated bone reabsorption	
_____ m. produces painful deformities of femur, tibia, lower spine	
_____ n. posterior rounding of the thoracic spine	
_____ o. severe pyogenic infection of bone and surrounding tissue	
_____ p. common foot deformity involving first metatarsal and great toe	

APPLYING SKILLS

5. Diagnosis of osteoarthritis may be confirmed by: (Select all that apply)
   1. radiographic changes.
   2. absence of osteophytes.
   3. narrowed joint space on xray.
   4. erosion of articular cartilage.

6. What symptoms would likely be prominent in a 68-year-old male with osteoarthritis? (Select all that apply)
   1. worsening pain, stiffness increase with activity
   2. crepitus, joint enlargement
   3. mild tenderness in area of joint
   4. deficits in range of motion
   5. rough, reddened skin over joints

7. An 80-year-old female is scheduled for a total hip replacement due to osteoarthritis. The most common serious complication would be:
   1. venous thrombus embolism.
   2. creptius of the hip.
   3. gastrointestinal bleeding.
   4. osteomyelitis.

8. Surgery on any joint carries a risk for neurological or vascular impairment. What assessment finding would cause the nurse to report possible nerve damage to the physician?
   1. pallor
   2. numbness
   3. bleeding
   4. dislocation

9. What laboratory test will be ordered to confirm the diagnosis of gout?
   1. serum calcium
   2. serum uric acid
   3. BUN
   4. bilirubin

BEST PRACTICES

10. When developing a teaching plan for a client with osteoarthritis, the nurse must include: (Select all that apply)
    1. pain management.
    2. strenuous exercise program.
    3. nutrition and weight loss.
    4. self-care strategies.

11. A client with osteoarthritis can minimize stress on a painful joint by
    1. becoming less physically active.
    2. eating green and yellow vegetables.
    3. maintaining normal weight.
    4. increasing intake of fruits and bread.

12. A 58-year-old female with osteoarthritis is scheduled for an arthroplasty with insertion of an artificial joint. The physician has ordered a continuous passive motion (CPM) machine during the postoperative period in order to:
    1. strengthen leg and calf muscle.
    2. reduce food and toe swelling.
    3. restore joint function and range of motion with good muscle control.
    4. reduce knee swelling.

13. What beverage should the clients with gout avoid even in small amounts?
    1. soda
    2. alcohol
    3. coffee
    4. tea

KEEPING DRUG SKILLS SHARP

14. The client with osteoarthritis has been prescribed 1 gram of acetaminophen PO every 6 hours for pain because acetaminophen: (Select all that apply)
    1. is the drug of choice for hip and knee osteoarthritis.
    2. is effective, safe, and low-cost.
    3. is less likely to cause gastrointestinal, hepatic, or renal damage over non steroidal anti-inflammatory drugs.
    4. improves circulation to the bone and reduces RBC formation.

15. True or False

    _____ An erythrocyte sedimentation rate (ESR) is useful only if systemic manifestations are present.

16. Pharmacologic agents routinely given to decrease risk of DVT include all of the following except
    1. aspirin.
    2. low dose heparin.
    3. low molecular weight heparin.
    4. warfarin.
    5. chlormycetin.

17. What laboratory tests do clients taking warfarin undergo to monitor its effects?
    1. platelet count
    2. prothrombin time (reported as INR)
    3. CBC
    4. ESR

18. Medications used to treat gout by reducing uric acid include: (Select all that apply)
    1. mercurial diuretics.
    2. allopurinol.
    3. probenecid.
    4. salicylates.

19. A 58-year-old male is being treated for an acute inflammation of gout. What body part or structure is most likely to be affected?
    1. great toe
    2. index finger
    3. TMJ
    4. vertebral coccyx

20. During an acute attack of gout, the physician prescribes colchicines to reduce pain and inflammation. What sign indicates toxicity from this drug?
    1. headaches
    2. elevated temperature
    3. vomiting
    4. dizziness

Management of Clients with Musculoskeletal Trauma or Overuse

OBJECTIVES

29.1 Identify the stages of bone healing.

29.2 Describe the clinical manifestations that patients with musculoskeletal injuries exhibit.

29.3 Compare and contrast the different types of fractures most commonly seen with musculoskeletal injuries.

29.4 Describe nursing management for patients with skin and skeletal traction.

29.5 Explain the common complications associated with musculoskeletal surgeries.

UNDERSTANDING PATHOPHYSIOLOGY

1. Which of the following conditions would slow the rate of healing in an elderly patient with a lower leg fracture?
   1. osteoporosis
   2. thyroid
   3. scleroderma
   4. gastroenteritis

2. Nerve damage to an extremity due to injury or fracture may result in which of the following clinical signs and manifestations? (Select all that apply)
   1. pallor
   2. coolness of affected extremity
   3. changes in client's ability to move digits/extremity
   4. paresthesia
   5. increasing complaints of pain

APPLYING SKILLS

3. Match the type of fracture with correct description or definition.

Type of Fracture	Description/Definition
_____ a. Impacted	1. Multiple pieces of bones, occurs at bone ends
_____ b. Burst	2. Breaks across entire section of bone, in fragments
_____ c. Comminuted	3. Multiple fracture lines, two bone fragments, splintered
_____ d. Complete	4. Fragments out of normal position at fracture site
_____ e. Linear	5. Fracture line intact, caused by force to bone
_____ f. Incomplete	6. Telescoped fracture with one fragment forced into another
_____ g. Displaced	7. Fracture through one cortex of bone, non-displaced
_____ h. Oblique	8. Fracture line from twisting force, spiral encircling bone
_____ i. Non-displaced	9. Fragments aligned at fracture site
_____ j. Spiral	10. Fracture line at 45-degree angle/long axis of bone
_____ k. Longitudinal	11. Fracture line extends in direction of bone's long axis
_____ l. Transverse	12. Bone fragments torn from body/site ligament/tendon
_____ m. Stellate	13. Bone buckles, due to unusual force to long axis
_____ n. Avulsion	14. Fracture line at 90-degree angle to long axis
_____ o. Compression	15. Fracture lines radiate from one central point
_____ p. Greenstick	16. Incomplete fracture, one side of cortex is broken

4. Which of the following best describes a greenstick fracture of the right ulna?
   1. incomplete fracture of bone with one side flexed and splintered
   2. bone fractured at different sites
   3. complete dislocation of the bone
   4. fracture across the child's growth plate

5. A _____ is a possible early complication of a compound or crushing fracture of a long bone.

6. True or False

   _____ Osteoporosis is a decrease in porosity of a bone.

   _____ In displaced fractures, the bone ends are separated at fracture lines.

   _____ Skeletal traction uses pulleys/ropes attached to bones with weights.

   _____ A complication of a fracture or a surgery on long bones is fat embolus.

   _____ Arthroplasty is fusion of a bone.

7. The greatest swelling to an extremity with a cast is likely to be evident in the first _____ to _____ hours.

8. _____ is a late sign of compartment syndrome.

9. The nurse can best assess circulation to an extremity of a patient with a lower leg fracture by:
   1. asking the patient to wiggle his toes.
   2. checking skin color.
   3. checking skin temperature.
   4. examining the leg for deformity.

10. While assessing a lower leg cast of a 12-year-old boy, the nurse detects an unusual odor. This is a sign of:
    1. limited areas for healing.
    2. infection under the cast.
    3. the skin being dirty and in need of washing.
    4. the cast drying to the skin.

11. When fracture fragments heal in improper alignment, the nurse would expect to see:
    1. external deformity of involved extremity.
    2. the fracture healing has not occurred.
    3. the client complains of bone pain and tenderness.
    4. enlarged bone fragments.

BEST PRACTICES

12. What details are helpful in determining the type of fracture and associated injuries to clients with musculoskeletal injuries? (Select all that apply)
    1. Was patient in MVA?
    2. Did patient have seat belt on?
    3. What was the angle of impact?
    4. Was patient pulled from car postcollision?
    5. Did the injury occur as result of a fall?

13. A client recently had a left hip fracture repair with an ORIF (Open Reduction Internal Fixation). The affected extremity should be maintained in a position of:
    1. abduction.
    2. internal rotation.
    3. external rotation.
    4. adduction.

14. Following hip surgery, the nurse is instructed to ambulate the patient. These patients must: (Select all that apply)
    1. use a walker for balance.
    2. not bear weight on affected side.
    3. not dangle legs or sit in a chair.
    4. avoid flexion on the hips.
    5. avoid positions with 60 to 90 degree flexion.

15. To prevent or relieve swelling in clients with casts, the nurse should elevate the extremity with the cast _____ for the first 24 to 48 hours.

KEEPING DRUGS SKILLS SHARP

16. A 29-year-old carpenter is admitted to the hospital after a falling off a ladder and breaking his left arm. In the emergency room, the nurse begins to medicate him with Toradol (NSAID) for pain. Prior to administering this drug, the nurse must know:
    1. if the patient is taking any steroid medication.
    2. if the patient has a history of ulcers or GI problems.
    3. if there is a history of cataracts in his family.
    4. if the patient has had any recent surgeries on the opposite arm.

17. The client with orthopedic injuries is at high risk for thromboembolic conditions such as deep vein thrombosis and pulmonary embolism. Given the patient's condition, what pharmacological agents will be used during treatment? (Select all that apply)
    1. oral anticoagulants
    2. subcutaneous or IV heparin (fixed dose)
    3. antibiotics
    4. steroids

18. The client has just returned from surgery where a cast has been applied to the right lower leg. In assessing his neurovascular status, the nurse must be aware of: (Select all that apply)
    1. circulation/color of affected extremity, pulse, capillary refill.
    2. movement of affected extremity.
    3. sensations of affected extremity.
    4. edema.
    5. pain (rate on pain scale 0-10).

Assessment of Nutrition and the Digestive System

OBJECTIVES

30.1   Discuss the importance of nutrition in maintaining client health status.

30.2   Describe the process for determining nutritional status of a client.

30.3   Identify nursing responsibilities in completing a thorough nutritional assessment of a client.

30.4   Describe the process for completing a physical assessment of the upper GI system.

30.5   Identify common diagnostic tests used for clients with disorders of the upper GI system.

ANATOMY & PHYSIOLOGY REVIEW

1. Label the structures of the digestive system.

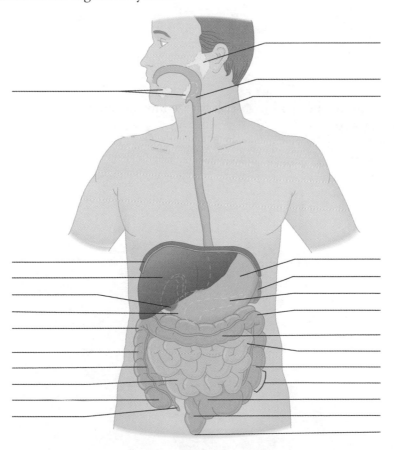

UNDERSTANDING PATHOPHYSIOLOGY

2. To meet the body's nutrient requirements, nutrients must be metabolized and used at the _____ level.

3. Identify the alterations in RDA that must be made for the following disease processes, and state the rationale for each:
   a. Client who is experiencing fever:

   b. Kidney or liver failure:

   c. Pancreatic exocrine dysfunction:

   d. Pancreatic endocrine dysfunction:

4. Identify the two main causes for the epidemic of obesity in America.
   a.

   b.

5. Differentiate between primary and secondary starvation.

6. Conditions that can place clients at high risk for malnutrition and potential nutritional deficit include: (Select all that apply)
   1. fat malabsorption.
   2. short-bowel syndrome.
   3. pressure ulcers.
   4. cancer.
   5. AIDS.
   6. gastric surgery.

7. Identify diseases which have a familial or genetic link.

8. Compare and contrast the characteristics of different causes of abdominal pain.

Etiology	Characteristics of Pain
Bowel Obstruction	
Peritoneal inflammation	
Vascular catastrophe (aortic aneurysm)	

APPLYING SKILLS

9. Identify the quickest way to begin collecting information about dietary intake.

10. In addition to the types of foods consumed, factors the nurse should consider when evaluating nutritional status include all of the following except:
    1. the amount of food or drink consumed.
    2. how the food was prepared.
    3. where the food was obtained.
    4. the time of day food or drink was consumed.

11. Compare and contrast between marasmus and kwashiorkor:

	Protein Intake	Calorie Intake	Appearance
Marasmus			
Kwashiorkor			

12. Explain how evaluation of albumin and prealbumin can determine nutritional status of the client.

13. List the components of an anthropometric measurement of a client:
    a.
    b.
    c.
    d.
    e.

14. The _____ is better standard for determining ideal body weight than conventional tables because it standardizes weight for the height of the individual.

15. True or False

    _____ A client with a BMI or 18.5 is in the acceptable range for weight.

    _____ Calculations for BMI are the same for males and females.

    _____ Bone and muscle are less dense than fat and count less with BMI.

    _____ Frame size of client can be determined by measuring wrist circumference.

    _____ A muscular client can have a high BMI and not be considered overweight.

16. Upon assessment of a client's mouth, the nurse notes an oral lesion. The client says that the lesion has been present for some time and is not causing any pain. Identify the appropriate nursing action for this situation and state the rationale.

17. Pain at _____ may suggest acute appendicitis.

18. True or False

    _____ Sitting at eye level with the abdomen, the nurse should see peristaltic movements.

    _____ Diastasis recti is a true herniation just below the diaphragm and will require surgical correction.

    _____ The nurse should apply the diaphragm of the stethoscope over the abdomen to listen for bowel sounds.

    _____ Normal bowel sounds occur irregularly at a rate of 5-35 per minute.

    _____ Clients with gastroenteritis will experience borborygmi.

19. Turbulent blood causes a _____ sound, which may indi-

cate an aneurysm or partial obstruction of a blood vessel.

20. State the rationale for the nurse asking the client to take a sip of water and then observing the client swallowing.

BEST PRACTICES

21. State the rationale for maintaining NPO status for a client who will undergo a xylose absorption test.

22. State the rationale for maintaining NPO status for a client who has undergone a modified barium swallow.

23. During an endoscopy the nurse should place the client in the _____ position.

KEEPING DRUG SKILLS SHARP

24. Explain how medications affect the elderly client's nutritional status:

25. List four common over-the-counter (OTC) medications which can interfere with GI function or cause complications:

a.

b.

c.

d.

26. Explain the hidden danger for clients using OTC supplements or herbs.

27. Nutrients in addition to iron that are needed for normal hematologic functioning include: (Select all that apply)
    1. protein.
    2. vitamin B$_{12}$.
    3. zinc.
    4. copper.

28. _____ medications are given to a client scheduled for an endoscopy because they decrease oropharyngeal secretions and prevent reflex bradycardia.

Management of Clients with Malnutrition

OBJECTIVES

31.1 Discuss the difference between malnutrition and protein-energy malnutrition including clinical manifestations.

31.2 Identify nursing care and medical management of clients experiencing malnutrition.

31.3 Discuss nursing responsibilities while providing nutritional support to clients experiencing malnutrition.

31.4 Discuss nursing care and medical/surgical management of clients with eating disorders.

UNDERSTANDING PATHOPHYSIOLOGY

1. Differentiate between malnutrition and protein-energy malnutrition (PEM).

2. Explain why each category of client is at risk for PEM.
    a. infants:

    b. pregnant/lactating women:

    c. elderly:

3. Secondary malnutrition is caused by all of the following except:
    1. decreased food intake.
    2. decreased nutrient absorption.
    3. increased nutrient losses.
    4. decreased nutrient requirements.

4. Socioeconomic factors that have a negative effect on nutrition include: (Select all that apply)
    1. social isolation.
    2. limited access to food.
    3. emotional depression.
    4. substance abuse.
    5. poverty.

5. True or False

_____ The functional status of the GI tract determines the site of the enteral feeding tube placement.

_____ The larger the diameter of the tube, the more likely the problems with infusing formulas and medications.

_____ Jejunostomy and gastrostomy tubes are used for long-term enteral feedings.

_____ Percutaneous endoscopic gastrostomy tubes must be placed surgically and require the client to receive anesthesia.

6. List four factors that increase the incidence of obesity:
   a.
   b.
   c.
   d.

7. Health risks associated with obesity include all of the following except:
   1. type I diabetes.
   2. cardiovascular disease.
   3. hypertension.
   4. hyperlipidemia.
   5. stroke.
   6. sleep apnea.
   7. arthritis.
   8. some cancers.

APPLYING SKILLS

8. _____ screening for nutritional problems obtains information from the client through the use of a questionnaire or admission form.

9. State the rationale for having the nurse to assess nutritional status of any client, rather than other types of health care workers.

10. Identify a possible physical diagnosis that could cause of each common manifestation that may lead to the nursing diagnosis of Self-care deficit, feeding.
    a. impaired motor function:

    b. impaired cognitive function:

    c. sensory-perceptual alterations:

    d. decreased appetite:

11. When visiting a rural village in a underdeveloped country, the nurse notes that all the young infants look healthy and robust, while the older children have thin arms and legs, swollen abdomens, and are lethargic. Explain the difference in nutritional status between the two groups of children.

12. Upon assessment of an elderly client admitted from a long-term care facility, the nurse would note which of the following clinical manifestations of protein malnutrition? (Select all that apply)
    1. hair loss
    2. oily skin
    3. brittle nails
    4. pale skin tone
    5. periodontal disease or bleeding gums
    6. muscle wasting/weight loss

BEST PRACTICES

13. Provide examples of the three phases of nursing interventions to help the client prevent or restore nutritional status.
    a. Health promotion:

    b. Health maintenance:

    c. Health restoration:

14. Nursing strategies to improve client nutritional status include: (Select all that apply)
    1. allowing the client to choose from a menu.
    2. reducing noxious odors.
    3. consistently offering the same foods/beverages.
    4. oral care.

15. The nurse can assist the blind client to ensure adequate food intake by: (Select all that apply)
    1. maximizing use of other senses: smell and taste.
    2. describing food to visually impaired client.
    3. arranging food in clock-face pattern and describing positions to client.
    4. not placing food on client's blind side.
    5. making sure client is wearing corrective lenses.
    6. using a highly patterned set of food dishes.

16. The nurse can assist the client with neuromuscular impairments to obtain adequate nutrition and maintain independence by: (Select all that apply)
    1. positioning the client at 45-degree angle.
    2. consulting with occupational therapy for assistive devices.
    3. ensuring privacy to avoid embarrassment.
    4. allowing adequate time for eating.

17. _____ equipment must be kept available when feeding a client with impaired swallowing function.

18. True or False

    _____ If the client has an obstruction in the GI tract, the enteral feeding tube can be placed proximal to the site.

19. List four nursing responsibilities when administering enteral feedings to a client and state the rationale for each:
    a.

    b.

    c.

    d.

20. After administering the medication via an enteral feeding tube and flushing the tube with water, the nurse should clamp the tube for _____ hour(s) to allow the medication to be absorbed.

KEEPING DRUG SKILLS SHARP

21. The main components of TPN include all of the following except:
    1. carbohydrates: 50-70% caloric supply.
    2. fat emulsion: 30-50% caloric supply.
    3. amino acids: 3-15%: source of protein.
    4. fluids, electrolytes, vitamins, trace elements.

22. _____ aids in weight loss by preventing the breakdown of dietary fat for absorption.

23. Identify samples for each classification of enteral nutrition products.

Classification	Sample Product
Low residue	
Standard protein	
Fiber supplemented	
Intermediate	
High protein	
Concentrated	
Pulmonary	
Renal failure	

Management of Clients with Ingestive Disorders

OBJECTIVES

32.1 Identify common clinical manifestations of clients experiencing disorders of the oral cavity.

32.2 Describe nursing care and medical management of clients with disorders of the oral cavity.

32.3 Describe nursing care and medical/surgical management of clients with malignant tumors of the oral cavity.

32.4 Describe nursing care and medical/surgical management of clients with disorders of the esophagus and stomach.

UNDERSTANDING PATHOPHYSIOLOGY

1. How does periodontal disease lead to tooth loss?

2. List the two mechanisms for developing stomatitis.
   a.

   b.

3. Compare and contrast primary and secondary stomatitis:

Classification	Etiology	Examples
Primary		
Secondary		

4. Common precipitating factors for Vincent's Angina include: (Select all that apply)
   1. poor oral hygiene.
   2. increased age.
   3. nutritional deficiencies.
   4. lack of rest/sleep.

5. Only a _____ can positively confirm oral cancer.

6. The pain that occurs with difficulty swallowing is called _____.

7. Differentiate between the pain of "heartburn" and the pain of cardiac origin (angina).

8. _____ develops when the lower esophageal sphincter (LES) fails to relax normally with swallowing, resulting in a buildup of food and fluid in the lower esophagus.

9. Compare and contrast the three surgical procedures to correct GERD.

Name	Procedure	Result
Nissen fundoplication		
Hill operation		
Belsey (Mark IV) repair		

10. Explain why esophageal cancer metastasizes so quickly.

APPLYING SKILLS

11. Describe the difference in clinical manifestations between a hiatal hernia and a rolling hernia.

12. A client has undergone surgery to remove a cancerous lesion from the oral cavity. In addition to monitoring nutritional and fluid intake, what other changes within the oral cavity should the nurse be alert to?

13. True or False

_____ Hemorrhage is a critical postoperative concern for the oral surgery client due to the large blood vessels that supply the mouth and oral area.

BEST PRACTICES

14. State the rationales for each of the following nursing actions to provide postoperative care to the client following a tooth extraction:
    a. instruct client to bite down gently on gauze pad:

    b. apply ice over jaw:

    c. monitoring bleeding from site:

    d. avoid hot/cold foods for several days:

e.   gentle mouth rinses/avoid tooth brushing:

f.   medicate for pain:

g.   maintain fluid intake:

15. Prior to discharge, the nurse should instruct the client with oral lesions to: (Select all that apply)
    1. use gauze or sponge pads instead of toothbrush.
    2. use cold saline mouth rinses.
    3. swish antifungal medications around mouth and then swallow; do not drink fluids or rinse mouth afterwards.
    4. drink plenty of orange juice.
    5. report any signs of infection to physician promptly.

16. Nursing interventions for the diagnosis: Impaired oral mucosa related to irritants include teaching the client to: (Select all that apply)
    1. avoid oral irritants (tobacco, alcohol).
    2. notify physician of lesion that does not heal in 2-3 days.
    3. perform careful oral hygiene daily.
    4. request medications if needed for nausea secondary to chemotherapy or radiation.
    5. see dentist about ill-fitting dentures.

17. True or False

    _____ After local excisions of oral tumors, the client should rinse gently with ½ saline – ½ peroxide solution.

    _____ Oral suctioning may be done 48 hours after oral surgery if there is no bleeding noted.

    _____ Clients who undergo oral surgery may begin tube feedings after 48 hours if no nausea or vomiting is present.

KEEPING DRUG SKILLS SHARP

18. Treatment of the herpes does not include _____ medications.

19. Medications used to treat stomatitis include: (Select all that apply)
    1. amlexanox (Aphthasol).
    2. corticosteroids.
    3. acyclovir.
    4. hydrourea (Hydraea).

20. Common chemotherapeutic agents used in treatment of oral cancer include all of the following except:
    1. bleomycin (Blenoxane).
    2. cisplatin (Platinol).
    3. cyclophosphamide (Cytoxan).
    4. diphenhydramine (Benadryl).
    5. doxorubicin (Adriamycin).
    6. 5-fluorouracil (5-FU).
    7. hydrourea (Hydraea).
    8. methotrexate (Folex).
    9. vincristine (Oncovin).

21. Identify the categories and actions of the medications a physician may order when treating a client with *H. pylori* bacteria.

Medication	Category	Action
Biaxin or amoxicillin		
Flagyl		
Prevacid		
Protonix		
Prilosec		

22. _____, a mucosal barrier fortifier, stimulates mucus production and accelerates peptic ulcer healing.

23. Identify the mechanism of action for H_2-receptor antagonists such as Zantac and Tagamet.

Management of Clients with Digestive Disorders

OBJECTIVES

33.1   Identify common clinical manifestations of clients experiencing gastric disorders.

33.2   Describe nursing care and medical/surgical management of gastric disorders.

33.3   Identify and discuss the purpose of various types of gastric intubation.

33.4   Describe nursing care and medical/surgical management of gastric disorders.

33.5   Develop and implement nursing care, medical, and surgical management of gastric neoplasms.

UNDERSTANDING PATHOPHYSIOLOGY

1.   Identify two common causes of gastric pain.
      a.
      b.

2.   _____ are the major cause of upper GI bleeding.

3.   The major electrolyte lost through NG tube suctioning is _____.

4.   Dietary habits that can lead to acute gastritis include consumption of excessive amounts of: (Select all that apply)
      1.   tea or coffee.
      2.   mustard.
      3.   ketchup.
      4.   paprika.
      5.   cloves.

5.   Chronic gastritis leads to an increased risk for _____ by causing a decrease in the production of stomach acid.

6.   Chronic gastritis can cause _____ by decreasing acid secretion, resulting in the loss of intrinsic factor and reducing the ability to absorb vitamin B_{12}.

7.   Explain the difference in etiology between duodenal ulcers and gastric ulcers.

8. A serious complication that can develop secondary to stress ulcers is _____
   _____.

9. Compare and contrast common gastric surgical procedures and the indications for each procedure:

Procedure	Indication
Vagotomy	
Vagotomy with pyloroplasty	
Gastroenterostomy	
Antrectomy	
Subtotal gastrectomy	
Total gastrectomy	

10. _____ develops secondary to pyloric obstruction because the persistent vomiting causes the loss of large quantities of acid gastric juice, altering the acid-base balance.

11. Causative factors in the development of gastric cancer include: (Select all that apply)
    1. cigarette smoking.
    2. *E. coli.*
    3. pernicious anemia.
    4. chronic atrophic gastritis.
    5. a diet of raw fish or meats.
    6. achloryia.
    7. metalcraft worker, coal miner, baker (dusty, smoky environment).

APPLYING SKILLS

12. Common clinical manifestations of gastric disorders include: (Select all that apply)
    1. nausea and vomiting.
    2. acute pain.
    3. acid reflux.
    4. anorexia.
    5. indigestion.
    6. bleeding.
    7. diarrhea.
    8. belching/flatulence.

13. Identify the clinical significance of vomiting coffee ground-like material.

14. Explain how the nurse would assess electrolyte losses for the client with a NG tube to low suction.

15. True or False

    _____ Clients with duodenal ulcers have pain with an empty stomach.

    _____ Gastric ulcer pain usually radiates toward the right side of the abdomen and upward toward the neck.

    _____ Vomiting occurs more often with gastric ulcers than with uncomplicated duodenal ulcers.

    _____ The major diagnostic test for gastric ulcers is an EGD with an upper GI tract x-ray series.

16. Complications resulting from a gastric ulcer perforation include all of the following except
    1. chemical peritonitis.
    2. bacterial septicemia.
    3. septic shock.
    4. paralytic ileus.

17. A client recovering from gastrojejunostomy is not tolerating her diet due to the increased rate of food emptying into the jejunum without mixing and duodenal digestive processing. When should the nurse assess for problems and what clinical manifestations would be present?

BEST PRACTICES

18. Important client teaching points for management of Dumping syndrome include (Select all that apply)
    1. decreasing the amount of food taken at one time.
    2. maintaining a low-protein, low-fat, high-carbohydrate, dry diet.
    3. delaying gastric emptying by eating in a recumbent or semi-recumbent position.
    4. avoiding fluids 1 hour before, with, or 2 hours after meals.

19. To facilitate insertion of intestinal tubes through the pylorus, the nurse should instruct the client to lie on his or her _____ side.

20. True or False

    _____ Dietary alterations remain one of the basic interventions to help clients with gastric ulcers.

21. Identify the nursing action for a client who is experiencing melena.

22. A nurse caring for a client with a NG tube notices that the tube is not draining properly. She irrigates the tube with 30 ml of normal saline solution and then connects the tube back to suction. Is the 30 ml of saline added to the intake amount for that shift? Why or why not?

23. State the rationale for instilling room temperature saline through a NG tube into a client who is experiencing gastric hemorrhage.

24. Identify the critical nursing observation in addition to monitoring vital signs that must be made in the client with severe hemorrhage due to gastric ulcers.

25. Explain why the nurse should avoid repositioning the NG tube in a client who has had gastric surgery.

KEEPING DRUG SKILLS SHARP

26. The phenothiazine derivative _____ reduces vomiting by depressing chemoreceptor stimulation of the emetic center in the brain.

27. Describe how NSAIDs contribute to the development of stress ulcers in a client.

28. True or False

    _____ Heptavax is a new vaccine being tested to prevent infection with *H. pylori*, a major cause of gastric ulcers.

29. Explain why a client with gastric ulcers must be cautious in using over-the-counter cold remedies.

30. Identify the indications for use for each the following common medications for treatment of gastric problems.

Medication	Indication for Use
Enteric-coated aspirin	
Cytotec	
Histamine receptor antagonists	
Proton pump inhibitors	

Chapter 34

Assessment of Elimination

OBJECTIVES

34.1 Identify nursing responsibilities when obtaining a complete history and physical examination of the gastrointestinal (GI) tract.

34.2 Describe nursing care of the client undergoing diagnostic testing for common disorders of the GI tract.

34.3 Discuss nursing responsibilities when obtaining a complete history and physical examination of clients with urinary disorders.

34.4 Describe nursing of the client during invasive and noninvasive diagnostic testing of the urinary system.

ANATOMY & PHYSIOLOGY REVIEW

1. Label the missing parts of the kidney in the diagram below.

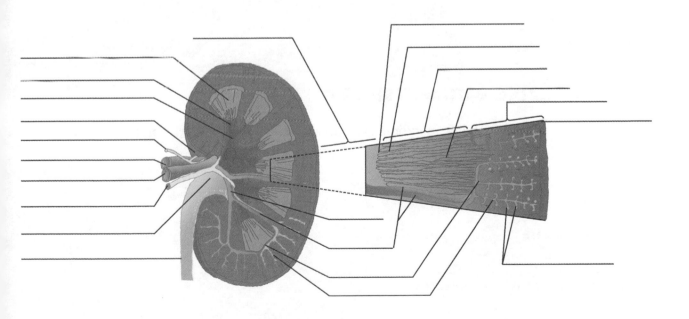

2. Label the missing parts of the nephron in the diagram below.

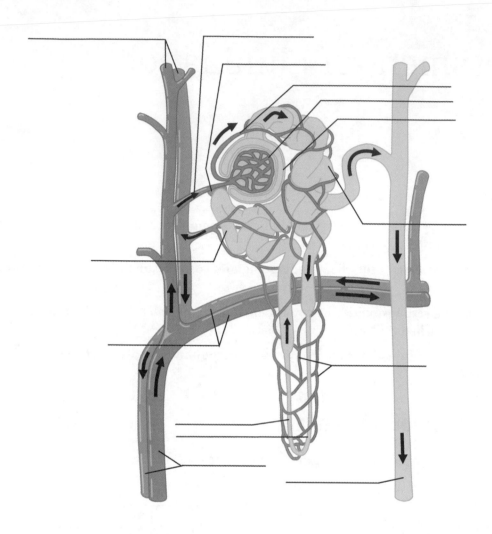

UNDERSTANDING PATHOPHYSIOLOGY

3. High levels of CEA (carcinoembryonic antigen) are detected with which conditions? (Select all that apply)
   1. proctitis
   2. colon cancer
   3. lung cancer
   4. breast cancer
   5. liver disease
   6. cirrhosis
   7. appendicitis
   8. inflammatory bowel disease

4. Compare and contrast the differences in urinary volume and their associated conditions and/or diseases.

Urine Output	Associated Conditions
Anuria	
Oliguria	
Polyuria	

5. Discuss the etiology, manifestations, and treatment of acute urinary retention.
   a. Etiology:

   b. Manifestations:

   c. Treatment:

6. Match each type of incontinence with the appropriate definition.

	Type of Incontinence	Definition
_____	a. urge incontinence	1. combination of stress or urge incontinence; typically in older women, less control
_____	b. stress urinary incontinence	2. involuntary loss of urine with a strong desire to void; diseases of spinal cord above S2-S4
_____	c. mixed urinary incontinence	3. chronic overdistention of bladder due to impaired bladder contractility or outlet obstruction; frequent or constant dribbling
_____	d. overflow urinary incontinence	4. cognitive or physical impairment outside the urinary tract; nursing home clients
_____	e. functional urinary incontinence	5. leakage of urine with physical exertion or increase in intra-abdominal pressure

7. _____ may indicate a fistula formation between the bladder and bowel.

8. True or False

   _____ Urinary tract disease does not always cause pain.

   _____ Acute, agonizing pain is due to an enlarged prostate gland.

   _____ Foreign bodies can irritate the bladder wall causing spasms.

   _____ Prostate pain is not common in men.

   _____ GI manifestations such as nausea, vomiting, and diarrhea can signal "silent" urologic disease.

   _____ Specific gravity reflects the hydration status of the client.

_____ Hypospadias refers to the concentrating ability of the kidneys.

_____ Glycosuria occurs when the serum blood glucose exceeds 180 mg/dl.

_____ Nitrites in the urine strongly suggest the presence of bacteriuria.

9. Creatinine level in the urine is equivalent to the _____ filtration rate of the kidneys.

APPLYING SKILLS

10. Describe the components to be included when reviewing symptom analysis for clients with suspected elimination disorders:
    a. timing:

    b. quality and quantity:

    c. location:

    d. precipitating factor:

    e. aggravating/relieving factors:

    f. associated manifestations:

11. True or False

    _____ Borborygmi are hypoactive bowel sounds found in clients who are constipated.

    _____ The diaphragm of the stethoscope is used to listen to bowel sounds.

    _____ If a client's bladder is full, a dull sound will be heard with percussion.

    _____ The client should be positioned supine for examination of the abdomen.

12. During a rectal examination of a male client, the _____ can be palpated.

13. In a female client, the _____ may be felt during a rectal exam.

14. Incidents reported in a client's history that may have caused injury to the urinary system include: (Select all that apply)
    1. history of MVA.
    2. falls.
    3. straddle injuries.
    4. penetrating abdominal injury.
    5. contact sports injury.

15. Areas of the client's psychosocial history significant in relation to urinary problems include: (Select all that apply)
    1. impairments in vision.
    2. level of mobility.
    3. marital status.
    4. living and work environment.
    5. wetness of clothing/odor/overall hygiene.
    6. access to toilets.
    7. positive or negative childhood experiences with toilet training.
    8. variables in daily life; stressors.

16. When taking a history for urinary problems the nurse includes the following areas: (Select all that apply)
    1. occupation.
    2. allergies.
    3. geographical location.
    4. nutrition.
    5. exercise habits.
    6. alcohol and tobacco use.

17. When assessing a client with suspected renal trauma, polycystic kidneys, abdominal aortic aneurysm, or appendicitis, the nurse should use all of the following techniques except:
    1. auscultation.
    2. deep palpation.
    3. inspection.
    4. percussion.

18. Describe each of the diagnostic tests used for evaluating bowel function and the implication for their use.
    a. Computed tomography:

    b. Ultrasonography:

    c. Proctosigmoidoscopy:

    d. Colonoscopy:

BEST PRACTICES

19. Before testing a client for fecal occult blood, the nurse should advise the client to avoid: (Select all that apply)
    1. raw meat for 3 days before the test.
    2. raw fruits/vegetables for 3 days before test.
    3. aspirin.
    4. NSAID products.

20. Identify four nursing responsibilities in caring for the client undergoing a barium enema and state the rationale for each.
    a.

    b.

    c.

    d.

21. Nursing actions to prevent serious complications in the client who has received a barium enema include: (Select all that apply)
    1. administering a laxative or cleansing enema.
    2. encouraging client to increase fluid intake.
    3. encouraging client to limit fluid intake.
    4. monitoring client for any report of pain, bloating, absence of stool or bleeding rectally.

22. Compare and contrast nursing care of clients undergoing a proctosigmoidoscopy and colonoscopy:

	Proctosigmoidoscopy	**Colonoscopy**
Preparation		
Obtain consent		
Positioning		
Instrument		

Sedation		
Postprocedure		

23. State the rationale for restricting fluid intake on the client scheduled for an IVP in the morning.

24. Identify the nursing action that must be implemented immediately after performing a renal biopsy.

KEEPING DRUG SKILLS SHARP

25. Treatments that can interfere with the results of a fecal examination for ova and parasites include all of the following except:
    1. mineral oil or castor oil enemas.
    2. bismuth.
    3. products with magnesium.
    4. antidiarrheal medications.
    5. barium enemas.
    6. antibiotics taken within 21 days before test.

26. State the rationale for documenting an allergy to antibiotics, sulfonamides, and quinolones.

27. _____ can be given prior to a radiologic procedure to a client with a known allergy to iodine dyes.

28. _____ and _____ are administered to a client who has undergone a cystoscopy to relieve bladder spasms.

Chapter 35

Management of Clients with Intestinal Disorders

OBJECTIVES

35.1   Identify common clinical manifestations of clients experiencing disorders of the intestinal tract.

35.2   Describe nursing care and medical/surgical management of inflammatory disorders of the large and small intestines.

35.3   Describe nursing care and medical/surgical management of other disorders of the intestinal tract.

35.4   Develop and implement nursing care, medical, and surgical management of neoplasms of the intestinal tract.

UNDERSTANDING PATHOPHYSIOLOGY

1.   Compare and contrast the etiology for each of the major clinical manifestations of intestinal disorders:

Disorder	Etiology
Hemorrhage	
Pain	
Visceral	
Somatic	
Referred	
Nausea/Vomiting	
Distention	
Diarrhea	
Constipation	

2. Laboratory evaluation of stool specimens showing presence of fats indicates all of the following except:
   1. vitamin deficiency.
   2. tumor growth.
   3. GI bleeding.
   4. tenesmus.

3. True or False

   _____ *Clostridium difficile* is the most common cause of nosocomial infections in the hospitalized client.

   _____ Cooked foods are a source of *E. coli* bacteria.

   _____ Outbreaks of food-borne *viral* infections are almost always caused by contaminated shellfish.

   _____ Food can be a vehicle for transmitting actively growing microbes.

   _____ The incubation period for ALL viral and bacterial infections is 6 hours to 4-5 days.

   _____ Paralytic ileus can be caused by extensive surgical procedures in the bowel.

   _____ Abdominal angina refers to distention and bloating of the stomach.

   _____ Intestinal obstructions can divert large amount of circulating blood volume resulting in hypotension and shock.

   _____ Borborygmi is a symptom of obstruction of the colon.

   _____ The prime focus for treating intestinal obstructions is enemas and suppositories.

4. Common causes of appendicitis include: (Select all that apply)
   1. fecalith.
   2. kinking of the appendix.
   3. swelling of bowel wall.
   4. perforation of bowel wall.
   5. adhesions.

5. Common causes for the development of peritonitis include: (Select all that apply)
   1. ruptured or gangrenous gallbladder.
   2. fibrous condition of bowel wall.
   3. perforated peptic ulcer.
   4. perforated stomach.
   5. penetrating wounds.

6. Inflammatory bowel disease (IBD) includes two chronic disorders: Crohn's disease and ulcerative colitis. Using the chart below, compare and contrast the two diseases:

	Crohn's Disease	Ulcerative Colitis
Area affected		
Age of client		

Amount of diarrhea		
Appearance of stool		
Systemic symptoms		
Nutritional deficiencies		
Medical treatment		
Surgical intervention		
Prognosis		

7. _____ are the most commonly found benign tumors in the bowel.

8. Explain the difference between *diverticulosis* and *diverticulitis*.

9. Causes of obstruction in the small bowel include all of the following except:
   1. inflammation.
   2. neoplasms.
   3. adhesions.
   4. hernias.
   5. aneurysms.
   6. volvulus.
   7. intussusception.
   8. food blockage.
   9. compression from outside intestines.

10. Compare and contrast *blunt* and *penetrating trauma* to abdomen.

	Cause	Injuries	Treatment
Blunt trauma:			
Penetrating injury:			

APPLYING SKILLS

11. Physical assessment of the client who is experiencing diarrhea should focus on all of the following except:
    1. the abdomen.
    2. muscle weakness/signs of fatigue.
    3. mucous membranes.
    4. the skin (especially in the perineal area).

12. True or False

    _____ The confirmation of appendicitis is pain at the costovertebral angle.

13. State the rationale for assessing the following areas in the postoperative peritonitis client.
    a. Temperature:

    b. Blood pressure:

    c. Respiratory rate:

    d. Bowel sounds:

    e. Urine output:

    f. Skin turgor/mucous membranes:

    g. Laboratory tests (CBC, electrolytes):

14. The nurse will assess for all of the following in a client who has returned from colon surgery except:
    1. return of peristalsis.
    2. colostomy output.
    3. stoma appearance.
    4. bowel sounds.
    5. dressings/drains.

BEST PRACTICES

15. State the rationale for the following treatment interventions for the client with gastroenteritis.
    a. Rest:

    b. NPO status:

    c. Fluids:

    d. Electrolytes in fluids/IV:

    e. Perineal/skin care:

16. To prevent the spread of disease from infectious diarrhea, the nurse should: (Select all that apply)
    1. isolate the patient in a private room.
    2. observe contact isolation precautions.
    3. provide separate equipment (BP cuff, thermometer).
    4. follow facility protocol for cleaning surfaces/equipment.

17. For each of the following nursing diagnoses for the client with appendicitis, identify an appropriate outcome and two interventions.
    a. Acute pain related to inflammation
       OUTCOME:

       INTERVENTION #1:

       INTERVENTION #2:

    b. Risk for infection related to rupture of appendix
       OUTCOME:

       INTERVENTION #1:

       INTERVENTION #2:

18. State the rationale for each of the following procedures to prepare the client for surgery to remove cancerous growths in the colon.
    a. Diet high in calories, protein, and carbohydrates:

    b. Diet low in residue/liquid diet:

c.   Cathartics, such as GoLYTELY or Fleet Prep Kit:

d.   Administration of antibiotics:

e.   Administration of enemas:

f.   Blood transfusions (if needed):

g.   Enterostomal nurse consult:

19. State the rationale for each nursing intervention for care of the client with an intestinal obstruction.
    a.   Insertion of a nasogastric tube:

    b.   NPO status:

    c.   IV fluids with electrolytes:

    d.   Monitor vital signs frequently:

KEEPING DRUG SKILLS SHARP

20. Antidiarrheal medications are used for clients with Crohn's disease and ulcerative colitis but *not* clients with _____.

21. Morphine is *not* used for pain control with diverticulitis because _____
_____.

22. Compare and contrast common medications used to treat inflammatory bowel disease (IBD).

Medication	Indication for Use	Action
5-ASA		
Azulfidine		
Asacol/Rowasa		
Dipentum		
steroids		
antacids		
antihistamines		
budesenide		
Purinethol		
methotrexate		
Imuran		
Sandimmune		
Remicade		
Antegren		
anticholinergic		
antidiarrheals		
antispasmodic		
Flagyl		
Cipro		

Management of Clients with Urinary Disorders

OBJECTIVES

36.1 Discuss etiology, pathophysiology, and clinical manifestations of selected disorders of the urinary system.

36.2 Describe nursing care and medical/surgical management of clients with disorders of the urinary system.

36.3 Develop nursing care plans and medical surgical management of clients with bladder cancer.

36.4 Identify nursing care and medical/surgical management of obstructive urinary disorders.

36.5 Describe nursing care and medical management of clients with chronic disorders of the urinary system.

UNDERSTANDING PATHOPHYSIOLOGY

1. A urinary tract infection (UTI) is confirmed on the basis of _____ in the urinary system, usually at a count greater than _____.

2. Identify two reasons why urinary tract infections are uncommon in men.
   a.

   b.

3. Common causes for urinary tract infections in female clients include: (Select all that apply)
   1. sexual intercourse.
   2. poorly fitting contraceptive diaphragm.
   3. spermicides.
   4. synthetic hormones.
   5. tight jeans/wet bathing suits.
   6. feminine hygiene sprays/bubble baths.
   7. perfumed toilet paper/sanitary napkins.

4. The most accurate diagnostic tool for a UTI is a _____.

5. A serious complication that can develop from cystitis is _____ _____ from an ascending infection.

6. _____ is commonly associated with sexually transmitted disease.

7. Identify the two main causes of urolithiasis.
   a.

   b.

8. Compare and contrast the etiologies of the different types of calculi.

Type of Calculi	Etiology
Calcium	
Oxalate	
Struvite	
Uric acid	
Cystine	
Xanthine	

9. True or False

   _____ Visceral pain from renal calculi can be manifested with nausea and vomiting.

   _____ Stones smaller than 4-5 mm can pass through the urethra.

10. After age 50, the incidence of urinary reflux increases in male clients due to

    _____.

11. Common causes of urinary retention include all of the following except:
    1. detrusor failure in women.
    2. enlarged prostate in men.
    3. urethral strictures.
    4. medications.
    5. calculi.
    6. aneurysms.
    7. tumors.
    8. neuropathies from diabetes, stroke.

APPLYING SKILLS

12. Clinical manifestations of urinary tract infection include: (Select all that apply)
    1. dysuria.
    2. cloudy urine.
    3. complete emptying of bladder.
    4. hematuria.
    5. abdominal distention.
    6. frequency.
    7. urgency.
    8. inability to void.
    9. rebound tenderness RLQ.
    10. nausea/diarrhea.

13. Other complaints from female clients that may be confused with urinary tract infections include: (Select all that apply)
    1. vaginal candidiasis.
    2. Chlamydia.
    3. trichomonas.
    4. gonorrhoeae.
    5. herpes simplex.

14. Identify the signs of postoperative complications in a new stoma.

15. Clinical manifestations that would be noted for a client who is developing septic shock from urosepsis include: (Select all that apply)
    1. fever.
    2. altered mental status.
    3. increased blood pressure.
    4. hyperventilation.

16. True or False

    _____ Peristalsis will return soon after bladder reconstruction surgery as the bowel is not involved in the process.

    _____ Urine never stops after surgery is done to remove bladder cancer.

    _____ A new stoma must be assessed every hour for the first 24 hours postoperatively.

    _____ The site for a stoma must be clearly visible to the client and avoid the umbilicus, pubis and iliac crests.

    _____ A client with bladder cancer must complete a bowel prep before surgery.

    _____ Pain of kidney stones will be intermittent, meaning the renal stone may have moved.

BEST PRACTICES

17. To successfully treat a urinary tract infection, the nurse should instruct the client to discontinue antibiotics after:
    1. 10 days.
    2. 2 weeks.
    3. manifestations disappear.
    4. the full antibiotic course is completed.

18. State the rationales for each of the health promotion interventions to prevent further urinary tract infections.
    a. Encourage fluid intake at least 3 liters per day:

    b. Avoid caffeinated beverages/alcohol:

    c. Learn risks associated with spermicides:

    d. Remind client to void every 2-3 hours:

    e. Instruct female clients to void before and after coitus:

19. Identify an appropriate outcome and two interventions for a client with the nursing diagnosis Impaired urinary elimination related to irritation and inflammation of the bladder mucosa.
    OUTCOME:

    INTERVENTION:

    INTERVENTION:

20. Identify an appropriate outcome and three interventions for a client with the nursing diagnosis Risk for injury from BCG instillation and/or radiation therapy related to side effects.
    OUTCOME:

    INTERVENTION:

    INTERVENTION:

    INTERVENTION:

21. A client should be instructed to avoid using a _____ skin barrier when replacing the appliance for a urinary diversion, due to the urine's eroding effect.

22. Critical nursing interventions for the treatment of autonomic dysreflexia include: (Select all that apply)
    1. removing triggering stimuli.
    2. re-establishing urine flow.
    3. removing fecal impaction.
    4. inserting urinary catheter or irrigating existing catheter.
    5. monitoring vital signs every hour.
    6. raising head of bed to semi-Fowler's position.

KEEPING DRUG SKILLS SHARP

23. _____ is often prescribed with antibiotics for the acute pain associated with cystitis.

24. Identify two considerations for administering medications to older clients with UTIs.
    a.

    b.

25. _____ is used to treat interstitial cystitis because it decreases the permeability of the bladder mucosa, so that the causative agent cannot penetrate the lining.

26. Explain how the chemotherapeutic agent bacille Calmette-Guérin (BCG) is used in treating the client with bladder cancer.

27. Identify medications used for treating the different types of urinary incontinence and the action for each.

Type	Medication	Action
Urge incontinence		
Stress incontinence		
Urinary incontinence		

Management of Clients with Renal Disorders

OBJECTIVES

37.1 Identify common clinical manifestations of clients experiencing renal disorders.

37.2 Describe nursing care and medical management of extrarenal conditions affecting the renal system.

37.3 Identify nursing care and medical management of intrarenal disorders.

37.4 Describe nursing care and medical/surgical management of renal cancer and renal trauma.

37.5 Discuss nursing care and medical/surgical management of clients with renal vascular abnormalities and congenital renal disorders.

UNDERSTANDING PATHOPHYSIOLOGY

1. Kidneys regulate which of the following functions in the body? (Select all that apply)
    1. body's fluid levels
    2. electrolyte levels
    3. acid-base balance
    4. removal of toxic substances
    5. erythropoietin synthesis
    6. prostaglandin production
    7. renin-angiotensin-aldosterone system

2. Decreased renal function causes _____ due to retained excess sodium and water causing increased vascular volume.

3. Compare and contrast acute and chronic pyelonephritis.

	Acute	Chronic
Etiology		
Manifestations		
Testing		
Medical treatment		

4. An elderly client has undergone a procedure to relieve urinary obstruction with the placement of a ureteral stent. Explain how correcting this problem can result in fluid and electrolyte imbalance.

5. True or False

_____ Hypertension can cause or be affected by renal disease.

_____ Clients with independent diabetes mellitus [IDDM] have a greater likelihood to develop end stage renal disease [ESRD].

_____ Hypotension is a classic symptom of glomerulosclerosis.

_____ The damage caused by rhabdomyolysis is irreversible and fatal.

_____ Blood flow to the kidneys decreases with normal aging.

_____ Most renal tumors are benign.

_____ There is a probable association between renal cancer and smoking.

_____ After undergoing a nephrectomy to remove renal cancer, the remaining kidney can meet the body's needs.

_____ The lungs and mediastinum are the most frequent sites for metastasis for renal cancer.

_____ Adenocarcinoma is the most common tumor type of renal cancer.

6. List the classic triad of manifestations of renal cancer.
   a.
   b.
   c.

7. Compare and contrast acute and chronic tubulointerstitial disease.

	Acute	Chronic
Cause		
Onset		
Manifestations		
Prognosis		

8. Compare and contrast acute and chronic glomerulonephritis.

	Acute	Chronic
Onset		
Manifestations		

9. Identify the five categories of traumatic injury to the kidney.

a.

b.

c.

d.

e.

10. _____ is a cardinal manifestation of renal injury and found in approximately 80% of cases.

11. Identify six anomalies involving the kidney and description of effect on renal function.

Disorder	Effect on Renal Function
a.	
b.	
c.	
d.	
e.	
f.	

APPLYING SKILLS

12. Assessment of the client with hydronephrosis includes: (Select all that apply)
    1. monitor for presence, location, and intensity of pain.
    2. urine output.
    3. CVA tenderness.
    4. reports of renal failure (oliguria, anorexia, lethargy).

13. _____ may occur after nephrectomy, observable as sudden shortness of breath and loss of breath sounds on the affected side.

14. When obtaining a history from a client with glomerulonephritis, why is a history of upper respiratory infections, skin infections, or recent invasive procedures of particular concern?

BEST PRACTICES

15. Explain the rationale for each of the following nursing interventions for clients with altered renal function:
    Rhabdomyolysis: IV fluids and bed rest

    Hypertension: medication and diet changes

16. Nursing interventions to reduce renal damage when contrast x-ray studies are ordered include all of the following except:
    1. thorough history and physical before procedure.
    2. use non-dye studies whenever possible.
    3. limit client fluid intake.
    4. monitor client's urine output after study.

17. Identify an appropriate outcome and two interventions for a client with the nursing diagnosis Fluid volume deficit related to fever, nausea, vomiting, and possible diarrhea.
    OUTCOME:

    INTERVENTION #1:

    INTERVENTION #2:

18. Identify an appropriate outcome and two interventions for a client with the nursing diagnosis Acute pain related to an inflammatory process in the kidney and possible colic.
    OUTCOME:

    INTERVENTION #1:

    INTERVENTION #2:

19. State the rationale for each of the following nursing interventions for a postoperative nephrectomy client:
    a. Use narcotic analgesia, including patient controlled analgesia [PCA]:

    b. Teach client to support chest and abdomen with pillow or hands:

    c. Assess urine output:

    d. Monitor bowel sounds:

20. The primary focus for treatment of nephritis is to heal the glomerular membrane, stop the loss of protein, and break the cycle of edema. Identify four pertinent nursing plans and interventions to achieve these goals.

Plan	Intervention(s)
a.	
b.	
c.	
d.	

KEEPING DRUG SKILLS SHARP

21. Decreased renal function in a diabetic patient requires a _____ in the level of insulin administered.

22. Common analgesics found to cause renal damage as nephrotoxins include: (Select all that apply)
    1. opioids.
    2. acetaminophen.
    3. phenacetin.
    4. NSAIDs.

23. Clients with hypertension are often prescribed diuretics as part of the medical treatment regimen. Explain how diuretics, which help lower blood pressure, can also cause renal damage.

24. Identify two reasons to make modifications for older clients who are prescribed antibiotics for pyelonephritis.
    a.

    b.

25. The inflammatory condition that results in interstitial nephritis or "tubulointerstitial disease" can be caused by use of: (Select all that apply)
    1. NSAIDs.
    2. hydrochlorothiazide.
    3. Captopril.
    4. cephalosporins.
    5. acetaminophen.
    6. sodium bicarbonate.
    7. aspirin.
    8. sulfonamide.

Chapter **38**

Management of Clients with Renal Failure

OBJECTIVES

38.1 Compare and contrast clinical manifestations of clients experiencing acute and chronic renal failure.

38.2 Describe nursing care and medical/surgical management of chronic renal failure.

38.3 Compare and contrast nursing care and medical management of clients receiving peritoneal and hemodialysis.

38.4 Describe nursing care and medical/surgical management of clients who receive a renal transplant.

UNDERSTANDING PATHOPHYSIOLOGY

1. Common manifestations of acute renal failure (ARF) include: (Select all that apply)
   1. abrupt loss of kidney function.
   2. hematuria.
   3. elevation in serum creatinine and urea nitrogen levels.
   4. a decrease in urine production below normal 400ml/24hrs.

2. List the three main classifications of ARF:
   a.

   b.

   c.

3. Describe the causes for acute tubular necrosis and give examples:
   a.

   b.

4. True or False

   _____ Once renal failure has begun, the ability to reverse the mechanism will depend on the level of destruction of the basement membrane.

   _____ The client diagnosed with diabetes mellitus is protected from renal failure due to high blood glucose levels.

_____   Hypertension is a major cause of chronic renal failure.

_____   Oliguria refers to a urine output which exceeds 1500 ml/day in a normal healthy client.

_____   Unless treated properly, the client with acute renal failure will develop chronic renal failure and require dialysis in the future.

_____   Chronic renal failure (CRF) causes more degenerative changes throughout the body than does acute renal failure.

_____   Pericarditis is usually related to increased amounts of uremic toxins related to CRF not from a source of infection.

5. Compare and contrast the two types of acute renal failure:

	Nonoliguric Renal Failure	Oliguric Renal Failure
Urine output		
Urine		
Clinical signs		
Prognosis		

6. Causes of chronic renal failure include all of the following except:
   1. diabetes insipidus.
   2. hypertension.
   3. chronic glomerulonephritis.
   4. acute renal failure.
   5. polycystic kidney disease.
   6. obstruction.
   7. repeated episodes of pyelonephritis.
   8. nephrotoxins.

7. Identify the five stages of chronic renal failure and clinical manifestations:
   a.
   b.
   c.
   d.
   e.

8. The accumulation of _____ may lead to gastrointestinal complications in clients with chronic renal failure.

9. Differentiate between ultrafiltration and diffusion.

10. Identify the cause of dialysis disequilibrium syndrome.

APPLYING SKILLS

11. Monitoring the client with ARF includes review of lab data. Discuss the implication for these abnormal lab values:
    a. Increasing BUN level:

    b. Low RBC, Hct, Hgb:

    c. Low platelets:

12. Chronic renal failure affects every system in the body. For each of the identified areas, give examples of manifestations:
    Electrolyte imbalances:

    Metabolic changes:

    Hematologic changes:

    Gastrointestinal changes:

Immunologic changes:

Changes to medication metabolism:

Cardiovascular changes:

Respiratory changes:

Musculoskeletal changes:

Integumentary changes:

Neurologic changes:

Reproductive changes:

Endocrine changes:

Psychosocial changes:

13. Clients who do not respond to conservative treatment for ARF may require dialysis to resolve the problem. Clinical manifestations that require dialysis include: (Select all that apply)
    1. significant volume overload.
    2. hypovolemia.
    3. progressive uremia (rising BUN and creatinine levels).
    4. altered central nervous system functioning.
    5. pericarditis.

14. Identify the critical nursing assessments that must be performed for a dialysis graft site and explain the implications of the findings.

BEST PRACTICES

15. For each of the following interventions for the treatment of ARF, give the rationale behind the action:
    a. Careful replacement of fluids:

    b. Replacement of other fluid losses:

    c. Cautious use of diuretics to reduce fluid overload:

    d. Electrolyte replacement based on lab data:

    e. Electrocardiograph monitors:

    f. Dietary restrictions:

16. Identify the dietary modifications for the client with ARF. Give a rationale for each action:
    a. High calorie:

    b. Low protein:

    c. Low sodium/magnesium/phosphate/potassium:

    d. TPN:

    e. Adequate/balanced fluids:

17. Identify an appropriate outcome and interventions for a client with the nursing diagnosis Excess fluid volume related to inability of kidneys to produce urine secondary to acute renal failure.
    OUTCOME:

    INTERVENTIONS:

18. Identify an appropriate outcome and interventions for a client with the nursing diagnosis Imbalanced nutrition: Less than body requirements related to anorexia and altered metabolic state.
    OUTCOME:

    INTERVENTIONS:

19. Constipation is a common problem for the client with CRF. The nurse should advise the client to avoid OTC laxatives because they contain _____ which cannot be excreted when kidneys have failed.

20. List the four basic goals of dialysis therapy.
    a.

    b.

    c.

    d.

21. The nurse should instruct the dialysis patient to avoid salt substitutes because they contain _____ which is not excreted in renal failure.

KEEPING DRUG SKILLS SHARP

22. The diuretic _____ is not prescribed for clients with acute renal failure because it can be nephrotoxic and increase risk of further kidney damage.

23. Before beginning dialysis, the client's dosage of the anticoagulant _____ must be reduced to reduce risk of bleeding during the procedure.

24. Explain why medications for the elderly renal client must be adjusted.

25. Adjustments that must be made for the diabetic client who also has chronic renal failure include all of the following except:
    1. lowering of insulin dosages.
    2. administering mannitol.
    3. fewer injections of insulin.
    4. close monitoring of client's blood glucose.

26. A client with acute renal failure has a dangerously high laboratory value of potassium. This is a life-threatening situation because of the risk of cardiac arrest. Treatment of the hyperkalemia can include administration of which of the following medications? (Select all that apply)
    1. calcium
    2. insulin
    3. normal saline
    4. vitamin C
    5. Kayexalate
    6. sodium citrate
    7. sorbitol
    8. sodium bicarbonate

27. The hormone _____ can be administered either intravenously after hemodialysis or subcutaneously.

CONCEPT MAP EXERCISES

The following questions are based on the concept map *Understanding Chronic Renal Failure and Its Treatment* in your textbook.

28. When the kidneys suffer damage resulting in a decreased glomerular filtration of the blood, what two lab values will be noted initially?

29. What initial clinical manifestations develop when the nephrons of the kidney can no longer concentrate urine?

30. When a client develops CRF, many systems of the body are affected. How is the client with CRF at greater risk for infection?

31. Decreased sodium reabsorption leads to water retention and which common manifestations?

32. What are the treatments for hyperkalemia?

33. A client diagnosed with CRF presents with changes in level of consciousness and pruritus. What is the mechanism for the development of these changes?

Chapter 39

Assessment of the Reproductive System

OBJECTIVES

39.1 Identify essential elements of a comprehensive gynecologic assessment.

39.2 Describe diagnostic exams used for women with gynecologic and reproductive disorders.

39.3 Describe key elements of a health assessment for men with reproductive disorders.

39.4 Identify diagnostic exams used for men with reproductive disorders.

39.5 Discuss primary, secondary, and tertiary prevention related to reproductive disorders.

ANATOMY & PHYSIOLOGY REVIEW

1. Label the structures of the female pelvis.

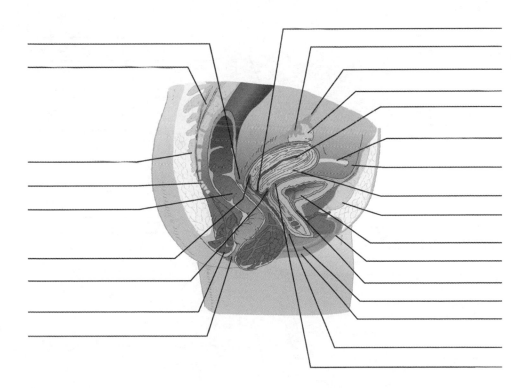

2. Label the lymph nodes near the female breast.

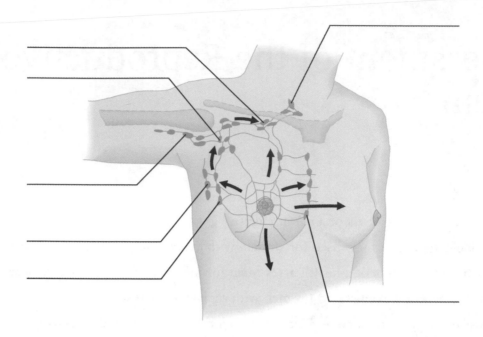

3. Label the structures of the male pelvis and genitalia.

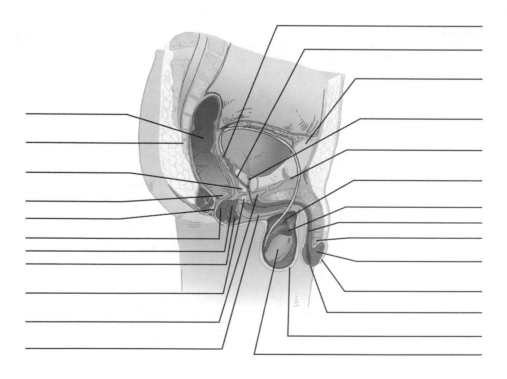

UNDERSTANDING PATHOPHYSIOLOGY

4. The most serious childhood infectious disease that can affect a woman of childbearing age is:
   1. viral pneumonia.
   2. hepatitis.
   3. endocarditis.
   4. rubella.

5. A 54-year-old female with a history of breast cancer is concerned about "hot flashes" and wants to know if she should be taking hormones, specifically estrogen. Which of the following statements is true regarding estrogen and women with a history of breast cancer?
   1. Estrogens are contraindicated in women who have had breast cancer or cancer of the reproductive tract.
   2. Estrogen will cause your cervix to swell.
   3. Estrogen can only be taken for a short period of time.
   4. Breast cancer has to be in remission before you can take estrogen.

6. The American Cancer Society (ACS) recommends that women who are or have been sexually active and have reached 18 years of age should have annual _____ and _____.

7. A mammogram _____ used to detect _____.

8. A 45-year-old African American male would be at risk for
   1. adenocarcinoma of the prostate.
   2. testicular cancer.
   3. benign prostatic hypertrophy.
   4. enlarged structures of the glans penis.

9. Which childhood infection can affect male fertility?
   1. chicken pox.
   2. measles.
   3. mumps.
   4. hepatitis.

10. Match the description or definition to the correct male reproductive disorders.

	Description/Definition	Disorder
_____	a. Antigen found in the serum of men with prostate cancer	1. Alkaline phosphatase
_____	b. Enzyme found in the serum of men with advanced prostate cancer	2. Prostate-specific antigen (PSA)
_____	c. Enzyme found in the serum of men whose prostate cancer has metastasized to the bone	3. Semen analysis
_____	d. Studies which measure pressure from bladder or urethra, urinary flow, and muscle activity	4. Serum acid phosphatase
_____	e. Analysis of sperm for fertility, the effectiveness of a vasectomy, to test DNA, or establish paternity	5. Urodynamic assessment

APPLYING SKILLS

11. As part of the reproductive assessment, what information should be included in the data obtained from the client? (Select all that apply)
    1. client's lifestyle
    2. health habits
    3. self perceptions
    4. body image
    5. developmental stage
    6. cultural, religious factors
    7. socioeconomic and educational background

12. What type of gloves should the nurse use for a routine gynecological examination on a client who is allergic to latex?
    1. latex
    2. vinyl
    3. rubber
    4. cloth

13. The nurse should instruct a client prior to a pelvic examination to: (Select all that apply)
    1. not douche.
    2. not have sexual intercourse.
    3. take a bath.
    4. not use vaginal products for 2-3 days.

14. The best time to performing a breast exam on a 55-year-old female is:
    1. 7-10 days before menses.
    2. 2-3 days before menses.
    3. 7-10 days after onset of menses.
    4. during menses.

15. If, during a pelvic examination, abnormal cervical or vaginal tissue or a mass is discovered, what other procedures may need to be performed? (Select all that apply)
    1. bimanual exam
    2. colposcopy or biopsy
    3. lithotrypsy
    4. wet smear

16. An enlargement of the breasts is called _____.

17. _____ is an examination in which one or two fingers are placed in the vagina and the other hand is placed on the abdomen to palpate the pelvic contents.

18. Bulging of the rectum into the vagina is called _____.

19. The _____ is the upper outer quadrant of the breast.

20. A curved ridge along the inferior breast is called _____.

BEST PRACTICES

21. During a pelvic examination of a 40-year-old female, the nurse should also take the opportunity to discuss which of the following health maintenance measure with the client: (Select all that apply)
    1. breast self-examinations
    2. risk factors associated with gynecologic cancer and heart disease
    3. menstrual hygiene
    4. lifestyle factors (diet, exercise, sleep, stress)
    5. protection against STD

22. A rectal prostate examination should be performed: (Select all that apply)
    1. in men over the age of 50.
    2. in men over the age of 45 with increased risk.
    3. to detect changes in size, consistency of prostate gland.
    4. to denote tumors or acute or chronic infections.

KEEPING DRUGS SKILLS SHARP

23. Medications that may cause impotence include: (Select all that apply)
    1. clonidine.
    2. hydralazine.
    3. methyldopa.
    4. guanethidine.

24. True or False

    _____ Tranquilizers can interfere with sexual performance.

25. Herbal medications commonly used to treat reproductive disorders include: (Select all that apply)
    1. saw palmetto.
    2. yohimbe.
    3. St. John's wort.
    4. milk thistle.

26. Recreational and illegal substances that may affect sexual behaviors and increase risk for exposure to STDs include: (Select all that apply)
    1. alcohol.
    2. amphetamines.
    3. barbiturates.
    4. marijuana.

Management of Men with Reproductive Disorders

OBJECTIVES

40.1 Describe the essential elements of nursing assessment of males with reproductive disorders.

40.2 Discuss disorders of infertility and impotence, and their medical, surgical, and nursing management.

40.3 Describe disorders of the prostate and their medical, surgical, and nursing management.

40.4 Describe medical, surgical, and nursing management of clients with testicular disorders.

UNDERSTANDING PATHOPHYSIOLOGY

1. The nurse examines a 72-year-old African American male who has been complaining of frequent trips to the bathroom at night and difficulty and pressure when urinating. Current history and physical data along with a diagnostic evaluation show that he has benign prostatic hypertrophy (BPH). The nurse explains to the client that BPH is:
   1. hypertrophy of periurethral glands.
   2. hyperplasia of periurethral glands that compresses the normal prostate gland.
   3. dysplasia of prostatic cells that begins in the periphery of posterior gland.
   4. inflammation of prostate glands that compresses the urethra.

2. The cause of testicular cancer is unknown. However, it has been associated with:
   1. prostatitis at an early age.
   2. sexual activity with many partners.
   3. undescended testicles.
   4. cancer of the prostate.

3. Match the following terms with the correct definition or description:

Terms	Definition/Description
_____ a. Orchitis	1. acute testicular inflammation caused by a viral infection
_____ b. Testicular torsion	2. testicle is mobile; spermatic cord twist
_____ c. Epididymitis	3. prolonged and painful erection
_____ d. Hydrocele	4. urethral meatus opens dorsally on the top of penis
_____ e. Varicocele	5. urethral meatus opens ventrally on the side of penis
_____ f. Cryptorchidism	6. penile foreskin constriction
_____ g. Phimosis	7. dilated testicular vein
_____ h. Epispadias	8. undescended testicles
_____ i. Hypospadias	9. inflammation of the epididymis
_____ j. Priapism	10. painless collection of clear, yellow fluid in scrotum

APPLYING SKILLS

4. During a physical assessment, a client with BPH would likely report having which symptoms?
   1. downward force of stream
   2. painful urination
   3. difficulty starting the flow of urine
   4. pain in lower abdomen

5. Digital rectal examinations are performed on male patients with BPH in order to:
   1. assess prostate size and to differentiate BPH from prostate enlargement.
   2. determine the size of cells.
   3. release a closed stricture above the testes.
   4. allow urine to flow freely.

6. A client with BPH will have which of these symptoms? (Select all that apply)
   1. frequency of urination
   2. urgency, hesitancy
   3. change in stream of urine
   4. urinary retention
   5. nocturia

7. Cancer of the prostate has which of the following diagnostic markers? (Select all that apply)
   1. hard nodules, unilateral enlargement of outer prostate
   2. elevated PSA greater than 10 ng/m, DRE exam positive
   3. increased acid phosphatase levels
   4. positive transrectal ultrasound and biopsy

8. The nurse examines a 28-year-old male with a testicular nodule that is highly suspicious for testicular cancer. What laboratory exam would provide further evidence to support this diagnosis?
   1. elevated testosterone level
   2. alpha-fetoprotein (AFP), human chorionic gonadotropin (HCG)
   3. carcinoembryonic antigen (CEA)
   4. antinuclear antibodies (ANA)

BEST PRACTICES

9. A 65-year-old male is scheduled for a TURP. The nurse explains to the client that in this procedure:
   1. a low abdominal incision is made in order to approach the prostate without entering the bladder.
   2. an incision is made into the area between the anus and the prostate.
   3. a transurethral incision of the prostate is made, followed by balloon dilation of the stricture.
   4. a lighted tube is placed in the urethra and excess prostatic tissue is removed.

10. What is a common nursing diagnosis for a client with TURP in the postoperative phase? (Select all that apply)
    1. Ineffective tissue perfusion related to deep vein thrombosis
    2. Altered comfort related to pain of bladder spasm
    3. Disturbed body image related to disfiguring surgery
    4. Imbalanced nutrition less than body requirement

11. Discharge teaching for clients with TURP should include:
    1. use enemas to avoid straining.
    2. increase intake of coffee, tea, and sodas.
    3. avoid heaving lifting, heavy climbing, driving, and prolonged sitting.
    4. do not have more than 2 glasses of alcohol per day.

KEEPING DRUGS SKILLS SHARP

12. Because they may aggravate his condition, clients with BPH should avoid taking these medications: (Select all that apply)
    1. antipsychotic medications, antidepressants
    2. calcium channel blockers
    3. cold medicines, diet pills (they contain alpha and adrenergic agonists which can cause urinary retention)
    4. topical agents for urinary constriction

13. Clients with BPH should be encouraged to drink fluids because concentrated urine acts as an irritant to the _____.

14. True or False

    _____ The use of phototherapeutic agents such as herbs to help control BPH has been increasing.

    _____ The most commonly used herbal agent in treating BPH is saw palmetto.

Chapter 41

Management of Women with Reproductive Disorders

OBJECTIVES

41.1 Discuss common menstrual disorders and menopause, and their medical, surgical, and nursing management.

41.2 Identify infectious and inflammatory uterine disorders, and their medical, surgical, and nursing management.

41.3 Describe and differentiate malignant and nonmalignant tumors of the uterus, and their medical, surgical, and nursing management.

41.4 Discuss common disorders of the uterus, and their medical and nursing management.

41.5 Discuss nursing care and management for ovarian disorders.

41.6 Describe medical, surgical, and nursing management of vaginal disorders.

41.7 Define gynecologic cancers.

UNDERSTANDING PATHOPHYSIOLOGY

1. A 35-year-old female complains of irritability, depression, frequent crying spells, migraine headaches, and abdominal bloating—all before her menses. These symptoms are probably related to:
   1. taking medications for extreme psychosis.
   2. iron and vitamin deficiency.
   3. PMS syndrome relating to hormonal imbalance.
   4. excessive retention of TSH.

2. Match the following terms with the correct description:

   _____ a. cystocele   1. descent of urinary bladder
   _____ b. vaginal prolapse   2. inflammation of the vulva
   _____ c. urethrocele   3. protrusion of vaginal wall musculature
   _____ d. enterocele   4. inflammation of the vagina
   _____ e. vaginitis   5. abnormal tube-like passage from the vagina to bladder
   _____ f. toxic shock syndrome   6. prolapse of the urethra
   _____ g. vaginal fistulae   7. toxins of *Staphylococcus aureus*
   _____ h. vulvitis   8. descent of the bowel/protrusion of posterior wall of vagina

3. A 45-year-old female has just had a hysterectomy and is anxious about experiencing severe symptoms of menopause. The nurse can respond appropriately by saying:
   1. "Only older women have this problem."
   2. "Menopausal symptoms occur when the ovaries are removed."
   3. "You must wait until symptoms are severe."
   4. "This surgery is unique and symptoms only start when you are 55 years and older."

4. More than 50% of women with history of PID have difficulty becoming pregnant after an infection of PID due to:
   1. fallopian tubes enlargement, which allows the harboring of more bacteria.
   2. cervical canal stretched by past infections.
   3. scarring by inflammatory process and subsequent closing and scarring of fallopian tubes.
   4. ruptured fallopian tubes being unable to hold eggs.

5. A total hysterectomy is the removal of the _____ and the _____.

6. Total hysterectomy with bilateral salpingo-oophorectomy is a total hysterectomy along with the removal of the _____ and the _____.

APPLYING SKILLS

7. The clinical symptoms of PID that a patient would be present with are: (Select all that apply)
   1. malaise, fever, chills.
   2. nausea and vomiting.
   3. acute sharp severe pain on both sides of abdomen.
   4. heavy, purulent vaginal discharge.

8. What is the most serious long-term complication that can result from endometriosis?
   1. infertility
   2. cancer of the uterus
   3. prolapsed uterus
   4. cervical cancer

9. List clinical manifestations of vasomotor instability associated with menopause:
   a.
   b.
   c.
   d.

10. When a Foley catheter is discontinued after a hysterectomy, the nurse should report which of the following to the physician? (Select all that apply)
    1. voiding frequently in small amounts
    2. inability to void
    3. bladder distention
    4. hematuria

BEST PRACTICES

11. A 26-year-old female has been complaining of persistent dysmenorrhea for the past 6 months. In providing patient education, the nurse should: (Select all that apply)
    1. encourage exercise, including swimming.
    2. tell her to decrease sodium and increase vitamin B_6, calcium, Mg, and protein in her diet.
    3. discuss oral contraceptives to relieve menstrual discomfort.
    4. encourage use of narcotics for extreme pain.

12. Diet and nutrition are important in helping to alleviate some of the symptoms of PMS. What nutritional advice would be helpful to a client with PMS? (Select all that apply)
    1. Reduce salt and refined carbohydrates.
    2. Eat small frequent meals to stabilize blood sugar.
    3. Take 1000 mg of calcium per day.
    4. Reduce alcohol and caffeine.

13. What are the priority nursing actions for a client who has just had a vaginal hysterectomy?
    1. Assist with tub and shower bath.
    2. Provide a high carbohydrate diet.
    3. Teach client exercises to strengthen chest and stomach.
    4. Observe client for decreased urine output.

14. The primary diagnostic tool for cervical cancer is:
    1. gram stain and culture.
    2. Pap smear.
    3. cervical ovulation.
    4. c-reactive protein.

15. During evaluation of the client with cervical cancer, the nurse would expect the client to have which of the following assessment findings? (Select all that apply)
    1. vaginal discharge
    2. metrorrhagia and bleeding
    3. painful intercourse
    4. pressure in bladder and bowel
    5. abdominal pain

16. When providing care for a client being treated at home for PID, the nurse should instruct the client to:
    1. continue to take medications for blood pressure elevations.
    2. avoid sexual contact with partner, no douching.
    3. ambulate at least 3-4 times per day.
    4. resume vaginal cleansing.

17. To promote drainage and comfort, a client with PID should: (Select all that apply)
    1. maintain semi-Fowler's position to promote downward drainage.
    2. take a sitz bath or apply heat to lower back and abdomen.
    3. maintain reverse Trendelenburg position for comfort.
    4. only take pain medication every 8 hours.

18. A 26-year-old female is admitted for a workup up PID. This condition is also associated with: (Select all that apply)
    1. bacterial vaginal infections (untreated).
    2. sexually transmitted diseases.
    3. lack of condom use with high incidence of passing bacteria between partners.
    4. recent viral infections of the lung.

19. While preparing discharge instructions for the client after an abdominal hysterectomy, the client asks when she can return to work. The nurse should respond:
    1. "It's possible to return to normal activities with in 4-6 weeks."
    2. "When the abdomen incision has healed in about 3-4 months."
    3. "In 2 weeks if she has no pain."
    4. "Following your next visit to the doctors' office."

KEEPING DRUGS SKILLS SHARP

20. A client scheduled for discharge after an abdominal hysterectomy with removal of ovaries and fallopian tubes wants information regarding hormone replacement therapy. What hormone will be most likely prescribed by the physician?
    1. thyroxin
    2. estrogen
    3. testosterone
    4. lactin

21. A 55-year-old female client diagnosed with cancer of the uterus is to receive radioactive implants. Where would you place the client on the clinical unit?
    1. while radioactive implants are in place, the client can be placed in a ward
    2. a private room with adjoining bathrooms
    3. far away from the nurses' station
    4. private room with radiation precautions

22. Commonly prescribed prostaglandin inhibitors include: (Select all that apply)
    1. Motrin.
    2. Ponstel.
    3. Indocin.
    4. Naprosyn.

23. Side effects of Motrin and Indocin that the client needs to be aware include: (Select all that apply)
    1. sodium and water retention.
    2. rashes.
    3. potential allergic reactions.
    4. pain in the back.

24. A client who is experiencing premenstrual discomfort should be advised to eliminate _____ from her diet and take _____.

Management of Clients with Breast Disorders

OBJECTIVES

42.1   Discuss the importance of breast self-examinations.

42.2   Describe diagnostic exams used to detect breast cancer.

42.3   Discuss breast cancer and its medical, surgical, and nursing management.

42.4   Describe benign breast disorders, their treatments, and nursing management options.

UNDERSTANDING PATHOPHYSIOLOGY

1.   The most important single risk factor for breast cancer is _____.

2.   The overall risk of breast cancer is greatest in women:
   1.   over 60 years of age.
   2.   who do not have breast changes.
   3.   who have BRCA1/BRCA2 genes.
   4.   who have tumor suppressor.

3.   While examining a female client, the nurse becomes alarmed when she palpates:
   1.   a painful reddened mass in the upper outer quadrant of breast.
   2.   a 3 cm movable mass in the axillary region.
   3.   a large, tender, movable mass in upper area of breast.
   4.   a hard, painless, immobile, non-tender lesion in an irregularly shaped mass in the upper outer quadrant.

APPLYING SKILLS

4.   The most accurate diagnostic test used for assisting in the diagnosis of breast cancer is:
   1.   fine needle aspiration.
   2.   closed biopsy.
   3.   mammography.
   4.   steriotactic core biopsy.

5. During the postoperative period for a client who has had breast surgery, possible complications include: (Select all that apply)
   1. lymphedema, infection.
   2. hematoma.
   3. cellulitis.
   4. seroma.

6. During the early postoperative period following a mastectomy, the nurse would encourage the client to:
   1. perform active elbow flexion and extension exercises on the affected side.
   2. perform full range of motion exercises.
   3. adduct the affected arm daily.
   4. keep affected arm straight and aligned for 24 to 48 hours.

7. What organization will be able to assist the mastectomy client who has had radiation and surgery with body image concerns?
   1. American Cancer Society
   2. Reach to Recovery
   3. National Cancer Foundation
   4. Society of American Mastectomy Society

8. Match these terms with the correct definition or description.

Term	Definition/Description
_____ a. tissue expanders	1. done to achieve symmetry, delayed for several months following breast reconstruction
_____ b. transverse rectus abdominal muscle flap	2. "tummy tuck"
_____ c. latissimus dorsi muscle flap	3. deflated saline envelope inserted under chest muscle that expands over 6-8 weeks
_____ d. gluteal muscle free flaps	4. large, fan-shaped muscle beneath the scapula that is used when inadequate skin is available at mastectomy site
_____ e. nipple areola reconstruction	5. breast construction involves use of gluteus muscle

BEST PRACTICES

9. Lifestyle changes that can to help reduce the potential risk for breast include:
   1. decreasing alcohol consumption.
   2. decreasing fat intake to 20% of dietary calories.
   3. exercising regularly.
   4. ingesting large quantities of niacin.

10. The National Cancer Advisory Board (NCAB) recommends to the National Cancer Institute (NCI) that women between 40-49 years of age:
    1. have mammograms every 5 years.
    2. have screening mammograms every 1-2 years if they are at average risk for breast cancer.
    3. only do manual breast self exams monthly.
    4. have diagnostic mammograms every 2-4 years.

11. Fine needle aspiration determines whether a solid lump is a _____ _____.

12. Stereotactic needle guided biopsy is used mainly to identify _____ _____.

13. A _____ is an en bloc removal of the breast, axillary lymph nodes, and overlying skin, with the muscles left intact.

KEEPING DRUG SKILLS SHARP

14. Additional treatments for clients who have breast cancer may include: (Select all that apply)
    1. chemotherapy.
    2. radiation therapy.
    3. hormone therapy.
    4. DNA screening.

15. True or False

    _____ Tamoxifen is an agent commonly used in clients who have breast tumors with receptors for estrogen.

16. Radiation therapy used to treat micrometastatic disease following a mastectomy:
    1. enables the healing process to adhere faster.
    2. successfully reduces the risk of local recurrence and distant metastasis.
    3. promotes skin graphs to become less infected.
    4. enhances the chemotherapy to be given in a shorter period of time.

17. Radiation therapy for breast cancer can be administered through which of these methods? (Select all that apply)
    1. external beams
    2. brachytherapy
    3. iridium implants
    4. intravenous via large bore needles

Chapter 43

Management of Clients with Sexually Transmitted Diseases

OBJECTIVES

43.1 Discuss common sexually transmitted diseases and their clinical manifestations.

43.2 Discuss the medical and nursing management of common sexually transmitted diseases.

43.3 Identify screening methods used to detect sexually transmitted diseases.

43.4 Discuss health prevention methods for sexually transmitted diseases.

UNDERSTANDING PATHOPHYSIOLOGY

1. Which of the following diseases are most commonly referred to as STDs? (Select all that apply)
   1. Chlamydia
   2. gonorrhea
   3. syphilis
   4. genital herpes
   5. genital warts

2. A _____ is a highly contagious infection caused by *Baullis haemophilus ducreyi.*

3. Lymphogranuloma is caused by strains of _____.

4. Individuals at high risk for acquiring STDs include: (Select all that apply)
   1. IV drug users.
   2. people involved in high risk sexual activity.
   3. adolescents who have unprotected sex.
   4. chronic renal failure patients.

5. The organism that causes Chlamydia is:
   1. genital herpes.
   2. *Chlamydia trachomatis.*
   3. human papilloma virus.
   4. *Neisseria gonorrhoeae.*

6. A female client who presents with a heavy, yellow-green, purulent vaginal discharge probably has:
   1. vaginitis.
   2. Chlamydia.
   3. syphilis.
   4. gonorrhea.

7. The principal clinical manifestation of primary syphilis is:
   1. enlarged lymph node.
   2. warts on the genitals.
   3. genital chancre sores.
   4. vaginal and rectal bleeding.

8. Women with genital herpes have an increased risk for:
   1. carcinoma of the cervix.
   2. sterility.
   3. fibroid tumors.
   4. Candida yeast infections.

APPLYING SKILLS

9. Male clients who present with mucopurulent discharge should have which initial exam done to confirm a preliminary diagnosis of Chlamydia?
   1. DFA (direct fluorescent antibody)
   2. urine culture
   3. GC culture and gram stain for gonorrhea
   4. clinical examination of pelvic pain

10. The most common complication of gonorrhea in women is:
    1. salpingitis that can progress to PID.
    2. reversible PID.
    3. meningitis.
    4. urethral enlargement.

11. Which laboratory studies can confirm a diagnosis of syphilis in its primary stages? (Select all that apply)
    1. DFA (dark field microscopy)
    2. culture and sensitivity of urethra
    3. serologic test for syphilis
    4. fluorescent treponemal antibody absorption test (FTA-ABS)

12. A young woman is newly diagnosed with genital herpes lesion, type 2. Which clinical manifestations would she present with? (Select all that apply)
    1. small vesicles with erythematous borders on genital regions
    2. burning sensation at site of inoculation
    3. anuria
    4. leukorrhea

BEST PRACTICES

13. A 16-year-old adolescent comes to the clinic for treatment of an STD and is concerned about her boyfriend. The nurse should provide which of the following information to the adolescent when she is being discharged from the clinic?
    1. All sexual partners need to evaluated and treated.
    2. You can return in 1 month for follow-up and see if he needs it.
    3. He will need to be treated only if he is having symptoms.
    4. His treatment will only start after you have completed the course of medications.

14. The most effective mechanical barriers to STDs are:
    1. oral contraceptives.
    2. IUDs (intrauterine devices).
    3. rhythm methods.
    4. latex condoms.

KEEPING DRUG SKILLS SHARP

15. The treatments of choice for Chlamydial infections include: (Select all that apply)
    1. gentamycin tid for 7 days.
    2. doxycycline (Vibramycin) for 7 days orally.
    3. azothromycin (Zithromax) in one dose.
    4. penicillin G for two doses IM.

16. The current recommended treatment regimen for uncomplicated gonorrhea is:
    1. amoxicillin.
    2. a single dose of IM rocephin (Ceftriaxine) or Cefixin.
    3. tetracycline tid for 7 days.
    4. gentamycin IM.

17. The recommended treatment for an acute primary infection of genital herpes is: (Select all that apply)
    1. streptomycin in two doses.
    2. penicillin G topical.
    3. zovirax (Acyclovir) for 7-10 days.
    4. famciclovir (antiviral agents).

Chapter 44

Assessment of the Endocrine and Metabolic Systems

OBJECTIVES

44.1   Understand current terminology relating to disorders of the endocrine and metabolic systems.

44.2   Describe detailed assessment information the nurse is required to understand when working with clients with endocrine and metabolic disorders.

44.3   List important information to be included in a history-taking session for clients with endocrine and metabolic disorders.

44.4   Identify current laboratory and diagnostic tests pertinent to clients with endocrine and metabolic disorders.

ANATOMY & PHYSIOLOGY REVIEW

1.   Label the diagram below with the name of each endocrine gland.

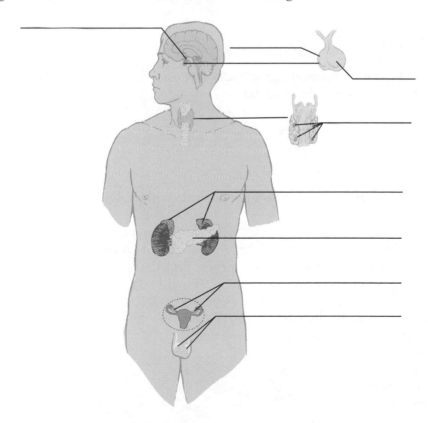

UNDERSTANDING PATHOPHYSIOLOGY

2. True or False

_____ Alcoholism often accompanies liver and pancreatic disease, causing fatty infiltration of the liver.

_____ Serum cortisol is measured in clients suspected of having hyperfunctioning or hypofunctioning adrenal glands.

3. Match the terms with the correct definition or description of clinical manifestations.

_____	a. Kussmaul's respirations	1. tetany
_____	b. pancreatic disorder	2. fatty, foul-smelling stools
_____	c. hyperthyroidism	3. dehydration
_____	d. glossitis	4. dark-colored, tarry stools
_____	e. biliary tract disorders	5. calcium stone formation
_____	f. gallbladder disorders	6. dark yellow, tea-colored urine
_____	g. aerophagia	7. right upper quadrant pain
_____	h. inadequate secretion of parathyroid hormone	8. excessive belching
_____	i. ADH suppression	9. red tongue
_____	j. steatorrhea (chronic pancreatitis)	10. elevation of body temperature/ exophthalmos
_____	k. hepatocellular disease	11. pain radiating to back
_____	l. hyperparathyroidism	12. deep, rapid breathing

APPLYING SKILLS

4. In evaluating a client with metabolic and endocrine disorders, which of the following areas should be explored? (Select all that apply)
   1. health history
   2. physical examination
   3. diagnostic tests
   4. family and social history

5. Family history is important when questioning clients with endocrine and metabolic disorders because: (Select all that apply)
   1. history of previous disorders increases risk for development.
   2. a number of disorders are inherited and tend to run in families.
   3. family members are not prone to inherit these disorders.
   4. most psychosocial concerns are limited.

6. When examining a client for hepatic or biliary pain, on which areas of the abdomen should the nurse concentrate? (Select all that apply)
   1. right lower quadrant
   2. mid abdomen
   3. lower back portion
   4. right upper quadrant

7. Which x-ray, used in diagnostic evaluation of clients with endocrine and metabolic disorders, provides vital and important information about liver and pancreatic and biliary conditions?
   1. abdominal ultrasound
   2. upper gastrointestinal series
   3. chest x-ray
   4. flat plate of the abdomen

BEST PRACTICES

8. True or False

   _____ Hepatic encephalopathy, caused by reduced tissue perfusion, is another complication resulting from drainage of ascitic fluid.

   _____ Hypovolemic shock can develop from dehydration.

9. _____ is a diagnostic procedure used to remove of a sample of living tissue for analysis.

10. _____ is the extraction of fluid accumulated in the peritoneum.

11. _____ is a major complication of paracentesis.

12. Contraindications to percutaneous liver biopsy include: (Select all that apply)
    1. thrombocytopenia.
    2. local infection of the lung base.
    3. prolonged prothrombin time.
    4. massive ascites.

KEEPING DRUG SKILLS SHARP

13. Many drugs and chemicals are hepatotoxic, including: (Select all that apply)
    1. alcohol.
    2. gold compounds.
    3. anabolic steroids.
    4. halothane.

14. True or False

    _____ Plasma levels of aldosterone can be decreased by infusion of saline.

    _____ Adrenal medullary secretion can be suppressed by administration of ganglionic blocking agents, which normally decrease the urine levels of catecholamines.

Chapter 45

Management of Clients with Thyroid and Parathyroid Disorders

OBJECTIVES

45.1 Describe the etiology of thyroid conditions along with risk factors.

45.2 Compare and contrast clinical signs and symptoms of hypo and hyperthyroidism.

45.3 Describe the nursing assessments used in identifying clients with thyroid and parathyroid disorders.

45.4 Identify the nursing interventions for pre and postoperative care of clients who have had thyroid surgery.

45.5 List the complications that the nurse must be aware of in the postoperative period following a thyroidectomy.

45.6 Discuss medication management for clients who experience thyroid and parathyroid disorders.

UNDERSTANDING PATHOPHYSIOLOGY

1. A normal functioning thyroid gland is referred to as _____.

2. Enlargement of the thyroid gland may be due to: (Select all that apply)
   1. lack of iodine.
   2. inflammation.
   3. benign tumors.
   4. malignant tumors.

3. Which of the following may cause primary hypothyroidism? (Select all that apply)
   1. antithyroid drugs
   2. surgery and treatment with radioactive agents for hyperthyroidism
   3. Hashimoto's disease
   4. defective hormone synthesis

4. The physiologic process of exophthalmos in hyperthyroidism is due to:
   1. accumulation of fluid in the fat pads and muscles that lie behind the eyeballs.
   2. increased venous pressure.
   3. retro-orbital dryness.
   4. excessive tearing from the duct.

5. What is likely to happen if a client has a diet lacking sufficient iodine or if production of thyroid hormone is suppressed?
   1. The thyroid decreases in size.
   2. The thyroid enlarges to compensate for hormonal defienciency.
   3. The gland uses more T$_3$.
   4. Positive feedback occurs.

6. Hypothyroidism results in a deficiency of thyroid hormones, causing: (Select all that apply)
   1. slowed body metabolism.
   2. decreased heat production.
   3. decreased oxygen consumption.
   4. increased appetite.

7. Hypothyroidism is also known as _____.

8. The thyroid gland needs iodine in order to:
   1. sybthesize and secrete thyroid hormones.
   2. enable the adrenal gland to operate.
   3. break down HCl.
   4. absorb trace elements on the system.

9. The reduction in thyroid hormones causes an increase in: (Select all that apply)
   1. ammonia levels.
   2. triglyceride levels.
   3. serum cholesterol.
   4. arteriosclerosis and coronary heart disease.

10. Hyperthyroidism is also known _____.

11. Hyperthyroidism may be due to: (Select all that apply)
    1. excessive stimulation of the adrenal gland.
    2. excessive levels of circulating TH.
    3. increased regulatory control.
    4. decreased metabolism.

APPLYING SKILLS

12. Laboratory values indicative of hypothyroidism in a client being admitted to the hospital would include: (Select all that apply)
    1. decreased TH level.
    2. increased TSH level.
    3. normal CBC.
    4. decreased AST.

13. Signs and symptoms most identifiable in a patient with hypothyroidism would include: (Select all that apply)
    1. sensitivity to cold.
    2. sensitivity to heat.
    3. dry skin or hair.
    4. weight gain.
    5. irregular menses.

14. Myxedema coma can be brought on by stressors from surgery or infections. When identifying common characteristics, the nurse would see certain clinical manifestations, including:
    1. decreased metabolic rate.
    2. hypoventilation.
    3. respiratory distress.
    4. hypothermia, hypotension.

15. In identifying thyrotoxicosis, the nurse will assess the following in the client: (Select all that apply)
    1. tachycardia.
    2. increased appetite, sweating.
    3. diarrhea.
    4. agitation and tremors.

16. Laboratory values indicative of hyperthyroidism include: (Select all that apply)
    1. increased TH levels.
    2. decreased cholesterol.
    3. normal hemoglobin and hematocrit.
    4. elevated AGT.

17. In assessing a patient with thyroid storm (thyrotoxicosis), the nurse will look for: (Select all that apply)
    1. increased fever.
    2. severe tachycardia.
    3. delirium.
    4. dehydration.
    5. extreme irritability.

18. The client having a thyroidectomy is at risk for which of the following complications? (Select all that apply)
    1. thyroid storm
    2. tetany
    3. respiratory obstruction
    4. laryngeal edema
    5. vocal cord injury

19. The major clinical and diagnostic manifestations of thyroid cancer are: (Select all that apply)
    1. a hard, irregular painless nodule.
    2. a "cold" nodule which does not take up radioactive iodine.
    3. greater than 10 cm mass.
    4. enlargement of the vocal area.

20. Hypercalcemia produces gastrointestinal symptoms such as: (Select all that apply)
    1. nausea.
    2. thirst.
    3. anorexia.
    4. constipation.
    5. abdominal pain, ileus.

BEST PRACTICES

21. To prevent negative nitrogen balance and weight loss, the hyperthyroid client must follow a: (Select all that apply)
    1. high calorie diet.
    2. high protein diet.
    3. 100 calorie diet.
    4. diet consisting only of meat intake for 48 hours.

22. Total thyroidectomy is performed to remove _____.

23. Subtotal thyroidectomy is performed to correct _____.

24. Immediate postoperative care for a thyroidectomy client includes: (Select all that apply)
    1. maintaining patent airway.
    2. minimizing strain on the suture line.
    3. relieving sore throat and tracheal irritation.
    4. relieving complications.

25. Clients experiencing gastrointestinal symptoms should avoid:
    1. meats.
    2. warm broths.
    3. milk, milk products.
    4. all fish products.

KEEPING DRUG SKILLS SHARP

26. Endemic goiter can be prevented by the ingestion of:
    1. fruits.
    2. potassium sparing diuretic.
    3. iodized salts.
    4. synthetic salt supplements.

27. Administration of low dose levothyroxine (Synthroid) helps improve: (Select all that apply)
    1. cardiac function.
    2. lipid profile.
    3. liver toxicity.
    4. respiratory adjuncts.

28. The major medications used to control hyperthyroidism are: (Select all that apply)
    1. iodide replacements.
    2. propylthiouracil.
    3. methimazole (Tapazole).
    4. Meganin.

29. The most serious toxic effect of propylthiouracil is:
    1. agranulocytosis.
    2. decreased RBCs.
    3. lymphedema.
    4. liver toxicity.

30. Iodine therapy is prescribed for which of the following reasons? (Select all that apply)
    1. decrease vascularity of the thyroid gland
    2. treat thyroid storm
    3. prevent release of TH
    4. increase amount of TH stored in the thyroid gland

31. The iodine medication of choice is _____.

32. The administration of I-131 will have which of the following effects on clients with hyperthyroidism? (Select all that apply)
    1. The thyroid gland will pick up radioactive iodine.
    2. Cells concentrating I-131 will make T_4 and destroy local irradiation.
    3. TH secretion will diminish.
    4. Oversecretion of gland will occur.

33. _____ is a major complication of I-131 administration

34. Drugs given to treat a thyroid storm include: (Select all that apply)
    1. sodium iodine.
    2. glucocorticoids.
    3. beta blockers.
    4. propylthiouracil.

35. What medication will be given to a client who is experiencing tetany after removal of a parathyroid gland?
    1. calcium chloride (IM)
    2. Synthroid
    3. Lasix
    4. calcium gluconate (IV)

Management of Clients with Adrenal and Pituitary Disorders

OBJECTIVES

46.1   Identify risk factors associated with adrenal and pituitary disorders.

46.2   Compare and contrast signs and symptoms of Addison's disease and Cushing's syndrome.

46.3   Describe complications associated with adrenal and pituitary disorders.

46.4   Discuss nursing responsibilities regarding adrenal function tests.

46.5   Describe nursing priorities for patients undergoing surgery for adrenal disorders.

46.6   Discuss possible complications of adrenal and pituitary surgery.

46.7   Discuss specific treatment protocols for adrenal surgery clients.

46.8   Describe the postoperative nursing care plan for adrenal and pituitary clients.

UNDERSTANDING PATHOPHYSIOLOGY

1. Risk factors for primary adrenal insufficiency include: (Select all that apply)
    1. a history of endocrine disorders.
    2. taking glucosteroids for 3 weeks and suddenly stopping.
    3. taking glucosteroids more than every other day.
    4. adrenalectomy and tuberculosis.

2. _____ is the most common cause of adrenal insuffiency.

3. Which of the following would be consistent with primary adrenal insufficiency? (Select all that apply)
    1. decreasing cortisol production rate
    2. increasing plasma adrenocorticptropic (ACTH)
    3. decreasing sodium concentration
    4. cachexia

4. Addisonian crisis or acute adrenal insuffiency may be brought on by: (Select all that apply)
    1. pregnancy.
    2. surgery.
    3. infections.
    4. emotional upsets.

5. Cushing's syndrome is caused by: (Select all that apply)
    1. overactivity of the adrenal gland.
    2. hypersecretion of the glucocorticoids.
    3. decreased circulating adrenal cortisol.
    4. diabetes insipidus.

6. _____ is hypersecretion of aldosterone resulting from an adrenal lesion.

7. _____ results from a variety of conditions that cause overproduction of aldosterone.

8. _____ is oversecretion of one or more of the hormones by the pituitary gland.

9. _____ is deficiency of one or more of the hormones produced by the anterior lobe of the pituitary.

10. A client with pheochromocytoma has an excessive amount of:
    1. renin.
    2. aldosterone.
    3. catecholamine.
    4. glucocortisol.

11. True or False

    _____ The diagnosis of Addison's disease depends on blood and urine hormonal assays.

APPLYING SKILLS

12. A client with adrenal crisis will experience which of the following clinical manifestations? (Select all that apply)
    1. pain
    2. hypoglycemia
    3. decreased fluid volume
    4. edema

13. A client with Addison's disease will exhibit which of these clinical menifestations?
    1. weight gain
    2. hunger
    3. lethargy
    4. muscle spasm

14. What findings would be normal with a client with Addison's disease?
    1. hyperglycemia
    2. hypoglycemia
    3. hypernatremia
    4. hypokalemia

15. A newly admitted 45-year-old male client reports a 20 lb weight gain and states, "My face and the middle section of my body are round and fat." The nurse also notes that his legs and arms are thin. Based on this assessment and the information the client has provided, what other clinical sign should the nurse look for in order to make a tentative diagnosis of Cushing's syndrome?
    1. bruises on the skin
    2. hypotension
    3. muscle hypertrophy of the extremities
    4. excessive hair on the head

16. The primary feature of pheochromocytoma's effect on blood pressure is:
    1. systolic hypertension.
    2. diastolic hypertension.
    3. hypertension resistant to drug management.
    4. muffled systolic sounds.

BEST PRACTICES

17. A nursing priority for a client with Addisonian crisis is to:
    1. promote anxiety.
    2. treat infections.
    3. prevent hypotension.
    4. control hypertension.

18. Nursing management of patients with Addison's disease includes: (Select all that apply)
    1. monitoring vital signs.
    2. monitoring for exposure to colds and infections.
    3. assessing physical vitality and emotional status.
    4. avoiding stress.

19. Clients with Cushing's disease need to modify their diets by increasing their protein intake and:
    1. restricting sodium.
    2. restricting potassium.
    3. reducing fat by 20%.
    4. increasing calorie consumption.

KEEPING DRUG SKILLS SHARP

20. When a client with Addison's disease develops hypoglycemia, it should be corrected with: (Select all that apply)
    1. IV D_5W.
    2. IV glucose push bolus.
    3. D_5NS 50%.
    4. normal saline 1000 cc.

21. Excessive use of glucocorticoids may lead to _____.

22. Prior to surgery for an adrenalectomy, the physician will order cortisol preparations IM or IV to be given to the client. The nurse knows that this preparation is given because:
    1. cortisol protects against the development of acute adrenal insuffiency.
    2. insulin per sliding scale will help regulate glucose uptake.
    3. antibiotics during surgery will need to be given.
    4. hormones will be readily decreased.

23. True or False

    _____ Kayexalate may be administered orally or as an enema, in combination with sorbitol, to release sodium ions in exchange for potassium ions.

Chapter 47

Management of Clients with Diabetes Mellitus

OBJECTIVES

47.1 Describe the pathophysiology of diabetes mellitus and its effect on carbohydrates, proteins, and fat in the body.

47.2 Identify the clinical signs and symptoms of diabetes mellitus.

47.3 Compare and contrast Type 1 and Type 2 diabetes mellitus.

47.4 Discuss the care goals for clients with diabetes mellitus.

47.5 List the actions, side effects, and nursing implications for oral hypoglycemic agents and insulin.

47.6 Describe the clinical manifestations of diabetic ketoacidosis, hyperglycemia, and hyperglycemic hyperosmolar nonketotic coma.

47.7 Discuss the long-term complications associated with diabetes mellitus.

47.8 Explain the special preoperative nursing care required for a diabetic patient.

UNDERSTANDING PATHOPHYSIOLOGY

1. Diabetes mellitus is a chronic systemic disease resulting from: (Select all that apply)
   1. deficiency of insulin.
   2. absent alpha cells distribution.
   3. decreased ability of the body to use insulin.
   4. abnormal glucose metabolism involving the spleen and muscle.

2. Type 1 diabetes mellitus is characterized by: (Select all that apply)
   1. destruction of pancreatic beta cells.
   2. absolute insulin deficiency.
   3. backup of liver and spleen distribution.
   4. abnormal cellular metabolism by the delta cells.

3. The most common form of diabetes mellitus is _____.

4. Gestational diabetes mellitus is discovered during:
   1. labor and delivery.
   2. pregnancy.
   3. delivery.
   4. a routine eye exam.

5. Type 1 diabetes is also referred to as _____.

6. Populations at greatest risk for developing diabetes mellitus are: (Select all that apply)
   1. Native Americans.
   2. Hispanics.
   3. African Americans.
   4. Asians.

7. Glucose in the urine is commonly referred to as _____.

8. Fat metabolism causes breakdown products called _____.

9. One major action of insulin is to:
   1. increase hepatic production of glucose.
   2. inhibit glucose storage as glycogen.
   3. promote breakdown of fat and glycogen.
   4. promote glucose uptake in skeletal muscle and adipose tissue.

10. Insulin increases:
    1. storage of glycogen and fatty acids.
    2. protein breakdown.
    3. breakdown of fats.
    4. blood glucose levels.

APPLYING SKILLS

11. Clients who would *not* need an oral glucose tolerance test would have a fasting glucose level of:
    1. between 140 and 200 mg/dl.
    2. above 110 mg/dl.
    3. between 60 and 100 mg/dl.
    4. above 120 mg/dl.

12. The classic clinical manifestations in clients with diabetes are: (Select all that apply)
    1. polyuria.
    2. polydipsia.
    3. polyphagia.
    4. postload glucose.

13. A diagnosis of diabetes is made when a client's fasting blood glucose level is:
    1. greater than 126 mg/dl.
    2. greater than 150 mg/dl.
    3. greater than 160 mg/dl.
    4. greater than 200 mg/dl

14. The best time to obtain a postprandial glucose level is _____.

15. The presence of protein in the urine (microalbuminuria) is an early sign of:
    1. liver toxicity.
    2. hepatic overload.
    3. kidney disease.
    4. peripheral liver destruction.

16. The polydipsia and polyuria related to diabetes are caused primarily by:
    1. the release of ketones from cells during fat metabolism.
    2. fluid shifts resulting from osmotic effects of hyperglycemia.
    3. damage to the kidneys from exposure to high levels of glucose.
    4. changes in RBCs resulting from attachment of excessive glucose to hemoglobin.

17. The primary difference between HHNK and ketoadicosis is that in HHNK there is:
    1. greater production of lactic acid.
    2. greater production of ketones.
    3. lesser production of lactic acid.
    4. no production of ketones.

18. Diabetic ketoacidosis and hyperglycemic hyperosmolar nonketotic (HHNK) coma are alike in that:
    1. both occur most often in insulin dependent (Type 1) diabetes.
    2. both may be caused by an infection or some other stress.
    3. metabolic acidosis is a prominent feature of both.
    4. serum glucose levels are usually greater that 800 mg/dl.

19. Factors that could cause hypoglycemia in a diabetic client are:
    1. decreased dose of insulin, too much exercise, eating too much carbohydrates.
    2. excessive dose of insulin, stress, injecting into an area of hypertropic lipodystrophy.
    3. excessive dose of insulin, too much exercise, eating too little.
    4. excessive dose of insulin, too little exercise, illness.

20. Which of the following would suggest to a nurse that a diabetic client is suffering from hypoglycemia?
    1. cold clammy skin, weakness, headache
    2. drowsiness, nausea, vomiting, soft eyeballs
    3. fruity smell to breath, warm dry skin
    4. intense thirst, abdominal pain

21. Which of these lab data would support the inference that a diabetic client is experiencing severe ketoacidosis?
    1. decreased pH, decreased Hct, decreased serum CO_2
    2. decreased pH, increased Hct, decreased serum CO_2
    3. increased pH, increased Hct, decreased serum CO_2
    4. increased pH, increased Hct, increased serum CO_2

BEST PRACTICES

22. A client who is hospitalized and recovering from an episode of diabetic ketoacidosis calls the nurse and reports feeling anxious, nervous, and sweaty. Based on the client's report, the nurse should:
    1. check the client's vital signs.
    2. administer 1 mg of glucagons SC.
    3. have the client eat a candy bar.
    4. give the client 4-6 ounces of orange juice to drink.

23. A diabetic client develops a sore throat, cough, and fever, then calls the nurse at the clinic to report that his blood glucose is 230mg/dl. According to the sick day rule for diabetics, the nurse should advise the client to:
    1. measure his urine output and test his urine for ketones.
    2. withhold both food and insulin until his fever is relieved.
    3. reduce his carbohydrate intake until his glucose level is about 130 mg/dl.
    4. monitor his blood glucose every 6 hours and notify the clinic if it rises above 300mg/dl.

24. Peripheral nerve degeneration is a chronic complication of diabetes that:
    1. may cause an inability to perceive pain.
    2. may cause urinary incontinence or impotence.
    3. may disturb the patient's sleep.
    4. tends to develop in stages.

25. In formulating an education plan with a new Type 2 diabetic client, it is important that the nurse encourage the client to become an active participant in the management of his or her diabetes. The first thing the nurse should do is:
    1. assess the client's perception of what it really means to have diabetes.
    2. assume the responsibility for all of the client's care to decrease his or her stress level.
    3. ask the client's family to participate in the diabetes education program with him or her.
    4. set goals for the client to be an active participant in the management of his or her diabetes.

KEEPING DRUG SKILLS SHARP

26. Humalog and Novolog are both available as premixed insulin and contain: (Select all that apply)
    1. rapid-acting insulin.
    2. intermediate-acting insulin.
    3. long-acting insulin.
    4. short-acting insulin.

27. _____ is a type of insulin that cannot be mixed with any other type of insulin.

28. Which type of insulin may be administered IV?
    1. Lente
    2. NPH
    3. Regular
    4. Ultralente

29. One action of medications such as Metformin, Avandia, and Actos is to:
    1. decrease fatty acid concentration in the bloodstream.
    2. increase production of beta cells.
    3. decrease the cell's resistance to insulin.
    4. increase the caloric requirement of the diabetic client.

30. The main purpose of giving insulin to a client with Type 1 diabetes is to:
    1. improve the functioning of the pancreas.
    2. replace the insulin not being produced by the pancreas.
    3. decrease the functioning of the pancreas.
    4. supplement the production of insulin by the pancreas.

Chapter 48

Management of Clients with Exocrine Pancreatic and Biliary Disorders

OBJECTIVES

48.1 Discuss clinical problems most frequently associated with the gallbladder.

48.2 Discuss the nursing and medical management of gallbladder disorders.

48.3 Describe clinical problems associated with pancreatic disorders.

48.4 Discuss nursing and medical management of pancreatic disorders.

UNDERSTANDING PATHOPHYSIOLOGY

1. Clients with pancreatic disorders may have problems with _____ and _____.

2. True or False

   _____ In the United States, alcohol abuse is the number one cause of acute pancreatitis.

   _____ Inflammation of the gallbladder may be acute or chronic.

3. Biliary pancreatitis occurs when: (Select all that apply)
   1. edema or an obstruction blocks the ampulla of Vater.
   2. there is reflux of bile into pancreatic ducts.
   3. there is direct injury to the acinar cells.
   4. there is blockage of spleen vats.

4. List seven risk factors for pancreatitis.
   a.
   b.
   c.
   d.
   e.
   f.
   g.

5. A cholecystectomy is the _____.

6. _____ appears only when common duct obstruction is present.

APPLYING SKILLS

7. Turner's sign is _____.

8. Cullen's sign is _____.

9. A client admitted to the clinic with a confirmed case of pancreatitis will show elevation of which of the following in the lab results? (Select all that apply)
   1. amylase
   2. glucose
   3. potassium
   4. trypsin

10. Early signs of shock in clients with acute pancreatitis can be difficult to diagnosis due to the:
    1. severity of intestinal problems.
    2. vasodilating effect of kinin enzymes.
    3. development of congestive heart failure.
    4. increase of tubular necrosis.

11. What symptoms would the nurse expect to see in a client with acute pancreatitis?
    1. diarrhea
    2. jaundice
    3. hypertension
    4. ascites

12. What conditions would be consistent with acute pancreatitis?
    1. leucopenia
    2. thrombocytopenia
    3. hyperkalemia
    4. hyperglycemia

13. What complication must the nurse watch for in a client with acute pancreatitis?
    1. congestive heart failure
    2. duodenal ulcer
    3. cirrhosis
    4. pneumonia

BEST PRACTICES

14. The overall management of a client with acute pancreatitis requires: (Select all that apply)
    1. replacing lost body fluids.
    2. correcting hypovolemia.
    3. restoring electrolyte balance.
    4. elevating the hemoglobin margins.

15. Dietary instructions for a client with pancreatitis being discharged from a clinic should include: (Select all that apply)
    1. eating frequent meals high in protein.
    2. following a low fat diet.
    3. ensuring moderate to high carbohydrate intake.
    4. avoiding alcohol.

16. The nurse must evaluate the client with pancreatitis for the development of:
    1. diabetes mellitus.
    2. hepatitis.
    3. cholelithiasis.
    4. irritable bowel syndrome.

17. Complications associated with cholecystectomy include: (Select all that apply)
    1. hemorrhage.
    2. pneumonia.
    3. thrombophlebitis.
    4. urinary retention and ileus.

KEEPING DRUG SKILLS SHARP

18. _____ is contraindicated in patients with pancreatitis because it causes spasms of the sphincter of Oddi.

19. When extreme hyperglycemia is present in clients with acute pancreatitis, which of the following medications will be ordered?
    1. oral agents
    2. insulin
    3. narcotic
    4. muscle relaxants

20. In the treatment of acute pancreatitis, _____ must be administered intravenously if there is evidence of hypocalcemia with tetany.

21. Pancreatic enzyme replacements should be taken:
    1. three times per day.
    2. with each meal.
    3. in the morning and at bedtime.
    4. every 4 hours.

Chapter 49

Management of Clients with Hepatic Disorders

OBJECTIVES

49.1   Discuss relevant terminology relating to hepatic disorders.

49.2   Discuss problems associated with hepatitis.

49.3   Describe the nursing management of selected liver disorders.

49.4   Identify the medical, nursing, and surgical management of clients with cirrhosis of the liver.

UNDERSTANDING PATHOPHYSIOLOGY

1. Jaundice is caused by:
    1. excessive accumulation of bile pigments in the blood.
    2. large amounts of ketones.
    3. intake of cellular hepatic cells.
    4. breakdown of carbohydrates in the cells.

2. Obstructive jaundice can also be caused by: (Select all that apply)
    1. stones.
    2. hepatic cellular damage.
    3. intake of excessive ketones.
    4. distribution of cellular wastes.

3. Hepatitis is an inflammation of the liver caused by which of the following? (Select all that apply)
    1. viruses.
    2. toxins.
    3. chemicals.
    4. drugs.

4. Portal vein hypertension develops in severe cirrhosis due to: (Select all that apply)
    1. a retrograde increase in pressure resistance.
    2. ascites due to osmotic or hydrostatic shifts.
    3. incomplete clearing of protein metabolic wastes.
    4. increase in ammonia levels.

5. Match the type of hepatitis with the correct description or definition. (More than one answer may apply.)

    a. Hepatitis A
    b. Hepatitis B
    c. Hepatitis C
    d. Hepatitis D
    e. Hepatitis E
    f. Toxic hepatitis

1. always found with hepatitis B
2. also known as infectious hepatitis
3. spread by carriers
4. spread by blood
5. primary prevention by careful handwashing
6. primary prevention by active immunity
7. caused by benzene and chloroform
8. health care workers at risk
9. spread by contaminated shellfish, water, and milk
10. contracted through travel in high incidence areas

APPLYING SKILLS

6. An extremely dangerous complication of portal hypertension is _____.

7. Clinical manifestations of alcoholic hepatitis include: (Select all that apply)
   1. anorexia.
   2. nausea.
   3. abdominal pain, jaundice.
   4. spleen enlargement.

8. Complications of cirrhosis of the liver include: (Select all that apply)
   1. ascites.
   2. bleeding esophageal varices.
   3. hepatic encephalopathy.
   4. renal failure.

BEST PRACTICES

9. Clients who have cirrhosis of the liver have high ammonia levels. If ammonia levels rise, the diet should be restricted in:
   1. protein.
   2. carbohydrates.
   3. fats.
   4. calcium.

10. The most appropriate candidates for a liver transplant are those: (Select all that apply)
    1. with severe liver disease with no alternative medical/surgical treatment.
    2. with end-stage liver disease.
    3. experiencing life-threatening complications.
    4. experiencing neurologic effects of liver damage.

KEEPING DRUGS SKILLS SHARP

11. Clinicians administer very few medications to clients with hepatitis because of hepatotoxicity. Medications that should be avoided include: (Select all that apply)
    1. aspirin.
    2. acetaminophen.
    3. various sedatives.
    4. chlorpromazine.

12. Clients with cirrhosis of the liver who are receiving thiazide diuretics should maintain a diet high in:
    1. potassium.
    2. sodium.
    3. calcium.
    4. protein.

13. Medications may be given to clients with cirrhosis of the liver to improve clotting factors. The medication that will be ordered is:
    1. heparin.
    2. vitamin K.
    3. calcium gluconate.
    4. dextran.

14. When a client has a rupture of esophageal varices, the physician will routinely order:
    1. vasopressin.
    2. Pitocin.
    3. oxytocin.
    4. Benadryl.

15. The purpose of administering vasopressin IV is to: (Select all that apply)
    1. achieve temporary lowering of portal pressure.
    2. reduce portal venous blood flow.
    3. constrict afferent arterioles.
    4. maintain liver functions.

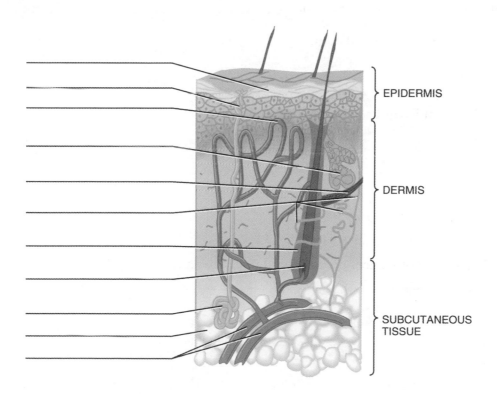

Chapter 50

Assessment of the Integumentary System

OBJECTIVES

50.1 Describe the assessment components for clients with integumentary system disorders.

50.2 Describe components of the physical examination of the integumentary system.

50.3 Discuss common diagnostic procedures for skin disorders.

50.4 Define common terms used to describe skin lesions and disorders.

ANATOMY & PHYSIOLOGY REVIEW

1. Label the specific parts of the three layers of the skin.

EPIDERMIS

DERMIS

SUBCUTANEOUS TISSUE

UNDERSTANDING PATHOPHYSIOLOGY

2. The clinical manifestation that most often brings a client to the health care provider is
    _____.

3. Differentiate between allergy and irritation.

4. List the dermatologic conditions that are genetically transmitted.
    a.

    b.

    c.

    d.

5. The skin disease that may be passed on to family members because of close and frequent expo-
    sure is _____.

6. Excess body hair is known as _____.

7. Nails indicate _____ and
    _____ status.

8. Pallor in the nail bed may be indicative of _____.

9. Differentiate between a callus and corn.

10. Differentiate between linear and satellite patterns.

11. True or False

    _____   A bulla is a secondary lesion.

    _____   An excoriation is a primary lesion.

    _____   Inflammation often goes unrecognized in Caucasians.

    _____   Skin turgor increases with age.

12. Identify the ABCDs of melanoma.
    A

    B

    C

    D

APPLYING SKILLS

13. Explain why it is important to ask clients about previous trauma or surgical interventions.

14. Explain the rationale for assessing occupational history in a client who presents with a skin disorder.

15. Match each dermatologic term with the appropriate description.

Dermatologic Term	Description
_____ a. circumscribed	1. spontaneously occurring wheals
_____ b. cytotoxic	2. lesion found in hives
_____ c. dermatome	3. scaling, peeling of epidermis
_____ d. erythema	4. hard (tissue)
_____ e. hives	5. wheals (hives)
_____ f. indurated	6. limited to a certain area by sharply defined border
_____ g. maceration	7. toxic to cells
_____ h. polymorphic	8. area of skin supplied by a single dorsal nerve root
_____ i. urticaria	9. tissue softening or disintegration from excessive moisture
_____ j. wheal	10. existing in many forms
_____ k. desquamation	11. redness

16. Explain the rationale for conducting a dermatologic assessment in a well-lit, private room with moderate temperature and neutral, white, or cream-colored walls.

17. Identify the body area where it is easiest to detect the following:
    a. pallor

    b. cyanosis

    c. jaundice

    d. jaundice in dark-skinned clients

18. Skin temperature should be assessed using the _____.

19. Identify the order used to assess and describe lesions.

20. In order to assess the contour and consistency of lesions, the nurse would need to _____ the lesions.

21. True or False

    _____ The location of lesions is described in reference to anatomic landmarks.

22. Label each assessment finding of the nails.

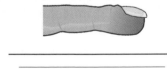

About 160°

_____   _____

_____   _____

_____
_____

BEST PRACTICES

23. Explain when a skin culture would be indicated.

24. Explain the purpose of a patch test.

25. Identify contraindications to a patch test.

26. Explain the rationale for instructing clients to avoid taking aspirin for 48 hours prior to a biopsy.

27. Explain the postprocedure care following a biopsy.

KEEPING DRUG SKILLS SHARP

28. The most common type of allergic drug reaction is _____.

29. Describe the type of reaction that may occur when taking a photosensitizing drug.

30. Match each type of reaction to the medication.

Type of Reaction	Medication
_____ a. maculopapular without blistering	1. prednisone
_____ b. sunburn-like rash	2. penicillin
_____ c. eczematous rash	3. tetracycline
_____ d. acne breakout	4. diphenhydramine hydrochloride

Chapter 51

Management of Clients with Integumentary Disorders

OBJECTIVES

51.1 Discuss the skin and types of topical applications and therapies for common skin disorders.

51.2 Discuss skin disorders including outcome management and nursing interventions.

51.3 Discuss skin cancer.

51.4 Discuss therapeutic benefits of cosmetic and plastic surgery and associated care of clients who have these procedures.

51.5 Discuss body image.

51.6 Discuss care of clients who have traumatic injuries of the face or extremities.

51.7 Discuss nail disorders.

UNDERSTANDING PATHOPHYSIOLOGY

1. Match each example of eczema or dermatitis with the correct description.

Eczema or Dermatitis	Description
_____ a. atopic dermatitis	1. eruptions from allergy to poison ivy, sumac, or oak or a proven allergen
_____ b. seborrheic dermatitis	2. eruption from direct contact with irritating substances, which can be almost anything including cosmetics, chemicals, dyes, or detergents
_____ c. irritant dermatitis	3. characteristic distribution of eczema in person with a family history of asthma, hay fever, or eczema
_____ d. allergic contact dermatitis	4. eruption resulting from peripheral venous disorders
_____ e. nummular eczema	5. yellowish-pink scaling of the scalp, face, and trunk
_____ f. stasis dermatitis	6. appearance of coin-shaped, oozing, crusting patches

2. The major clinical manifestation of atopic dermatitis that causes the greatest morbidity is
   _____.

3. Differentiate between irritant and allergic contact dermatitis.

4. The most common cause of intertrigo is contamination with _____
   _____.

5. The length of time it takes for normal skin cells to grow, move to the surface and slough off is
   _____; however, in psoriasis this cycle speeds up and
   takes only _____.

6. List the most common sites for psoriasis eruptions:
   a.
   b.
   c.
   d.

7. Acne rosacea occurs most often between the ages of _____ and _____.
   _____ are affected more frequently than
   _____.

8. Differentiate first-degree from second-degree sunburn.

9. List the three most common types of skin cancer:
   a.
   b.
   c.

10. The greatest risk for skin cancer would be found in a client who:
    1. never burns and always tans.
    2. burns once or twice and then tans.
    3. always burns.

11. List the five risk factors for malignant melanoma:
    a.
    b.
    c.
    d.
    e.

12. List the four changes in a skin lesion that are suspicious of malignant melanoma:
    a.
    b.
    c.
    d.

13. Survival for clients with malignant melanoma is directly related to the _____ _____ of tumor invasion.

14. The malignant disease involving the T helper cells is _____.

15. The two major complications of herpes zoster are _____ and _____.

16. The two types of plastic surgery are _____ and _____.

17. The most common cause of free flap failure is _____.

18. True or False

    _____ Pruritus is a skin disease.

    _____ Xerotic skin lacks moisture in the top layer of the skin and is common in the younger population.

    _____ Stasis dermatitis results from venous insufficiency.

    _____ Changes in physical and emotional health can precede flares of psoriasis.

    _____ Skin tears are most common in older adults due to thinning of the epidermis.

    _____ It is believed that pressure ulcers are a specific indicator of malnutrition.

    _____ Actinic keratosis is the most common epithelial precancerous lesion caused by sun exposure.

    _____ Basal cell carcinoma almost always metastasizes.

    _____ Unlike other skin cancers, squamous cell carcinoma occurs frequently in dark-skinned clients.

    _____ Malignant melanoma is the deadliest form of skin cancer.

    _____ Pemphigus vulgaris is an autoimmune disease caused by circulating immunoglobulin G autoantibodies.

    _____ A person who has never had chickenpox cannot get it from someone who has herpes zoster.

    _____ Clients who have had a traumatic amputation have dreams that depict the tragedy and should be counseled that these are normal.

    _____ Unguis incarnates is one of the most common nail conditions and is caused by not trimming the nail.

    _____ Paronychia is an infection under the nail.

    _____ Onychomycosis is a fungal infection of the nail.

APPLYING SKILLS

19. Explain why a quantitative culture versus a swab culture is used to diagnose an ulcer infection.

20. A score below _____ on the Braden Scale indicates a client is at high risk for pressure ulcer development.

21. An assessment finding that may indicate that the rhinoplasty client is experiencing excessive bleeding is _____.

22. True or False

_____   For a client with a nursing diagnosis of impaired skin integrity related to pressure ulcer, an appropriate outcome statement is "Stage IV ulcer will heal to Stage III."

BEST PRACTICES

23. Explain how the care of pruritus is altered for the older client.

24. Management of contact dermatitis begins with identification of the _____
_____.

25. Match each type of ulcer care with the appropriate description.

	Type of Ulcer Care (Debridement)	Description
_____	a. mechanical debridement	1. use of synthetic dressings to cover an ulcer, allowing enzymes in the wound bed to digest the devitalized tissues
_____	b. biodebridement	2. use of wet-to-dry dressings, hydrotherapy, and high-pressure wound irrigation to soften and remove devitalized tissues
_____	c. sharp debridement	3. use of topical debriding agents to dissolve the collagen anchors that hold the necrotic slough tissue to the wound bed
_____	d. autolytic debridement	4. debridement is carried out at the bedside using a scalpel and forceps to remove loose necrotic tissue
_____	e. enzymatic debridement	5. use of sterile larvae (maggots), which secrete enzymes that digest wound tissue
_____	f. conservative sharp debridement	6. use of a scalpel to excise devitalized thick, adherent eschar; this is completed in the operating room

26. Explain the benefit of cool tap water soaks for the treatment of superficial, partial-thickness sunburn.

27. An appropriate nursing intervention for a client with an altered body image is to:
    1. be sensitive to the client's feelings and needs.
    2. reassure the client that plastic surgery will change everything.
    3. empathize with the client and tell them you know exactly how he or she feels.
    4. ignore client statements about his or her feelings.

28. Match each facial resurfacing procedure with the appropriate description.

	Procedure	Description
_____	a. skin peel	1. products are used to fill in small wrinkles or depressed blemishes in the skin
_____	b. laser resurfacing	2. substance is injected to temporarily improve the appearance of moderate to severe frown lines between eyebrows
_____	c. dermabrasion	3. various products are used to lift superficial layers of skin and remove fine wrinkles from the skin
_____	d. dermal fillers	4. treatment creates a shallow burn injury to the skin
_____	e. botulinum injection	5. process of sanding the surface layers of skin on cheeks and forehead with an electric rotating brush to smooth out pitting and surface blemishes

29. The primary nursing responsibility for a client with a flap is to _____.

30. The most important emergency measure for a client who has sustained a traumatic amputation is to _____.

31. True or False

_____ Ultraviolet light is used to cause desquamation.

_____ Cryotherapy is common, painless therapy for the treatment of multiple lesions of actinic keratosis.

_____ Because of the risk of tumor spread during biopsy, clients who have malignant melanoma removed in a two-stage process (biopsy first followed by tumor removal in a separate procedure) have poorer outcomes than clients who have the procedure done in one step.

_____ A rhytidectomy is a procedure that restores youthful appearance and removes all of the wrinkles of the face.

_____ Clients can expect to see immediate results following liposuction.

_____ A client with intermaxillary wires should avoid alcoholic and carbonated beverages.

KEEPING DRUG SKILLS SHARP

32. List the factors that influence the absorption, penetration, and permeation of topically applied preparations:
    a.
    b.
    c.
    d.
    e.
    f.

33. Which of the following medications draw moisture into the cell structure of the stratum corneum? (Select all that apply)
    1. menthol
    2. urea
    3. camphor
    4. lactic acid

34. Psoralens should be taken:
    1. orally 3 hours before UVA irradiation.
    2. on an empty stomach.
    3. with food to minimize bloating.
    4. in a dosage determined by body weight.

35. Identify the two topical immunomodulators (TIMs) that are approved for the treatment of atopic dermatitis.
    a.
    b.

36. The most important thing to consider when using a short course of oral steroid therapy is to
    _____.

37. A client with psoriasis is being treated with methotrexate. What laboratory value should be monitored before and during treatment?
    1. lipids
    2. blood glucose
    3. creatinine
    4. CBC

38. A substance with an anti-inflammatory effect is:
    1. Balnetar.
    2. Burrow's solution.
    3. Domeboro.
    4. Betadine.

39. True or False

    _____ Absorption is increased in inflamed skin.

    _____ Cyclosporine is most often used as a rescue drug in the treatment of chronic plaque psoriasis.

Chapter 52

Management of Clients with Burn Injury

OBJECTIVES

52.1 Describe the different types of burn injuries.

52.2 Explore measures used to assess and classify burn injuries.

52.3 Discuss the medical and nursing interventions for burn clients during the emergent, acute, and rehabilitative phases of burn injury.

UNDERSTANDING PATHOPHYSIOLOGY

1. Match each term related to burn injury with the appropriate description.

	Burn Injury	Description
_____	a. zone of stasis	1. outer ring of tissue injury consisting of tissue that is inflamed and vasodilated
_____	b. zone of hyperemia	2. directly damaged skin is coagulated and fully destroyed
_____	c. zone of coagulation	3. consists of skin that initially is viable but may also eventually die of ischemia

2. List the three protective measures the body loses due to destruction of the skin in burn injury:

a.

b.

c.

3. Match each type of burn injury with the appropriate definition.

	Type of Burn Injury	Definition
_____	a. Partial-thickness	1. characterized by damage throughout the dermis and skin appears dry and may be black, brown, white or ivory
_____	b. Full-thickness	2. involves skin, fat, muscle, and sometimes bone and skin appears charred or may be completely burned away
_____	c. First-degree	3. involves injury to the epidermis and portions of the dermis
_____	d. Second-degree	4. damage throughout the dermis
_____	e. Third-degree	5. superficial and painful and skin appears red
_____	f. Fourth-degree	6. skin appears wet or blistered and is extremely painful

4. The clinical manifestations of CO poisoning do not usually occur until COHb levels reach

    _____.

5. Basal metabolic rates of the burn client are _____.

6. The two complications that inhibit the return of optimal physical functioning are

    _____ and _____.

7. True or False

    _____ Seventy-five percent of all burn injuries result from the actions of the victim.

    _____ Scalding liquids are the leading cause of burn injury.

    _____ Ignition from cigarettes is the nation's largest single cause of all fire deaths.

    _____ Immune function is increased in burn injury.

    _____ Donor sites for skin grafts can only be used one time.

APPLYING SKILLS

8. Differentiate between the causes of thermal, chemical, electrical, and radiation burns.

9. A 197 lb client's urine output is less than 0.5 ml/kg/hour after a burn injury. Calculate the urinary output that would be considered minimally adequate.

10. Following a major burn injury, the nurse would expect the bowel sound to be:
    1. hypoactive.
    2. hyperactive.
    3. absent.

11. Following a burn injury to the upper airway, the client is at risk for upper airway obstruction. Typically, the nurse would be vigilant of this complication between _____ and _____ hours.

12. When assessing a client for possible smoke exposure, the nurse would note:
    1. complaints of dizziness.
    2. soot in the nares.
    3. pallor.
    4. inflamed nares.

13. An assessment finding consistent with decreased cardiac output in the first 24 hours after burn injury is:
    1. increased urine output.
    2. bounding peripheral pulse.
    3. normal capillary refill.
    4. decreased blood pressure.

14. Differentiate between background and procedural pain experienced by burn victims.

15. Pulmonary assessment is performed every _____ to _____ hours during the first 24 hours after injury.

16. List the nursing assessments that are performed to determine adequacy of circulation in a client with a nursing diagnosis of ineffective tissue perfusion:
    a.

    b.

    c.

    d.

    e.

17. Using the Curreri formula, calculate the energy requirements for a 146 lb female with 36% TBSA.

18. Using a modified Brook's formula, calculate the fluid resuscitation requirements for the first 24 hours for a 212 lb man with a 45% TBSA burn.

19. On physical examination, a 33-year-old male has large, thick-walled blisters over deep red, wet, and shiny tissue over all his upper extremities and half of his face. The upper half of his face is red with small, thin blisters. His hands appear dry and deep red with some brown tissue. Compute the size of body surface area burned by using Berkow's formula with the chart provided below.

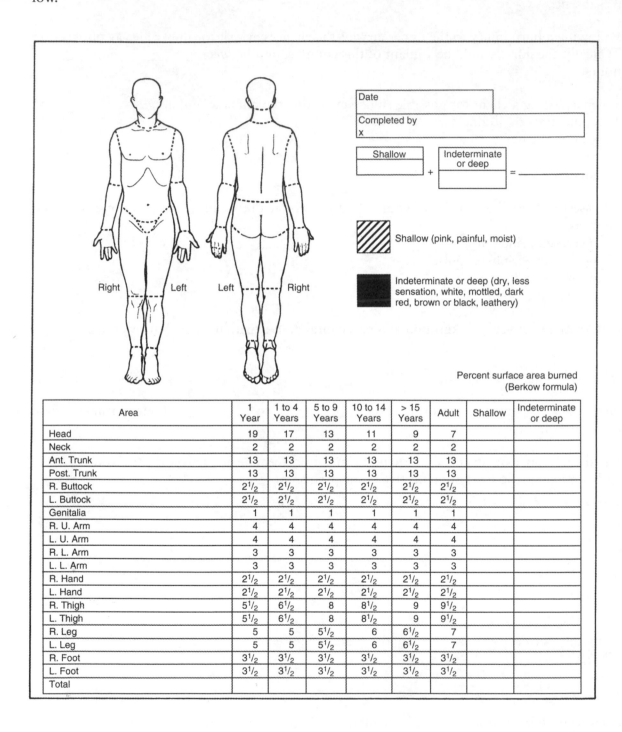

Percent surface area burned
(Berkow formula)

Area	1 Year	1 to 4 Years	5 to 9 Years	10 to 14 Years	> 15 Years	Adult	Shallow	Indeterminate or deep
Head	19	17	13	11	9	7		
Neck	2	2	2	2	2	2		
Ant. Trunk	13	13	13	13	13	13		
Post. Trunk	13	13	13	13	13	13		
R. Buttock	2½	2½	2½	2½	2½	2½		
L. Buttock	2½	2½	2½	2½	2½	2½		
Genitalia	1	1	1	1	1	1		
R. U. Arm	4	4	4	4	4	4		
L. U. Arm	4	4	4	4	4	4		
R. L. Arm	3	3	3	3	3	3		
L. L. Arm	3	3	3	3	3	3		
R. Hand	2½	2½	2½	2½	2½	2½		
L. Hand	2½	2½	2½	2½	2½	2½		
R. Thigh	5½	6½	8	8½	9	9½		
L. Thigh	5½	6½	8	8½	9	9½		
R. Leg	5	5	5½	6	6½	7		
L. Leg	5	5	5½	6	6½	7		
R. Foot	3½	3½	3½	3½	3½	3½		
L. Foot	3½	3½	3½	3½	3½	3½		
Total								

BEST PRACTICES

20. A nursing intervention that can be initiated to decrease facial edema and facilitate lung expansion is to _____.

21. A client is at risk for acute tubular necrosis secondary to myoglobin and hemoglobin released from damaged muscles. The goal is maintain a urinary output of _____ to _____ ml/hr.

22. Explain why it is important to debride burn wounds of loose, nonviable tissue.

23. The single most important measure to prevent infection is _____
    _____.

24. A nursing consideration for a client using 0.5% silver nitrate for wound care is to:
    1. store the antimicrobial agent in a warm environment.
    2. assess adequacy of pain management.
    3. check serum electrolytes daily.
    4. assess for hypersensitivity.

25. List the measures used to prevent wound contracture:
    a.

    b.

    c.

    d.

26. The therapeutic position that should be used when the burn injury involves the hip is
    _____.

27. An intervention that will help the client feel some control over his or her situation would be to:
    1. provide passive ROM.
    2. provide dressing changes at a time the client specifies.
    3. allow the client to assist with wound care.
    4. apply splints and pressure garments before visitors arrive.

28. Meals provided during the acute phase of treatment should be high in
    _____ and _____.

29. Explain why burn clients scheduled for wound debridement are scheduled at the end of the day.

30. True or False

    _____ A static splint exercises the affected joint.

KEEPING DRUG SKILLS SHARP

31. The drug of choice in treating pain in the client with a moderate or major burn is IV
    _____.

32. If NSAIDs are used in the treatment of mild to moderate pain, measures need to be initiated to
    prevent _____.

33. True or False

    _____ Analgesic medications are given so that the client receives the benefit of the drug's peak
    effect immediately following dressing changes.

Chapter 53

Assessment of the Vascular System

OBJECTIVES

53.1   Discuss the important components required when obtaining a vascular history from a client.

53.2   Describe the process for performing a physical examination of the vascular system.

53.3   Identify common diagnostic tests used to assess the vascular system.

53.4   Describe nursing responsibilities when caring for a client undergoing invasive testing of the vascular system.

ANATOMY & PHYSIOLOGY REVIEW

1.   Label the structures of each type of blood vessel.

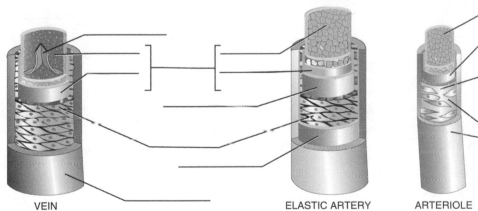

VEIN   ELASTIC ARTERY

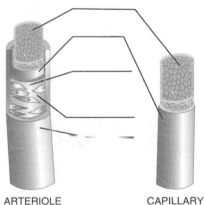

ARTERIOLE   CAPILLARY

UNDERSTANDING PATHOPHYSIOLOGY

2.   List the two classic characteristics for intermittent claudication:
   a.

   b.

3. Factors that may predispose a client to venous disorders include: (Select all that apply)
    1. positive family history of venous disorders.
    2. occupation requiring high levels of physical activity.
    3. multiple pregnancies.
    4. obesity.

4. _____ is discoloration of the skin from chronic venous disorders.

5. True or False

    _____ Dependent cyanosis is caused by venous pooling in the extremities.

    _____ Dependent rubor is caused by venous disorders affecting circulation.

6. _____ is caused by venous insufficiency, resulting in "spider veins" on the legs.

7. Explain the clinical significance of a pseudoaneurysm.

APPLYING SKILLS

8. Assessment of the vascular system includes biographic and demographic data. Identify the rationale for obtaining this information in relation to the vascular system.
    Age:

    Occupation:

9. When completing a medical history on a client, the nurse should inquire about *current* health status and the presence of any clinical manifestations to establish a _____ to aid in diagnosis and treatment.

10. True or False

    _____ Clients with arterial insufficiency will have shiny, hairless skin and thick, ridged toenails.

    _____ Edema is not usually present in clients with pure arterial insufficiency.

11. When assessing temperature in extremities, the nurse should compare one extremity with the _____ limb.

12. _____ is performed on a client with vascular problems to assess for blood flow in the arm prior to performing a stick for ABGs.

13. _____ studies for DVT are more accurate than the test for Homan's sign.

BEST PRACTICES

14. List two nursing actions to assist the client with an incompetent vein to reduce interstitial fluid buildup:

    a.

    b.

15. State the rationales for each of the following nursing actions prior to a physical examination of a client with vascular disorders.

    a. natural lighting:

    b. warm the room temperature:

    c. quiet the exam room:

16. A 76-year-old client with vascular problems has just returned from the radiology department after undergoing an angiography. Potential complications the nurse should observe for following this procedure include: (Select all that apply)

    1. allergic reaction to contrast dye.
    2. development of thrombus.
    3. vessel wall perforation.
    4. aneurysm.
    5. renal failure (due to contrast dye).

Management of Clients with Hypertensive Disorders

OBJECTIVES

54.1   Discuss the incidence of hypertension in the United States and its impact on the health care system.

54.2   Differentiate between the major classifications of hypertension.

54.3   Discuss pathophysiology of primary and secondary hypertension including modifiable and non-modifiable risk factors.

54.4   Identify potential complications from primary hypertension.

54.5   Describe nursing care and medical management of clients with primary hypertension, including pharmaceutical interventions.

54.6   Discuss nursing role in community-based prevention programs to address hypertension.

UNDERSTANDING PATHOPHYSIOLOGY

1. Despite the advances made in detection and treatment of hypertension, there is a trend of *increasing* mortality rates for heart disease and strokes among all of the following except:
   1. older adults.
   2. Asian Americans.
   3. African Americans.
   4. lower socioeconomic groups.

2. The most common complication of untreated hypertension is _____
   _____.

3. The elevation in blood pressure in hypertension is caused by persistent and progressive _____
   _____.

4. Compare and contrast between primary and secondary hypertension.

Type	Characteristics
Primary (essential)	
Secondary	

5. List the steps in the renin-angiotensin-aldosterone system to control blood pressure:
   a.

   b.

   c.

   d.

   e.

6. The increase in _____ seen in Cushing's causes increases in sodium retention and angiotensin II levels, resulting in increased blood pressure.

7. Untreated hypertension causes damage to which of the following "target organs"?
   1. brain
   2. liver
   3. eyes
   4. kidneys

APPLYING SKILLS

8. The diagnosis of hypertension is made when the average of two or more separate blood readings is _____ or higher for the systolic blood pressure and _____ or higher for the diastolic blood pressure.

9. List the factors that should be used to evaluate whether a treatment regimen for controlling hypertension is effective:
   a.

   b.

   c.

10. True or False

    _____ When completing a physical assessment, the nurse notes a client to be overweight with increased fat around the midriff, waist and abdomen. This body shape has been shown to be associated with the development of hypertension.

_____ Clients should have blood pressure readings taken immediately upon arrival at the clinic to reflect normal pressures at home.

_____ Clients who report complaints of persistent headaches, fatigue, dizziness, blurred vision, or epistaxis may have undiagnosed hypertension.

_____ If a blood pressure reading is classified as "prehypertension" category, measures should be taken to address modifiable risk factors immediately.

_____ Visible changes to the blood vessels of the eye can be seen resulting from untreated hypertension.

BEST PRACTICES

11. For each *modifiable* risk factor for hypertension, discuss what actions the nurse should advise the client to take to reduce effect on blood pressure:

Risk Factor	Action
Stress	
Obesity	
Nutrients	
Substance abuse	

12. State the critical nursing action that should be implemented prior to taking a blood pressure in a client.

13. For each of the following lifestyle factors contributing to hypertension, discuss what specific actions the nurse should advise the client to take.
    a. Weight reduction:

b. Sodium restriction:

c. Dietary fat modification:

d. Exercise:

e. Alcohol restriction:

f. Caffeine restriction:

g. Relaxation techniques:

h. Smoking:

i. Potassium supplement:

14. List the two key aspects to dietary intervention in clients with hypertension:
    a.

    b.

15. In planning treatment regimens, the nurse recognizes that _____
    usually improves when the client understands the reasons for treatment and consequences of in-
    adequate interventions.

16. List the nursing interventions that can be implemented to prevent injury from syncope:
    a.

    b.

KEEPING DRUG SKILLS SHARP

17. List the first line choices for drug therapy to treat hypersion:
    a.

    b.

18. It would be appropriate to evaluate reducing the number and amounts of antihypertensive medications for a client if the client's blood pressure has been controlled effectively for _____.

19. A client newly diagnosed with hypertension is concerned about "remembering all the information" related to medications and monitoring her blood pressure at home. The nurse develops the diagnosis of: Risk for Ineffective Management of Therapeutic regimen related to lack of knowledge. Identify outcomes to meet the learning needs of this client.

20. Explain the phrase "start low and go slow" in relation to medication for older clients with hypertension.

CONCEPT MAP EXERCISES

The following questions are based on the Concept Map *Understanding Hypertension and Its Treatment* in the textbook.

21. Combination therapy is often used to control hypertension, including ACE inhibitors and diuretics. How do ACE inhibitors affect elevated blood pressure?

22. A 67-year-old client with hypertension has been prescribed a new medication, which is a calcium channel blocker. She doesn't understand how a "calcium" drug helps with blood pressure. How would the nurse explain the effect of this medication in treating her hypertension?

23. Increased pressure detected by the baroreceptors in the carotid arteries causes what clinical manifestation?

24. When is secondary prevention of hypertension instituted?

Chapter 55

Management of Clients with Vascular Disorders

OBJECTIVES

55.1 Identify the etiology and risk factors for the development of vascular disorders.

55.2 Describe clinical manifestations of peripheral vascular disease.

55.3 Discuss nursing care and medical/surgical management of clients with peripheral vascular disease.

55.4 Discuss nursing care and medical/surgical management of clients with arterial vascular disorders.

55.5 Discuss nursing care and medical/surgical management of clients with acute and chronic venous disorders.

55.6 Describe nursing care and medical management of clients with lymphatic disorders.

UNDERSTANDING PATHOPHYSIOLOGY

1. Peripheral arterial occlusive diseases are caused primarily by _____
   _____.

2. List the primary risk factors for the development of athcrosclerosis:
   a.

   b.

   c.

3. Physical manifestations of peripheral vascular disease (PVD) include: (Select all that apply)
   1. lack of pulses in brachial artery.
   2. pallor of legs.
   3. thick, brittle nails.
   4. hairy shins.
   5. poorly healing ulcers.
   6. mottling color.
   7. paralysis.
   8. lack of pulse in dorsalis pedis artery.

4. The most successful grafting material used today for bypass surgery is
    _____.

5. The major indication for the "open" or guillotine type of amputation over a "flap" amputation is
    _____.

6. List the classic manifestations of acute ischemia caused by peripheral thrombus or embolism
    ("The 6 P's"):
    a.

    b.

    c.

    d.

    e.

    f.

7. List the risk factors for development of an aneurysm:
    a.

    b.

8. Ruptures occur most often in abdominal aortic aneurysms larger than _____.

9. Color changes to the hands are a classic manifestation of a Raynaud's vasospasm. Describe the
    physiologic reason for each of the stages of the spasm:

Stage	Physiologic changes
Pallor (white) color in hands	
Cyanotic (blue) color in hands	
Rubor (red) color in hands	

10. List the three conditions of Virchow's triad for the development of venous thrombosis and their
    etiologies:
    a.

    b.

    c.

11. True or False

_____ A dissecting aneurysm is not a true aneurysm.

_____ The classic sign for an abdominal aortic aneurysm is colicky pain.

_____ A client can feel a pulsating mass in the abdomen, with or without pain, from an abdominal aneurysm.

_____ Abdominal aortic aneurysms (AAA) are the most common type of aneurysm.

_____ If the aneurysm is smaller than 4-5 cm and asymptomatic, it is safe to surgically correct it.

_____ Repair of AAA requires an incision from the xiphoid process to the symphysis pubis.

_____ If a client has cardiac disease, he or she will undergo a coronary artery bypass before repairing an aneurysm.

_____ The spinal cord can become ischemic, resulting in paraplegia, if an AAA ruptures.

_____ The client who undergoes AAA repair faces the greatest risk of cardiac and pulmonary complication during the 4 hours of surgery under anesthesia.

_____ A client's sexual functioning will be greatly improved after correction of an AAA, due to increased blood flow.

APPLYING SKILLS

12. List the three characteristics of intermittent claudication:
    a.
    b.
    c.

13. Mr. Thomas, a 78-year old construction worker, has had PVD for a number of years. He now tells the nurse that his sleep is being interrupted by pain in his legs that requires him to get up and walk around. He states that the pain used to occur when walking but now it hurts when he is stationary. State the clinical significance of "pain at rest" for the client with intermittent claudication.

14. When evaluating vascular disorders, a _____ can determine the quality of blood flow of the vessels.

15. List four anatomical areas where pulses should be assessed in a client with a possible peripheral vascular disorder:
    a.
    b.
    c.
    d.

16. A nurse assesses a postoperative client who has undergone a bypass grafting of a lower extremity. Manifestations that would indicate a clot blocking blood flow include that the limb has become: (Select all that apply)
    1. cool.
    2. pale in appearance.
    3. painful.
    4. pulseless.

17. List the critical nursing assessments that should be performed in the *preoperative* time period for a client who will undergo a bypass grafting for an extremity with PVD:
    a.

    b.

    c.

18. A change in urine color from yellow to rusty brown indicates a critical postoperative complication of _____.

19. True or False

    _____ Tachypnea is the most frequent manifestation of a pulmonary embolism

BEST PRACTICES

20. For each medical management goal, identify specific client teaching areas for the nurse to discuss:

Goal	Specific Teaching Area
a. Reduce risk	
b. Promote arterial flow	
c. Save the limb of clients with intermittent claudication	

21. A nursing intervention for a client with arterial insufficiency would be to place the client in _____ positioning to aid blood flow through gravity.

22. Identify the priority nursing action for the client with a nursing diagnosis of Risk for impaired skin integrity related to decreased peripheral circulation.

23. When planning an exercise program for a client with vascular disorders, the nurse should exclude clients who have: (Select all that apply)
    1. leg ulcers.
    2. gangrene.
    3. cellulitis.
    4. DVT.

24. When teaching a client about phantom sensations, the nurse would explain that: (Select all that apply)
    1. the sensations are often felt immediately after surgery but gradually decrease over the next 2 days.
    2. the client may feel warmth, cold, itching, or pain, which is caused by intact peripheral nerves above the amputation site.
    3. most phantom pain occurs in clients who had pain prior to amputation.
    4. phantom sensations are unusual and may indicate a complication from the amputation surgery.

25. To prevent edema at the stump postoperatively, the nurse would elevate the stump only for the first _____ and then place it flat.

26. Compare and contrast the types of nursing care required for a client who has undergone a traumatic amputation and for a client who has undergone a planned amputation.

    Traumatic:

    Planned:

27. List the activity restrictions the nurse should instruct a client who has undergone AAA repair to follow as part of discharge teaching:
    a.

    b.

    c.

    d.

28. True or False

    _____ Clients at risk for DVT should not position pillows under the knee for comfort.

    _____ Clinical manifestations of DVT include bilateral swelling of the legs.

    _____ Homans' sign is not considered an accurate test for DVT anymore.

    _____ Venous duplex scanning is the primary diagnostic test for DVT.

    _____ Elastic wraps applied to the legs of clients with venous stasis should be rewrapped once a day to assess the skin.

    _____ Nurses do not need to document the lack of manifestations of pulmonary embolism in clients with DVT if they are stable.

KEEPING DRUG SKILLS SHARP

29. Compare and contrast common medications used for anticoagulant therapy in clients:

Medication	Indication	Route	Nursing Considerations
Coumadin			
heparin			
low-molecular-weight heparin			
heparin			

30. The calcium antagonist _____ is the first choice for decreasing the frequency, duration, and intensity of vasospastic attacks.

31. True or False

_____ Anticoagulant agents do not break up or dissolve clots; prevent new clots from forming

_____ Heparin therapy requires monitoring of a client's PTT levels but low-molecular-weight heparin does not.

Chapter 56

Assessment of the Cardiac System

OBJECTIVES

56.1   Describe the risk factors that are predominant for cardiovascular disease.

56.2   Elicit a health history of clients that focuses on cardiovascular disease.

56.3   Identify clinical manifestations that coexist with cardiovascular disease.

56.4   Discuss medications relevant to cardiovascular disease.

56.5   Identify relevant diagnostic procedures utilized to diagnosis cardiovascular disease.

56.6   Describe nursing responsibilities for care of clients with cardiovascular disease.

ANATOMY & PHYSIOLOGY REVIEW

1. Label the structures of the heart and trace the flow of blood through the heart systemic circulation.

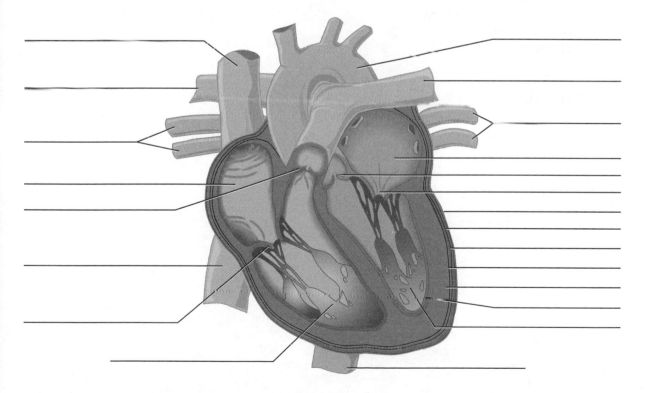

UNDERSTANDING PATHOPHYSIOLOGY

2. True or False

_____ Chest pain is one of the most important manifestations of cardiac disease.

_____ There are greater CVD risk factors among black and Mexican American women than among white women of comparable socioeconomic status.

_____ Murmurs are heard as a consequence of turbulent blood flow through the heart and large vessels.

3. Clients who smoke increase their risk for _____ and _____.

4. Nicotine, a major ingredient in cigarettes, causes: (Select all that apply)
   1. peripheral vasoconstriction.
   2. increasing resistance to left ventricular emptying.
   3. increased myocardial workload.
   4. no reduction in cardiac output.

5. The most common causes of fatigue include: (Select all that apply)
   1. anemia.
   2. anxiety.
   3. chronic diseases.
   4. depression.
   5. thyroid dysfunction.

6. The cardiac cycle is composed of: (Select all that apply)
   1. the first heart sound (S1).
   2. the second heart sound (S2).
   3. rhythm direct forces.
   4. cardiac noding.

APPLYING SKILLS

7. When evaluating chest pain, it is important to assess: (Select all that apply)
   1. timing.
   2. quality.
   3. quantity.
   4. location.
   5. any precipitating or aggravating factors.

8. True or False

_____ Tachycardia (rapid heart beat) can occur as a result of increased force of myocardial contraction caused by the ingestion of caffeine or emotional stress.

_____ Exertional dyspnea is the most common form of cardiac-related dyspnea.

_____ Syncope is a transient loss of consciousness related to inadequate cerebral perfusion.

_____ Clubbing of the fingernails is seen in clients with significant cardiopulmonary disease.

_____ Elevated serum cholesterol levels are associated with coronary artery disease.

_____ Neck vein distention can be used to estimate central venous pressure (CVP).

_____ Crackles frequently signal left ventricular failure and usually occur just after the onset of an S3 gallop.

_____ Blood-tinged sputum or pink frothy sputum may indicate acute pulmonary edema.

_____ Frank hemoptysis may be associated with pulmonary embolus.

9. Which sign indicates acute pulmonary edema?
   1. cough
   2. pink frothy sputum
   3. green sputum
   4. chills

BEST PRACTICES

10. The American Heart Association recommends that health care providers routinely assess a client's general risk of CVD beginning at age _____.

11. Auscultation of the precordium yields valuable information about: (Select all that apply)
    1. normal or abnormal heart rate and rhythm.
    2. ventricular filing.
    3. blood flow across heart valves.
    4. constant flux of arteries.

12. The most common diagnostic procedures used to diagnose CVD are: (Select all that apply)
    1. laboratory test.
    2. ECG.
    3. radiographic studies.
    4. hemodynamic studies.

13. Clients with chronic conditions such as cardiovascular disorders should be vaccinated against

_____.

KEEPING DRUG SKILLS SHARP

14. Oral contraceptives increase the incidence of _____.

15. Numerous medications can affect the cardiovascular system, including: (Select all that apply)
    1. antihypertensives.
    2. diuretics.
    3. cardiotonic drugs.
    4. bronchodilators.

16. Tricyclic antidepressants and other psychotropic medications can cause _____
    _____.

17. List seven herbs known to have antidysrhythmic action:
    a.

    b.

    c.

    d.

    e.

    f.

    g.

Chapter 57

Management of Clients with Structural Cardiac Disorders

OBJECTIVES

57.1 Describe the pathophysiology, etiology, and clinical manifestations for selected structural abnormalities.

57.2 Describe clinical manifestations and complications associated with selected structural abnormalities of the heart.

57.3 Identify medical management and nursing care for clients with cardiac conditions.

57.4 Define current terminology related to cardiac disorders.

57.5 Identify inflammatory disorders that cause cardiac problems.

UNDERSTANDING PATHOPHYSIOLOGY

1. Factors that can lead to the development of acquired valvular disease include: (Select all that apply)
   1. myocardial ischemia.
   2. rheumatic fever.
   3. infectious endocarditis.
   4. connective tissue disorders.

2. The most common cause of mitral stenosis that is preventable is _____
   _____.

3. Inflammation of the endocardium resulting from acute rheumatic fever or infectious endocarditis is caused by: (Select all that apply)
   1. inflammation causeing the valve leaflets and chordae tendinae to become fibrous.
   2. shortening of chordae tendinae, which narrows the outflow tract.
   3. abnormal respiratory reserve remains.
   4. rhythm disturbances.

4. Mitral valve prolapse occurs when:
   1. anterior and posterior cusps of the mitral valve billow upward into the atrium during systolic contraction.
   2. unable to detect current conduction of atrial valve.
   3. posterior centers of the heart relax and cause stress.
   4. upward flow of cardiac strain produces exertional dyspnea.

5. Myocardial oxygen consumption is higher in aortic stenosis due to:
   1. hypertrophy of the right ventricle.
   2. hypertrophy of the left ventricle.
   3. enlarged ventricular tissue.
   4. venous congestion.

6. Risk factors known to contribute to development of rheumatic fever include: (Select all that apply)
   1. poor hygiene.
   2. crowding.
   3. poverty.
   4. chronic infections.

7. Aortic regurgitation is most often a result of which of these infectious disorders? (Select all that apply)
   1. rheumatic fever
   2. syphilis
   3. infective endocarditis
   4. mild pneumonia

8. _____ is a syndrome resulting from inflammation of the pericardial and visceral pericardium

APPLYING SKILLS

9. Most clients with structural cardiac problems will present with a classic _____
   _____.

10. The organism responsible for rheumatic fever is:
    1. *Staphylococcus aureus.*
    2. group A beta-hemolytic *Streptococci* (GAS).
    3. nongroup *Streptococci.*
    4. *Candida albicans.*

11. Rheumatic fever directly impacts which areas of the body? (Select all that apply)
    1. layers of the heart
    2. joints
    3. subcutaneous tissue
    4. central nervous system
    5. skin

12. True or False

    _____ Atrial fibrillation is a common finding in clients with mitral stenosis.

13. Complications of rheumatic fever include: (Select all that apply)
    1. valvular disorders.
    2. cardiomegaly.
    3. heart failure.
    4. venous congestion.

14. The inflamed myocardium of the heart in rheumatic fever has areas of necrosis called

_____.

15. The nurse needs to obtain which of the following to assist in confirming a diagnosis of rheumatic fever?
    1. urine culture
    2. blood culture
    3. throat culture
    4. immunoassay of stool

16. Additional diagnostic tests that will be ordered for a client with rheumatic fever include: (Select all that apply)
    1. CBC with WBC elevation.
    2. erythrocyte sedimentation rate (ESR).
    3. C-reactive protein.
    4. ECG.

17. Clinical signs that a client with cardiac tamponade will present with include: (Select all that apply)
    1. hypotension and muffled heart sounds.
    2. tachycardia and dyspnea.
    3. jugular venous distention.
    4. cyanosis of lips and nails.

18. Clinical manifestations of tricuspid stenosis include: (Select all that apply)
    1. dyspnea and fatigue.
    2. pulsations in the neck.
    3. peripheral edema.
    4. weight loss.

BEST PRACTICES

19. The primary focus of nursing management of valvular heart disease includes: (Select all that apply)
    1. helping the client maintain a normal cardiac output.
    2. preventing manifestations of heart failure.
    3. avoiding venous congestion.
    4. preserving tissue perfusion.

20. Most clients treated in the hospital for rheumatic fever are put on the bed rest because it: (Select all that apply)
    1. reduces myocardial oxygen demands.
    2. reduces cardiac effort.
    3. helps inflammation around the heart to subside.
    4. aids in promoting rest.

21. When teaching a client being discharged from the hospital with rheumatic fever, it is important to stress avoidance of exposure to streptococcal infections. To do this, the nurse would encourage the client to: (Select all that apply)
    1. avoid people who have upper respiratory infections.
    2. avoid people who have had a recent strep infection.
    3. notify physician if any symptoms of sore throat or pharyngitis develops.
    4. guard against infections for the rest of his or her life to avoid development of heart disease.

22. The emergency intervention of choice for treating cardiac tamponade is _____ _____.

KEEPING DRUG SKILLS SHARP

23. The drug of choice for treatment of rheumatic fever is:
    1. oral penicillin.
    2. oral diuretics.
    3. beta blockers.
    4. angiotensin releasing agents.

24. Clients with rheumatic fever will be given prophylactic antibiotics for an extended period of time post-treatment. How long would the nurse tell a client he would be taking oral penicillin?
    1. 10 years or more
    2. up to 5 years after the initial attack
    3. no more than 1 year
    4. up to 6 months

25. Digitalis is useful for slowing the ventricular heart rate in clients with _____.

26. _____ are helpful in reducing the risk of embolus.

27. Which of the following medications bring about significant hemodynamic changes in clients with chronic mitral regurgitation? (Select all that apply)
    1. angiotensin converting enzymes
    2. nitrates
    3. digitalis
    4. sulfonamides

28. _____ has been given to prevent transient ischemic attacks.

29. Prophylactic antibiotics may be given on an individual basis for invasive medical or dental procedures in order to prevent _____ in persons who have rheumatic heart disorders.

Chapter 58

Management of Clients with Functional Cardiac Disorders

OBJECTIVES

58.1 Discuss the etiology and clinical manifestations of coronary artery disease and congestive heart failure.

58.2 Describe diagnostic studies used to assess clients with coronary artery disease and congestive heart failure.

58.3 Describe medical and nursing management for clients with coronary artery disease and congestive heart failure.

UNDERSTANDING PATHOPHYSIOLOGY

1. True or False

   _____ In coronary heat disease (CHD), atherosclerosis develops in the coronary arteries, causing them to become narrowed or blocked.

   _____ Exercise and low fat, low cholesterol diets increase the amount of HDL in the blood.

   _____ Heart failure is a physiologic state in which the heart cannot pump enough blood to meet the metabolic needs of the body.

   _____ In chronic heart failure, the increased workload of the heart and the extreme work of breathing increases the metabolic demands of the body.

   _____ Dependent edema is one of the early signs of right ventricular failure.

2. List six modifiable risk factors for CHD:
   a.

   b.

   c.

   d.

   e.

   f.

3. When compared to the white population, the risk of coronary heart disease is greatest among which of the following groups? (Select all that apply)
   1. Mexican Americans
   2. American Indians
   3. Native Hawaiians
   4. Asians

4. The incidence of CHD markedly increases among women after _____.

5. Atherosclerosis primarily affects the _____ of the _____ and normally takes years to develop.

6. _____ is the presence of more than one artery supplying blood to a muscle.

APPLYING SKILLS

7. True or False

   _____ Elevated serum cholesterol levels increase as blood cholesterol levels increase.

   _____ High levels of HDL seem to protect against the development of CHD.

8. Diagnostic studies used to determine underlying causes and degrees of heart failure include: (Select all that apply)
   1. B-type natriuretic peptide (BNP).
   2. echocardiogram.
   3. chest x-ray.
   4. ECG.

BEST PRACTICES

9. True or False

   _____ The primary goals that guide the medical management of a client with CHD are reducing and controlling risk factors and restoring blood supply to the myocardium.

   _____ Coronary artery bypass graft surgery involves the bypass of a blockage in one or more of the coronary arteries using the saphenous veins, mammary artery, or radial artery.

10. Postoperative complications that are more prevalent in the older client who has had a CABG include: (Select all that apply)
    1. dysrhythmias related to aged sinoatrial node cells.
    2. drug toxicity associated with impaired hepatic and renal function.
    3. multiple drug interactions.
    4. decreased physical stamina.

11. Prior to discharge, the nurse will instruct the family of a client who has had a CABG regarding: (Select all that apply)
    1. medication actions and side effects.
    2. dietary restrictions.
    3. physical activity restrictions.
    4. incisional care.

12. Other terms used to denote heart failure include: (Select all that apply)
    1. cardiac decompensation.
    2. cardiac insufficiency.
    3. ventricular failure.
    4. heart pump syndrome.

KEEPING DRUG SKILLS SHARP

13. Which of the following are true regarding glycoprotein IIb/IIIa receptor antagonists? (Select all that apply)
    1. prevent platelet aggregation in the acute coronary syndromes
    2. when combined with aspirin, decrease the incidence of recurrent cardiac events
    3. help to smooth the lining of the heart
    4. decrease the need for heparin

14. Beta adrenergic antagonists are used to inhibit the effects of the _____ _____.

15. Diuretics are given to clients to: (Select all that apply)
    1. reduce circulating blood volume.
    2. diminish preload.
    3. lessen systemic and pulmonary congestion.
    4. relieve systemic threshold.

16. True or False

    _____ Hypokalemia can potentiate digitalis toxicity and cause myocardial weakness and cardiac dyshythmias.

17. Digoxin exerts which of the following effects? (Select all that apply)
    1. improves cardiac output; enhances kidney perfusion
    2. creates a mild diuresis of sodium and water
    3. helps in treating heart failure
    4. helps control to ventricular response in atrial fibrillation

Chapter 59

Management of Clients with Dysrhythmias

OBJECTIVES

59.1   Identify relevant terminology related to disorders of cardiac rhythms.

59.2   Identify critical components of the electrocardiogram (ECG) pattern.

59.3   Discuss assessment findings for abnormal rhythm determination.

59.4   Interpret selected rhythm strips for accuracy.

59.5   Discuss the medical management of selected abnormal rhythms.

59.6   Identify the course of treatment and nursing interventions for disorders of the cardiac rhythm.

UNDERSTANDING PATHOPHYSIOLOGY

1. The conduction and rhythm system of the heart is susceptible to damage by heart disease as a result of: (Select all that apply)
   1. ischemia of the heart tissue.
   2. decreased coronary artery blood flow.
   3. too much calcium in the chambers.
   4. inability of the vessels to return the blood.

2. Abnormal rhythms are referred to as: (Select all that apply)
   1. dysrhythmias.
   2. arrhythmias.
   3. abnormal sounds.
   4. irregular tones.

3. A heart rhythm that begins in the sinoatrial (SA) node is referred to as:
   1. normal sinus rhythm.
   2. normal conduction.
   3. atrial sinus pattern.
   4. ectopic rhythm.

4. The most serious complication of a dysrhythmia is _____.

5. Dysrhythmias result from disturbances in: (Select all that apply)
   1. automaticity.
   2. conduction.
   3. reentry of pulses.
   4. endocardial swings.

6. Automaticity is used to describe:
   1. alterations in the normal heart rates produced by various pacemaker cells in the myocardium.
   2. impulses driven from sinus activity.
   3. aberrant sounds that collect in the sinus nodes.
   4. abnormal gateway keeping of sounds from the ventricles.

7. Latent pacemaker cells can also fire at increased rates beyond their inherent rate. When rates exceed these values, the rhythm is _____.

8. _____ is the activation of muscle for a second time by the same impulse.

9. A _____ is a conduction delay that occurs between the sinus node and atrial muscle.

APPLYING SKILLS

10. The nurse will evaluate clients for dysrhythmias based on which of the following clinical observations? (Select all that apply)
    1. heart rate below 50 or above 140 beats per minute
    2. an extremely irregular heart rhythm or pulse
    3. a first heart sound that varies in intensity
    4. sudden appearance of heart failure, shock, and angina
    5. slow, regular heart rate that does not change with activity or medications

11. Sinus tachycardia has which of the following clinical characteristics? (Select all that apply)
    1. regular rhythm at a rate of 100-180 beats per minute
    2. normal P wave and QRS complex
    3. occurs in response to an increase in sympathetic stimulation
    4. occurs in response to a decreased vagal stimulation

12. _____ is a delay in passage of the impulse from the atria to the ventricles.

13. Which of the following characteristics describe ventricular tachycardia? (Select all that apply)
    1. a life-threatening dysrhythmia
    2. occurs when irritable ectopic focus in ventricles takes over
    3. occurs in significant cardiac disease
    4. mildly treated with aspirin

14. Which identifying features of ventricular tachycardia are evident on the ECG monitor? (Select all that apply)
    1. rapidly occurring series of PVCs (three or more)
    2. P waves are absent
    3. ventricular rate ranges between 100-220 beats per minute
    4. QRS complex is wide and bizarre

15. A client with ventricular tachycardia will be experiencing which of the following clinical manifestations? (Select all that apply)
    1. cerebral ischemia
    2. myocardial ischemia
    3. feels like impending death
    4. feeling faint, weak, and dizzy

16. Ventricular fibrillation is a life-threatening dysrhythmia characterized by: (Select all that apply)
    1. extreme, rapid, erratic impulse formation and conduction.
    2. abrupt cessation of effective cardiac output.
    3. bizarre fibrillatory wave patterns on ECG.
    4. impossible-to-identify P waves, QRS complexes or T waves.

17. Ventricular fibrillation can be either _____ or
_____.

18. Clients with sinus bradycardia must be evaluated for: (Select all that apply)
    1. hypotension.
    2. light-headedness.
    3. syncope.
    4. fatigue.

19. Sinus dysrhythmia is characterized by: (Select all that apply)
    1. changes in the automaticity of the SA node.
    2. firing at varying speeds.
    3. heart rate between 60-100 beats per minute.
    4. abnormal ECG.

20. A dysrhythmia arising in an ectopic pacemaker or the site of a rapid reentry circuit in the atria is called _____ or _____.

21. An atrial flutter appears on the ECG with which of these identifying characteristics? (Select all that apply)
    1. inverted P waves
    2. picket fences or sawtooth pattern
    3. rate generally around 220-350 beats per minute.
    4. no noted changes in the QRS complex

22. Patients with atrial flutter may experience which of the following clinical signs and symptoms? (Select all that apply)
    1. palpitations
    2. chest pains
    3. lightheadedness and dizziness
    4. hypertension

23. Atrial fibrillation can best be described as: (Select all that apply)
    1. rapid, chaotic atrial depolarization from a reentry disorder.
    2. impulses between 400-700 beats per minute.
    3. extremely slow response and reactivity.
    4. mechanical depolarization.

24. Atrial fibrillation has which of these identifying characteristics on an ECG?
    1. erratic or no identifiable P waves and an underlying ventricular rhythm that is irregular
    2. identifiable QRS complex
    3. P-P ratio is normal
    4. T wave high

25. Causes of atrial fibrillation include: (Select all that apply)
    1. sick sinus syndromes.
    2. hypoxia.
    3. increased atrial pressure.
    4. pericarditis.

26. Cardioversion is used to treat: (Select all that apply)
    1. SVT.
    2. atrial fibrillation.
    3. atrial flutter.
    4. ventricular tachycardia in an unstable client.

Using the information in Box 59-1 of the textbook, interpret the following ECG tracings.

27.

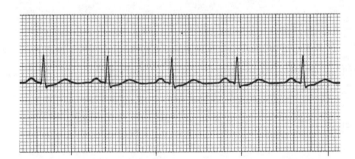

28.

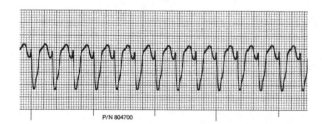

29.

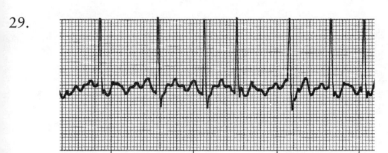

30.

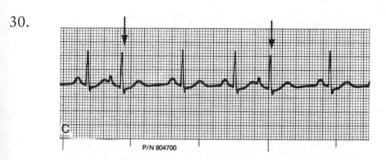

31.

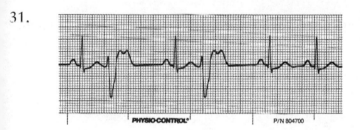

32.

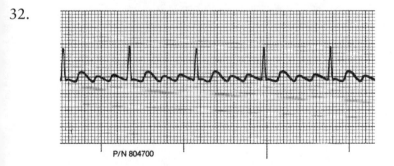

33.

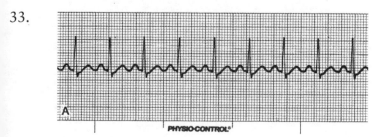

34.

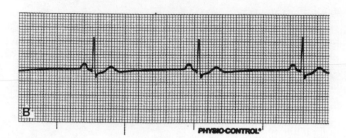

KEEPING DRUG SKILLS SHARP

35. Medications used in the treatment of atrial flutter in combination with cardioversion include: (Select all that apply)
    1. digitalis.
    2. quinidine.
    3. verapamil.
    4. Inderal and procainamide.

36. If the client has been taking digitalis preparations, a current therapeutic drug level must be obtained prior to cardioversion because:
    1. digitalis toxicity may predispose the client to ventricular dysrhythmias during cardioversion.
    2. abnormal heart rhythms will be noted.
    3. cardiac cycle will be slowed.
    4. QRS complexes will not be identifiable on the ECG.

Management of Clients with Myocardial Infarction

OBJECTIVES

60.1 Compare coronary artery disease, angina pectoris, and myocardial infarction.

60.2 Discuss associated risk factors pertaining to angina pectoris and myocardial infarction.

60.3 Describe clinical manifestations of angina pectoris and myocardial infarction.

60.4 Identify diagnostic and laboratory tests used to diagnosis angina and myocardial infarction.

60.5 Discuss the medical and nursing management for clients with angina pectoris and myocardial infarction.

UNDERSTANDING PATHOPHYSIOLOGY

1. Angina pectoris is associated with _____.

2. Myocardial ischemia develops when: (Select all that apply)
    1. blood supply through the coronary vessels is not adequate.
    2. oxygen content of the blood is not adequate to meet body demands.
    3. walls of the vessels are too thin.
    4. venous congestion exists.

3. _____ is paroxysmal chest pain or discomfort triggered by a predictable degree of exertion or emotion.

4. _____ is paroxysmal chest pain triggered by an unpredictable degree of exertion or emotion, which may occur at night.

5. _____ is chest discomfort similar to classic angina but of longer duration, and that may occur while the client is at rest.

6. The most common site of an MI is the _____.

APPLYING SKILLS

7. Clients with angina are likely to have which of the following symptoms? (Select all that apply)
   1. pain as retrosternal or slightly to the left of the sternum
   2. burning, pressing pain
   3. pain usually last 5 minutes
   4. dyspnea, pallor, sweating

8. The most common laboratory tests and non-invasive tests of clients suspecting of having angina are: (Select all that apply)
   1. resting ECG.
   2. chest x-ray.
   3. fasting glucose.
   4. fasting lipid profile.

9. The major clinical manifestation in a client who is experiencing a myocardial infarction is
   _____.

10. Symptoms that clients with MI are likely to describe upon admission to the hospital include: (Select all that apply)
    1. pain radiating to the neck, jaw and shoulder, back or left arm.
    2. some epigastric indigestion.
    3. nausea and dizziness.
    4. unexplained anxiety and weakness.

11. When blood flow to the heart is decreased, ischemia and necrosis of the heart muscle occur, causing which of the following ECG changes? (Select all that apply)
    1. altered Q waves
    2. ST segment changes
    3. T waves changes on a 12 lead ECG
    4. QRS changes

12. What laboratory findings would indicate that a client has just suffered a myocardial infarction? (Select all that apply)
    1. elevated levels of serum creatine kinase – MB
    2. cardiac troponin T elevated
    3. cardiac troponin I elevated
    4. LDH, AST, ESR are elevated

13. True or False

    _____ A client is at the highest risk of sudden death during the first 24 hours after an MI.

14. The most common cause of death after a myocardial infarction is _____
    _____.

BEST PRACTICES

15. When educating a client about weight reduction, it is important to explain that: (Select all that apply)
    1. weight reduction can reduce blood pressure.
    2. weight reduction can reduce cholesterol.
    3. weight reduction can decrease risk for diabetes mellitus.
    4. eating high calorie foods is important.

16. Nursing actions performed when a client is admitted to the emergency room with suspected MI include: (Select all that apply)
    1. beginning oxygen therapy.
    2. obtaining an ECG.
    3. establishing an intravenous line.
    4. obtaining serum cardiac markers.

KEEPING DRUG SKILLS SHARP

17. When treating angina, the physician will most likely prescribe:
    1. nitroglycerin.
    2. aspirin.
    3. heparin.
    4. lovenox.

18. Several different types of medications are used to treat acute angina pectoris, including: (Select all that apply)
    1. vasodilators.
    2. beta-adrenergic blockers.
    3. calcium channel blockers.
    4. vitamins and minerals.

19. Sublingual nitroglycerin is given to clients to: (Select all that apply)
    1. reduce pain.
    2. dilate coronary arteries.
    3. restore coronary blood flow.
    4. increase upper levels of cytokines.

20. When at home, clients who experience chest pain or suspect they are having an MI should: (Select all that apply)
    1. ingest aspirin.
    2. resume usual activity for 30 minutes to see if pain goes away.
    3. go to bed and wait until the pain subsides.
    4. ingest large quantities of glucose.

21. Not all clients are suitable candidates for thrombolytic therapy, including clients: (Select all that apply)
    1. with a history of recent cerebral vascular accident.
    2. who have had recent surgery.
    3. who are pregnant.
    4. who are taking anticoagulants.

Chapter 61

Assessment of the Respiratory System

OBJECTIVES

61.1 Discuss the important components required when obtaining a respiratory history from a client.

61.2 Describe the process for performing a physical examination of the respiratory system.

61.3 Identify common diagnostic tests used to assess the respiratory system.

61.4 Describe nursing responsibilities when caring for a client undergoing invasive testing of the respiratory system.

ANATOMY & PHYSIOLOGY REVIEW

1. Label the structures of the upper airway.

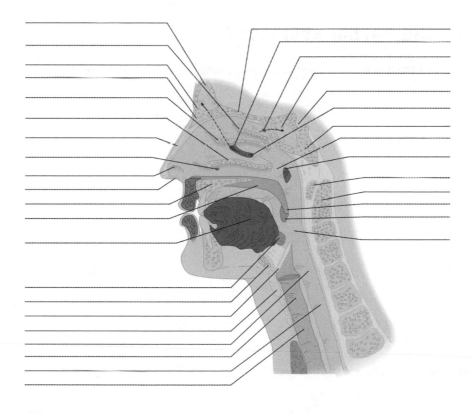

2. Label the structures of the lower airway.

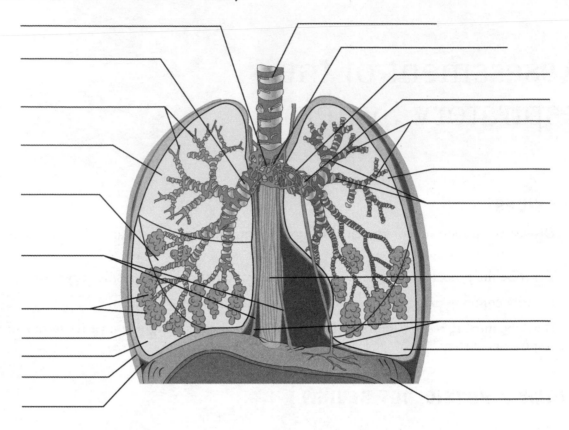

UNDERSTANDING PATHOPHYSIOLOGY

3. Compare and contrast pleuritic chest pain and complaints of angina pectoris.

4. Childhood illnesses associated with respiratory complications include all of the following except:
   1. bronchitis.
   2. influenza.
   3. asthma.
   4. pneumonia.
   5. frequency of lower respiratory infections.
   6. measles.
   7. cystic fibrosis.
   8. premature birth history.

5. The normal inspiration to expiration ratio is _____.

6. Identify the etiology for each type of abnormal breath sounds.
   a. Crackles:

   b. Rhonchi:

   c. Wheezes:

   d. Pleural friction rub:

APPLYING SKILLS

7. A client reports problems with foul taste in the mouth, nasal obstruction, and facial pain. These manifestations may be associated with _____.

8. The _____ assists the client to quantify their degree of dyspnea and aids in evaluating client status after interventions.

9. The nurse inquires whether the client has had any changes in voice character, hoarseness, difficulty swallowing, or sleep-related disorders, such as snoring. These changes are associated with _____.

10. Compare and contrast factors of a client's psychosocial history:

Factor	Area to be assessed
Occupation	
Geographic location	
Environment	
Habits	
Exercise	
Nutrition	

11. A nurse notes an increase in the anterior-to-posterior diameter of a client who has a history of cigarette smoking. This finding is consistent with a diagnosis of _____.

12. When examining the fingers of a client, the nurse notes clubbing, which occurs as a compensatory mechanism due to _____.

13. The nurse is assessing for tactile fremitus on the posterior chest wall. An increase in vibrations felt over an area may indicate _____.

14. Identify each type of chest deformity visible during assessment.

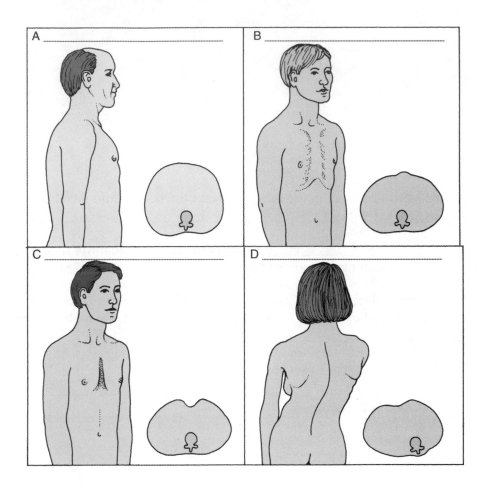

A _____

B _____

C _____

D _____

15. True or False

_____   Upon percussion of the chest wall, a resonant sound is heard. This is a normal finding.

_____   Hyperresonant sounds are normally heard in adults with good air exchange.

_____   If the nurse percusses an area and hears a flat note, the area is solid tissue such as bone.

_____   Tympanic notes can be heard when percussing over the stomach.

_____   Percussion is done over the entire chest wall, including ribs and sternum, to check for abnormalities.

16. Label each type of respiratory pattern illustrated below.

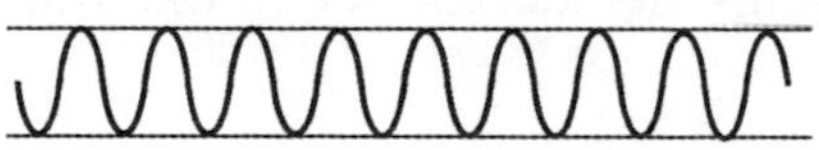

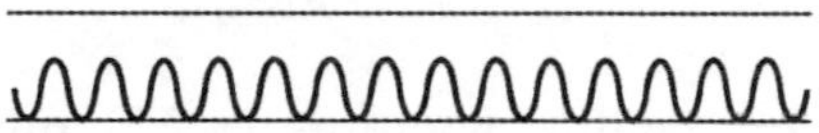

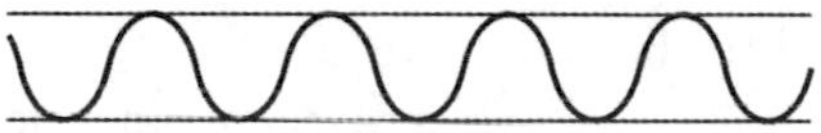

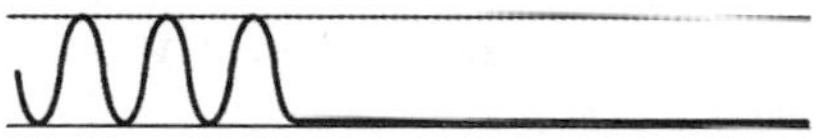

A. _____

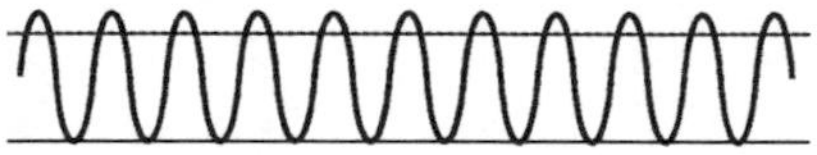

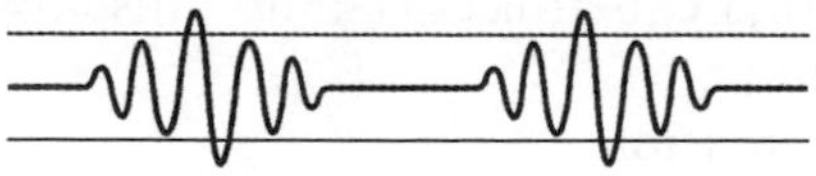

F. _____

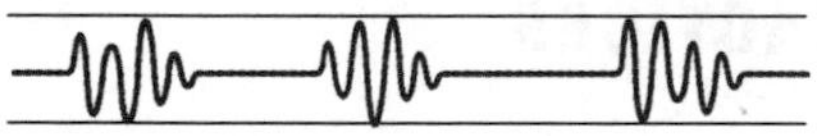

B. _____

G. _____

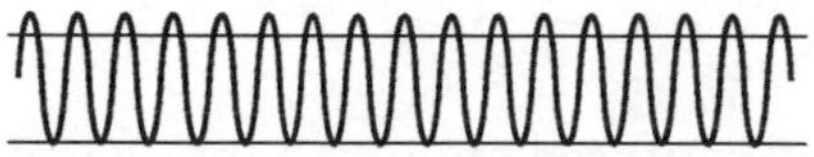

C. _____

H. _____

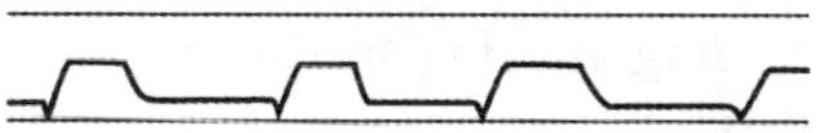

D. _____

I. _____

E. _____

17. When assessing a client's status, the _____ is considered the "fifth vital sign."

18. Factors that can affect accurate pulse oximetry readings include: (Select all that apply)
    1. motion.
    2. hypertension.
    3. hypothermia.
    4. vasoconstriction.
    5. inflated blood pressure cuff placed on same arm.
    6. dark nail polish (blue, green, black or brown-red).

BEST PRACTICES

19. A client is resting in bed. Upon assessment, the nurse notes a pulse oximetry reading of less than 90%. State the actions the nurse should take.

20. A client is confused about the frequency of vaccinations against pneumonia. The nurse explains that Pneumovax provides _____ immunity against pneumo-coccal pneumonia but "flu shots" must be received _____.

21. Prior to undergoing pulmonary function tests, a client should be instructed not to _____ or _____.

22. After obtaining an ABG specimen, pressure is applied to the puncture site for _____. If client is receiving _____ medications, pressure must be applied to the puncture site longer.

23. A client has undergone a ventilation-perfusion lung scan and the results show areas of the lung where there is ventilation but no perfusion. _____ may be the cause of this finding.

24. A 23-year-old male college student has been ordered to have a chest x-ray. After properly positioning the client for the x-ray, the nurse should make sure all _____ are shielded before beginning the procedure.

25. State the rationale for instructing clients to "take a deep breath and hold it" when taking a radiograph.

26. After completion of a thoracentesis, the client should be placed on the _____ side for 1 hour.

Chapter 62

Management of Clients with Upper Airway Disorders

OBJECTIVES

62.1 Discuss medical management and nursing interventions for clients with common upper airway disorders.

62.2 Describe types, purposes of, and nursing care of tracheostomy.

62.3 Describe pre and postoperative nursing care for clients having head and neck surgery.

62.4 Discuss clinical manifestations of airway obstruction and appropriate interventions.

UNDERSTANDING PATHOPHYSIOLOGY

1. A client has a nursing diagnosis of Risk for impaired gas exchange. List the three factors that affect removal of carbon dioxide:
   a.

   b.

   c.

2. The primary etiologic agent in laryngeal cancer is _____.

3. Risk factors for laryngeal cancer include: (Select all that apply)
   1. history of smoking.
   2. exposure to asbestos.
   3. chronic pharyngitis.
   4. concurrent alcohol and smoking use.

4. Factors that contribute to altered nutrition in clients with laryngeal tumors include: (Select all that apply)
   1. dysphagia.
   2. altered sense of taste.
   3. weight loss.
   4. loss of appetite.

5. Oral secretions accumulate in the client with a laryngectomy due to
   _____ and _____
   impairment.

6. All of the following are clinical manifestations suggestive of sinusitis except:
    1. fever and chills.
    2. pain in the lower teeth.
    3. headaches.
    4. purulent nasal discharge.

7. The most common infection organism in pharyngitis is _____.

8. All of the following are clinical manifestations of pharyngitis except:
    1. sore throat.
    2. difficulty swallowing.
    3. malaise.
    4. otalgia.
    5. fever.

9. All of the following are complications from streptococcal tonsillitis except:
    1. osteomyelitis.
    2. pancreatitis.
    3. nephritis.
    4. rheumatic fever.

10. The most frequent manifestation of chronic tonsillitis is recurrent
    _____.

11. Peritonsillar abscess is typically manifested several days after the onset of
    _____.

12. Rhinitis medicamentosa is caused by abuse or overuse of
    _____ or _____.

13. Hoarseness in clients with GERD is caused from the chemical irritation by
    _____ on the vocal cords.

14. Factors that contribute to the spread of diphtheria include: (Select all that apply)
    1. poor hygiene.
    2. crowding.
    3. limited access to medical care.
    4. poor nutrition.

15. Compare and contrast tonsillar and pharyngeal diphtheria.

16. When only one vocal cord is paralyzed, the primary clinical manifestation is
    _____.

17. Which of the following are the possible indications of a thyroid fracture?
    1. hoarseness
    2. stridor
    3. tender, swollen ecchymotic neck
    4. subcutaneous emphysema

18. True or False

    _____ Once the stoma of a permanent tracheostomy is healed, most clients do not need a tube.

    _____ Subcutaneous emphysema is a serious condition that requires treatment immediately.

    _____ It is harmless for others to smoke in a room with a client who has a tracheostomy.

    _____ It is safe to use room deodorizers in a room with a client who has a tracheostomy.

    _____ Cancer of the larynx most often occurs in women.

    _____ Metastasis is uncommon in subglottic tumors.

    _____ Voice quality is maintained in clients that have supraglottic laryngectomy.

    _____ The sense of smell is lost with total laryngectomy.

    _____ Blood-tinged sputum is not expected in tracheal secretions in the immediate postoperative period.

    _____ Viral and bacterial pharyngitis is contagious by droplet spread.

    _____ *Haemophilus influenzae* is the most common infection organism in tonsillitis.

    _____ Pain in the first 7 to 10 postoperative days is common after tonsillectomy.

    _____ Laryngitis may be the result of GERD.

    _____ Abnormal voice may be the result of vocal abuse.

    _____ Whispering can also cause excessive vocal cord strain.

    _____ Laryngeal injury most often results from trauma during a motor vehicle accident.

APPLYING CONCEPTS

19. Which of the following clients are not good candidates for a single-cannula tracheostomy tube? (Select all that apply)
    1. client with excessive secretions
    2. client who has difficult clearing secretions
    3. client with a thick neck
    4. client with an altered airway

20. The client's biggest concern about weaning is:
    1. the experience of pain.
    2. fear of not being able to breathe.
    3. inability to manage secretions on his or her own.
    4. fear of letting providers of care down.

21. List the clinical assessments that would indicate respiratory distress during the weaning process:
    a.

    b.

    c.

    d.

    e.

22. Following laryngectomy, clients are at risk for aspiration. Which of the following assessment findings indicate that interventions to prevent aspiration have been effective?
    1. adventitious breath sounds in both lung bases
    2. normal respiratory rate and rhythm
    3. clear secretions
    4. ability to cough effectively

23. _____ from the oral cavity, neck, or trachea might alert the nurse to impending carotid rupture.

24. An assessment finding that indicates to the nurse that interventions to prevent aspiration have been effective is:
    1. decreased breath sounds throughout the chest.
    2. increased respiratory rate and rhythm.
    3. chest secretions that are clear.
    4. decreased ability to cough.

25. List the nursing assessments that indicate a return of gastric functioning in the postoperative client:
    a.

    b.

    c.

26. List the critical nursing observations of manifestations of aspiration in a client with vocal cord paralysis:
    a.

    b.

    c.

    d.

27. True or False
    _____ Tracheostomy tubes are universally the same for each client.
    _____ A tracheostomy cuff holds the tube in place.

BEST PRACTICES

28. Place the following steps the nurse follows in order of their occurrence in the event that accidental deccanulation occurs in the client with a tracheostomy.

_____ a. auscultate for breath sounds

_____ b. call a respiratory arrest

_____ c. maintain ventilation and oxygenation by bag and mask

_____ d. call for help

_____ e. reinsert the tube, if possible

29. For the client scheduled for an elective tracheostomy, two essential areas for the nurse to discuss with the client preoperatively are the _____ and the
_____.

30. A nursing intervention used to minimize postoperative edema in the client who had sinus surgery is to place the client in either the _____ or
_____ position.

31. After surgery, the T&A client is placed in the _____ position until he or she is awake and alert.

32. List the interventions that promote comfort for the client with peritonsillar abscess:
a.

b.

c.

d.

e.

33. List the interventions used to decrease dryness and oral pharyngeal discomfort in a client with nasal packing:
a.

b.

c.

34. Immediately after a nasal fracture occurs, _____ should be applied.

35. True or False

_____ A tracheostomy provides the best route for long-term airway maintenance.

_____ A cuffed tracheostomy tube should always be deflated before the client uses the talking tracheostomy adapter.

_____ Ideally, the tracheostomy tube should be changed at least every 4 to 6 weeks.

_____ When a client with a tracheostomy is on a ventilator, the ventilator tubing should be coiled neatly on the bed next to the client.

_____ If the tumor is limited to the true vocal cord, without causing limitation of the cords, radiation therapy is the best treatment.

_____ Supraglottic tumors may be treated with radiation therapy or partial laryngectomy, with or without lymph node dissection.

_____ In the immediate postoperative phase, the inner cannula is cleaned after suctioning.

KEEPING DRUG SKILLS SHARP

36. During antitoxin therapy, the client should be observed for _____ and _____ kept at the bedside.

37. If acute laryngeal edema is precipitated by anaphylaxis, _____ is given subcutaneously.

Management of Clients with Lower Airway and Pulmonary Vessel Disorders

OBJECTIVES

63.1   Apply evidence-based concepts of care for clients with lower airway and pulmonary vessel disorders.

63.2   Assess, plan, implement, and evaluate nursing interventions for clients with lower airway and pulmonary vessel disorders.

63.3   Apply concepts of pharmacotherapy and other therapeutic interventions to care of clients with lower airway and pulmonary vessel disorders.

UNDERSTANDING PATHOPHYSIOLOGY

1. A late manifestation of hypoxia is:
    1. wheezing with exhalation.
    2. nasal flaring.
    3. use of intercostal muscles.
    4. cyanosis.

2. Characteristics of chronic bronchitis include: (Select all that apply)
    1. decreased ciliary function.
    2. destruction of bronchioles.
    3. increased number of goblet cells.
    4. isolated blebs in the lung periphery.
    5. increase in size of sub mucosal glands in the bronchi.
    6. polycythemia.

3. Which type of emphysema increases the client's risk for spontaneous pneumothorax?
    1. Centrolobular
    2. Panlobular
    3. Paraseptal (panacinar)

4. The types of emphysema most often associated with a history of smoking include: (Select all that apply)
   1. centrolobular.
   2. panlobular.
   3. paraseptal (panacinar).

5. Factors which contribute to the development of tracheobronchitis include: (Select all that apply)
   1. viral infections.
   2. exposure to noxious gases.
   3. smoking cessation.
   4. bacterial pneumonia.
   5. intermittent cough.
   6. suctioning.

6. Bronchiectasis is characterized by:
   1. inflammation of the trachea and bronchial tree.
   2. abnormal dilation of the bronchi.
   3. decreased perfusion of the bronchial tree.
   4. increased pulmonary vascular resistance.

7. Which of the following clients is at greatest risk for pulmonary embolus?
   1. client having laparoscopic cholecystectomy
   2. client having placement of gastric feeding tube
   3. client having lung biopsy
   4. client having total abdominal hysterectomy

8. The resulting hypoxemia that occurs following pulmonary embolus (PE) is due to _____
   _____.

9. Common clinical manifestations of PE include: (Select all that apply)
   1. bradycardia.
   2. dyspnea.
   3. anxiety.
   4. chest pain.
   5. tachycardia.
   6. wheezing.

10. Pulmonary hypertension is defined as an elevated pulmonary artery pressure above
    _____ at rest and above _____ during exercise.

11. The underlying pathophysiology which contributes to pulmonary hypertension is _____
    _____.

12. Factors which compromise the treatment of elderly clients with emphysema include: (Select all that apply)
    1. comorbid conditions.
    2. decrease exercise tolerance.
    3. decrease nutritional status.
    4. smoking history.
    5. drug–drug interactions.

13. True or False

_____ All pulmonary embolus originate from deep vein thrombus.

APPLYING SKILLS

14. The nurse is assessing a client with emphysema. Which assessment finding would indicate increasing hypoxia?
    1. decreased breath sounds
    2. bradycardia
    3. eupnea
    4. restlessness

15. The diagnostic measure that is replacing the V/Q lung scan to diagnose pulmonary embolus is
    _____.

16. Supplemental oxygen would be indicated for the client with asthma when the PaO_2 falls below:
    1. 90 mm Hg.
    2. 80 mm Hg.
    3. 70 mm Hg.
    4. 60 mm Hg.

17. What is an indication to the nurse that a client with asthma is approaching acute respiratory failure? Explain the rationale behind this indicator.

18. An indication that a client with asthma may need supplemental oxygen would be:
    1. PaO_2 of 63 mm Hg.
    2. O_2 saturation of 92%.
    3. respiratory rate of 24.
    4. PaO_2 of 56 mm Hg.

19. The client with a PE is receiving anticoagulant therapy. Which assessment finding would alert the nurse to signs of excess therapy?
    1. dark, yellow urine
    2. abdominal pain
    3. dark, tarry stool
    4. ecchymosis at the injection site

20. A nurse is reviewing the ABGs of a client with primary emphysema for 15 years. The nurse would expect the analysis to reveal that the client has:
    1. uncompensated respiratory acidosis.
    2. compensated respiratory acidosis.
    3. uncompensated respiratory alkalosis.
    4. compensated respiratory alkalosis.

21. The home care nurse is caring for a client with emphysema. Which of the following findings would indicate that treatment goals are being met?
    1. increase in severity of clinical manifestations.
    2. increase in ability to manage and remove secretions.
    3. increase in complications.
    4. increase in ventilatory problems.

22. Anticoagulant therapy is monitored through the International Normalized Ratio (INR). The nurse caring for the client receiving anticoagulant therapy achieves therapeutic levels when the INR is:
    1. 1 time the control.
    2. 2 times the control.
    3. 2.5–3 times the control.
    4. 4 times the control.

23. Clients with PE are at risk for developing right-sided heart failure. Assessment findings that would alert the nurse to developing complications include: (Select all that apply)
    1. increasing dyspnea.
    2. heart murmur.
    3. distended neck veins.
    4. peripheral edema.
    5. clear breath sounds.
    6. engorged liver.

BEST PRACTICES

24. A client uses a peak flow meter to monitor respiratory status and notices a fall in peak flow values. Explain what the nurse should teach the client about this finding and what actions the client should take.

25. The nurse is providing teaching for a client with asthma. The client asks, "What if I have an attack and I don't have my medications with me. What do I do?" The nurse should teach the client to perform _____ in this situation.

26. State the rationale for the following activities with the client who has asthma.

Activity	Rationale
a. Assess severity of dyspnea	
b. Return demonstration of spirometry	

c. Return demonstration of metered dose inhaler (MDI)	
d. Assess medication allergies	
e. Assess medication history	
f. History of triggers	
g. Ability to manage disease	
h. Assess family support	
i. Environmental assessment	

27. The nurse is teaching the client with emphysema about measures to improve his or her general health. The most effective measure would be for the client to:
    1. avoid high altitudes.
    2. move to a warm, dry climate.
    3. stop smoking.
    4. use supplemental oxygen.

28. List multiple measures that can be used to prevent pulmonary embolus:
    a.

    b.

    c.

    d.

29. Explain why the client with a PE who manifests with lower extremity edema should not have the lower extremities elevated.

30. The client with emphysema should be instructed to eat a:
    1. High carbohydrate, low fat diet
    2. Low carbohydrate, moderate fat diet
    3. High carbohydrate, high protein diet
    4. High protein, low fat diet

KEEPING DRUG SKILLS SHARP

31. Match the following drugs with their use for quick relief or long-term control of symptoms in asthma and then their mode of action. Answers may be used more than once.

Drug	Use	Action
a. albuterol nebulizer (Proventil)	___	___
b. cromolyn inhaler (Intal, Nasalcrom)	___	___
c. ipratropium inhaler (Atrovent)	___	___
d. beclomethasone inhaler (Vanceril)	___	___
e. montelukast (Singulair)	___	___
f. IV aminophylline	___	___
g. oral prednisone	___	___

Uses
1. long-term control
2. quick relief

Actions
i. beta agonist
ii. anticholinergics
iii. mast-cell stabilizer
iv. leukotriene inhibitor
v. steroid, anti-inflammatory
vi. methylxanthine bronchodilator

32.   A nurse administers Albuterol through the use of a nebulizer to decrease asthma symptoms. An expected outcome of this intervention would be:
1. O_2 saturation of 92%.
2. increased anxiety.
3. a self-report of dyspnea of 8 on a 1-10 scale.
4. continuous, non-productive cough.

33. The nurse is caring for a client receiving Atrovent. An adverse reaction to this drug is:
    1. tachycardia.
    2. increased energy.
    3. nausea.
    4. dry mouth.

34. The client is receiving aminophylline. Which of the following adverse effects would alert the nurse to possible toxicity?
    1. tachycardia.
    2. nervousness.
    3. nausea and vomiting.
    4. headache.

35. Adverse effects of corticosteroids include: (Select all that apply)
    1. hypotension.
    2. gastric burning.
    3. dysphoria.
    4. hypoglycemia.
    5. oral thrush.
    6. thin, sparse hair.

36. The medication most often administered to the client with PE to reduce anxiety is:
    1. valium.
    2. morphine sulfate.
    3. aspirin.
    4. Tylenol with codeine.

37. The first line drug of choice for the treatment of pulmonary hypertension is:
    1. calcium channel antagonists.
    2. diuretics.
    3. ACE inhibitors.
    4. peripheral vasodilators.

CONCEPT MAP EXERCISE

The following questions are based on the Concept Map *Understanding Asthma and Its Treatment* in the textbook.

38. Which of the following types of medications are given to the client with asthma to decrease IgE stimulation? (Select all that apply)
    1. mast cell stabilizers
    2. leukotriene modifiers
    3. anticholingergics
    4. steroids

39. Clinical manifestations of bronchospasm include: (Select all that apply)
    1. wheezing.
    2. non-productive cough.
    3. chest tightness.
    4. shortness of breath.
    5. peak flow variability.

40. Increased mucous secretion is a direct pathophysiologic response to
    1. IgE stimulation.
    2. mast cell degradation.
    3. airway hyper-responsiveness.
    4. bronchospasm.

Chapter 64

Management of Clients with Parenchymal and Pleural Disorders

OBJECTIVES

64.1 Define common terms associated with parenchymal and pleural disorders.

64.2 Discuss common parenchymal disorders including their clinical manifestations, outcome management, and associated nursing care.

64.3 Discuss common pleural disorders including their clinical manifestations, outcome management, and associated nursing care.

64.4 Describe closed-chest drainage and associated nursing care.

64.5 Discuss surgical interventions for parenchymal and pleural disorders.

64.6 Differentiate among lung carcinomas.

UNDERSTANDING PATHOPHYSIOLOGY

1. List the common clinical manifestations associated with influenza:
   a.
   b.
   c.

2. List the 10 major risk factors for pneumonia:
   a.
   b.
   c.
   d.
   e.
   f.
   g.
   h.
   i.
   j.

3. Which of the following clinical manifestations of pneumonia may not be present in older adults?
   1. fever
   2. pleuritic chest pain
   3. headache
   4. altered mental status

4. Match each type of pneumonia with the appropriate description.

Types of Pneumonia	Description
_____ a. segmental	1. death of a portion of lung tissue surrounded by viable tissue
_____ b. necrotizing	2. accumulation of fluid in lung's distal air spaces
_____ c. bronchopneumonia	3. involves inflammatory responses within lung tissue surrounding air spaces and vascular structures
_____ d. lobar	4. lobes of both lungs
_____ e. alveolar	5. involves terminal bronchioles and alveoli
_____ f. bilateral	6. one or more segments of the lung
_____ g. interstitial	7. lobes in both lungs

5. Tubercles heal over a period of months by forming scars and calcified lesions known as
_____.

6. List the nine factors that contribute to TB becoming an active disease:
a.
b.
c.
d.
e.
f.
g.
h.
i.

7. The only physical finding that is specific for disseminated TB is _____
_____.

8. The incubation period for SARS is typically _____ to _____ days.

9. List four major types of lung cancer:
a.
b.
c.
d.

10. The most important risk factor for lung cancer is _____.

11. List the two major categories of lung cancer:
a.
b.

12. Match the following types of lung cancer resection with the correct description.

	Type of Resection		Description
_____	a. wedge	1.	removal of entire lobe
_____	b. segmental	2.	removal of entire lung
_____	c. lobectomy	3.	removal of small localized area
_____	d. pneumonectomy	4.	removal of one or more segments

13. The term _____ is used to indicate that the interstitium of the alveolar walls in thickened and usually fibrotic.

14. The _____ results in hypoxemia and carbon dioxide retention in the client with ILD.

15. Compare and contrast transudates and exudates.

16. If there is a high WBC count and the pleural fluid is purulent, the effusion is called an
_____.

17. List the four processes that can lead to a subdiaphragmatic abscess:
a.

b.

c.

d.

18. True or False

_____ TB infection is acquired by inhalation of a particle small enough to reach the alveolus.

_____ A primary TB infection is said to be when the client is exposed for the first time.

_____ Most clients know when exposure to TB occurred.

_____ NTM is most prevalent in the northeastern United States.

_____ Person-to-person transmission of fungal lung infections is virtually unknown.

_____ Lung cancer is the leading cause of cancer deaths in the United States.

_____ Lung diseases are among the most common occupational health problems.

_____ Obesity may lead to restrictive lung disorders.

_____ Cystic fibrosis is the most common inherited genetic disease in Caucasians.

_____ The cause of sarcoidosis is unknown.

_____ Clinical manifestations of ILD are insidious and nonspecific.

_____ Clinical manifestations of a subdiaphragmatic abscess include pleuritic pain or pain referred to the shoulder on the same side as the abscess.

_____ A classic manifestation of bilateral paralysis of the diaphragm is decreased dyspnea when the client is lying flat on the back.

APPLYING SKILLS

19. When auscultating the chest of a client with pneumonia, bronchial breath sounds occur over _____.

20. List the respiratory assessments the nurse performs on a client with pneumonia:
    a.

    b.

    c.

21. _____, rather than erythema, indicates a positive TB test.

22. Definitive diagnosis of TB is accomplished with _____ and _____.

23. List the clinical assessments that would alert the nurse to possible hemorrhaging in a client with closed chest drainage:
    a.

    b.

24. Differentiate between intermittent and continuous bubbling in the water-seal compartment.

25. What does rapid bubbling in the water-seal compartment indicate?

26. True or False

    _____ A 5 mm of induration on a TB skin test is positive for clients in low-risk groups.

BEST PRACTICES

27. When caring for an unconscious client with pneumonia, the nurse places the client in a _____ position.

28. List the nursing actions that prevent the spread of pneumonia in hospitalized clients:
    a.

    b.

    c.

    d.

29. Explain the rationale for instructing a client with a closed-chest drainage to cough and deep breathe.

30. List the three primary nursing goals for providing care for a client with restrictive lung disease:
    a.

    b.

    c.

31. List the interventions that help clear tracheobronchial secretions in a client with CF:
    a.

    b.

    c.

32. True or False

    _____ Persons with NTM are isolated to control infection.

    _____ Survival rates are best for NSCLC if treated in the early stages.

    _____ Closed-chest drainage is used after pneumonectomy.

    _____ The lower the height of the water column in the suction chamber, the more suction.

    _____ Closed-chest drainage systems must always be placed lower than the client's chest.

    _____ In most situations, clamping of chest tubes is contraindicated.

    _____ The removal of chest tubes is a painful procedure.

KEEPING DRUG SKILLS SHARP

33. For anti-influenza medications to be effective, they must be administered within
_____ of onset.

34. When a TB program of treatment fails, how many medications are added?

35. The intravenous antibiotic typically used to treat pulmonary fungal infections is
_____.

36. _____ are medications are used to control inflammation in clients with ILD.

Management of Clients with Acute Pulmonary Disorders

OBJECTIVES

65.1   Discuss the pathophysiology, clinical manifestations, outcome management, and nursing care of clients with non-traumatic acute pulmonary disorders.

65.2   Discuss the pathophysiology, clinical manifestations, outcome management, and nursing care of clients with traumatic acute pulmonary disorders.

65.3   Discuss ARDS including underlying pathophysiology, clinical manifestations, outcome management, and nursing care.

UNDERSTANDING PATHOPHYSIOLOGY

1.   The most important function of the respiratory system is to provide the body tissues with _____ and to remove _____.

2.   Compare and contrast hypoxemic versus ventilatory failure.

Hypoxemic	Ventilatory

3.   List two underlying causes of elevated $PaCO_2$ related to alveolar hypoventilation in clients with acute respiratory failure:

a.

b.

4. A noncardiogenic cause of pulmonary edema is:
   1. mitral valve stenosis.
   2. shock.
   3. pneumonia.
   4. hypertension.

5. The hallmark of ventilatory failure is an elevated level of _____.

6. The phenomenon of systolic blood pressure falling more than 10 mm Hg during inspiration is called _____.

7. The most common physiologic change that occurs when a client is placed on mechanical ventilation is _____.

8. Which of the following may contribute directly to intensive care unit psychosis?
   1. respiratory acidosis
   2. respiratory alkalosis
   3. elevated vasopressin levels
   4. cerebral edema

9. Clinical manifestations of oxygen toxicity include: (Select all that apply)
   1. insomnia.
   2. weakness.
   3. nausea and vomiting.
   4. tachypnea.
   5. increased energy.
   6. hiccoughs.

10. Factors that contribute to the development of ARDS include: (Select all that apply)
    1. ischemia during shock.
    2. oxygen toxicity.
    3. inhalation of noxious fumes.
    4. inflammation from pneumonia.
    5. positive pressure ventilation.

11. Complete the following critical path that depicts the hallmark of ARDS.
    (↑ = increases, → = leads to, ↓ = decreases)

    Massive _____ by the lungs that
    _____ movement of fluid into the
    _____ and
    _____ spaces which
    _____ pulmonary edema which
    _____ and impairs
    _____.

12. Destruction of the _____ cells results in a decrease in _____ production.

13. Deposition of _____ into the lung contributes to pulmonary fibrosis in Phase 3 ARDS.

14. The two earliest clinical manifestations of ARDS are _____
    and _____ 12 to 24 hours after the initial injury.

15. Major dangers associated with chest injuries are _____
    and _____.

16. List the five potential causes of ventilation-perfusion imbalance in clients with chest trauma:
    a.

    b.

    c.

    d.

    e.

17. A clinical manifestation of rib fracture is:
    1. generalized pain and tenderness.
    2. deep respirations.
    3. client tendency to hold the chest protectively.
    4. clicking sensation during exhalation.

18. Pneumothorax is the presence of _____ in the
    _____ space that prohibits complete lung expansion.

19. The two classifications of pneumothorax are _____ and
    _____.

20. A risk factor for spontaneous pneumothorax is:
    1. thoracentesis.
    2. fall.
    3. motor vehicle accident.
    4. tuberculosis.

21. A clinical manifestation of moderate pneumothorax is:
    1. bradypnea.
    2. dyspnea.
    3. dull pain on the affected side.
    4. symmetrical chest expansion.

22. A clinical manifestation of severe pneumothorax is:
    1. distended neck veins.
    2. increased tactile fremitus.
    3. trachea in midline.
    4. dullness to percussion.

23. A clinical manifestations of a tension pneumothorax is:
    1. mild dyspnea.
    2. bradycardia.
    3. progressive cyanosis.
    4. bradypnea.

24. A risk factor that increases the potential of near drowning is:
    1. alcohol ingestion.
    2. hyperglycemia.
    3. hypoventilation.
    4. eating immediately before swimming.

25. True or False

    _____ Increased volume of fluid in the pulmonary arteries from obstruction of forward flow is the most common cause of pulmonary edema.

    _____ Subcutaneous emphysema is a risk of PEEP.

    _____ Positive pressure ventilation during the inspiratory phase can lead to a decreased blood flow to the splanchnic area and ischemia of the gastric mucosa.

    _____ Clinical manifestations of respiratory muscle fatigue include a respiratory rate more than 20 breaths per minute.

    _____ An additional benefit of the prone position is better draining of bronchial secretions.

    _____ The most probable cause of shock in the chest-injured client is hypovolemia.

    _____ A flail chest consists of fractures of two or more ribs on the same side and possibly the sternum.

APPLYING SKILLS

26. Which of the following two assessments verify correct ET tube placement? (Select all that apply)
    1. feeling air through the ET tube during exhalation
    2. client is unable to talk
    3. auscultation of breath sounds bilaterally
    4. chest x-ray

27. The amount of air required to seal an ET tube cuff is reflected by the cuff pressure, which is usually maintained at less than _____ mm Hg.

28. All of the following meet diagnostic criteria for ARDS except:
    1. delayed onset.
    2. bilateral infiltrates.
    3. ratio of PaO_2 and FiO_2 ≤ 200 mm Hg.
    4. PAWP ≤ 18 mg Hg.

29. List the priority assessments of any client with chest trauma:
    a.

    b.

    c.

30. In the client with flail chest, breath sounds are either _____
    or _____ on the affected side.

BEST PRACTICES

31. An intervention aimed at reducing preload is:
    1. oxygen therapy with continuous positive airway pressure.
    2. diuretic therapy.
    3. antihypertensive drugs.
    4. intra-aortic balloon pump.

32. Which of the following is an expected outcome for intervention for a client with a nursing diagnosis of impaired gas exchange related to capillary membrane obstruction from fluid?
    1. capillary refill $\geq$ 3 seconds
    2. decreased peripheral edema
    3. O_2 saturation > 90 %
    4. weight loss

33. State the rationale for keeping the client's legs in a dependent position when he or she has pulmonary edema.

34. Match each type of ventilator with the appropriate description.

Type of Ventilator	Description
_____ a. pressure-cycled	1. terminates when a preset inspiratory time has elapsed
_____ b. volume-cycled	2. triggered to stop when a preset flow rate has been achieved
_____ c. time-cycled	3. delivers a preset tidal volume of inspired gas
_____ d. flow-cycled	4. delivers a volume of gas to the airway using positive pressure during inspiration

35. Match each type of inhalation with the appropriate description.

Type of Inhalation	Description
_____ a. volume-triggered	1. used to manage clients who cannot breathe on their own
_____ b. flow-triggered	2. triggered by the initial negative pressure that begins inspiration
_____ c. negative pressure	3. occurs when the client can initiate a breath
_____ d. time-triggered	4. occurs when the ventilator completes the breath to maximize inhaled gas

36. Differentiate between CPAP and PEEP.

37. Compare and contrast the rapid versus gradual (slow) weaning process.

38. Explain the rationale for placing clients with ARDS in the prone position.

39. Essential nursing activities to keep the family of an ARDS client adequately informed include
_____ and _____.

40. The treatment of choice for the client with flail chest is intubation with mechanical ventilation. Indicate below if the therapeutic effect of ventilation is increased or decreased for each of the following parameters.
    a. hypoxia:
    b. hypercapnia:
    c. paradoxical motion:
    d. pain:

41. True or False

    _____ In the client with acute ventilatory failure, mechanical ventilation is an early intervention.

    _____ One criteria for a weaning trial is a tidal volume $\geq$ 325 ml.

    _____ Mechanical ventilation, ET intubation, and PEEP are usually required to maintain adequate blood oxygen levels.

    _____ Strapping the ribs is the treatment of choice for rib fracture.

KEEPING DRUG SKILLS SHARP

42. Which of the following medications is a beta$_2$ agonist given to reverse bronchospasm?
    1. ipratropium
    2. theophylline
    3. corticosteroid
    4. albuterol

43. The most common neuromuscular blocking agents given to clients on ventilation are
_____ and _____.

44. The actions of nitric oxide include: (Select all that apply)
    1. selective vasodilation in the pulmonary vascular system.
    2. bronchoconstriction.
    3. reduced pressure in the pulmonary arteries.
    4. increased systemic blood pressure.

45. A desired therapeutic effect of dobutamine in the ARDS client is:
    1. improved cardiac output.
    2. decrease in cardiac output.
    3. decrease in systemic blood pressure.
    4. decrease in preload.

46. Narcotics administered to the client with chest injury to control pain are most effective if administered via:
    1. PO.
    2. IM.
    3. per patch.
    4. IV.

47. True or False

    _____ Surfactant therapy has been successful in adults with ARDS.

    _____ Clinical trials have demonstrated the effectiveness of steroid administration in ARDS.

CONCEPT MAP EXERCISES

The following questions are based on the concept map *Understanding ARDS and Its Treatment* in the textbook.

48. Which of the following directly decrease lung compliance?
    1. ventilation-perfusion mismatch
    2. decreased surfactant production
    3. release of vasoactive substances
    4. atelectasis

49. Hemoptysis is a result of:
    1. ventilation-perfusion mismatch.
    2. increased permeability of alveolar membrane.
    3. damage to alveolar epithelium.
    4. protein movement into the alveoli.

50. Which position improves ventilation and perfusion in the client with ARDS?
    1. dorsal recumbent
    2. semi-Fowler's
    3. Sims' lateral
    4. prone

Assessment of the Eyes and Ears

OBJECTIVES

66.1 Discuss the important components required when obtaining an ophthalmic history from a client.

66.2 Describe the procedure for performing an ophthalmic examination.

66.3 Discuss common diagnostic tests used to assess both external and internal structures of the eye.

66.4 Discuss the important components when obtaining an otologic history from a client.

66.5 Describe the procedure for performing a physical examination of the ear.

66.6 Discuss common diagnostic tests for hearing and balance.

ANATOMY & PHYSIOLOGY REVIEW

1. Label the structures of the eye.

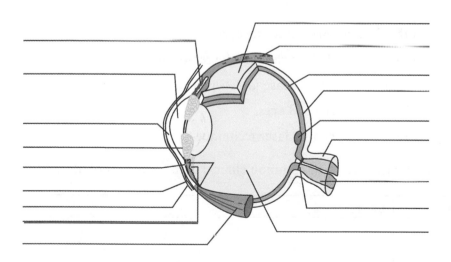

2. Label the structures of the ear.

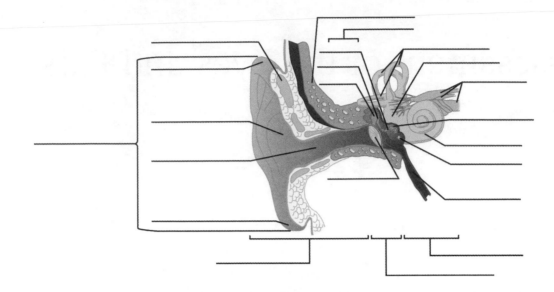

UNDERSTANDING PATHOPHYSIOLOGY

3. The three most common preventable causes of permanent vision loss are:
    1. nystagmus.
    2. amblyopia.
    3. diplopia.
    4. glaucoma.
    5. diabetic retinopathy.
    6. "floaters."
    7. age-related maculopathy.
    8. strabismus.

4. True or False

    _____ Reading in the dark is harmful to the eyes.

    _____ Cataracts must "ripen" before they can be removed.

    _____ Emotional stress does not increase intraocular pressure.

    _____ Children will outgrow crossed eyes.

    _____ Cataracts are not removed by laser technique.

5. Compare and contrast the causes of common clinical manifestations of abnormal vision.

Manifestation	Cause
Glare/halo	
Flashing/flickering lights	

Floating spots	
Diplopia	

6. Compare and contrast the possible causes of common hearing complaints.

Complaint	Possible Cause
Hearing loss	
Pain	
Ear drainage	
Tinnitus	
Loss of balance	

7. Exposure to noise at a level greater than _____ can cause cochlear damage and hearing loss.

8. _____ results from blockage of normal sound conduction through ear canal.

9. _____ results from damage to the acoustic nerve.

10. A client with normal hearing ability has _____% or more hearing, depending on age.

APPLYING SKILLS

11. A thorough ophthalmic assessment is different from the assessment of other body systems because many ophthalmic disorders are _____
_____.

12. State the clinical significance of each disorder when taking a client's ophthalmic history.
Hypertension:

Multiple sclerosis:

Myasthenia gravis:

Thyroid disorders:

Rheumatoid arthritis:

Diabetes mellitus:

13. During an examination of the eyelids the nurse notes that the upper lids rest at the top of the iris and the lower lids rest at the bottom, so that the sclerae is not visible. This finding is considered _____.

14. To test the functioning of the trigeminal cranial nerve, the nurse would perform the _____ test.

15. Upon examination of the cornea of an older client, the nurse notes *arcus senilis*. This finding is considered _____.

16. When examining the iris of the eye at an oblique angle, it should appear _____ and _____.

17. The pupil should _____ when the client looks at an object far away and _____ when the client looks at a near object.

18. The Hirschberg's test determines the _____ function of the eye.

19. _____ is used to assess intraocular pressure and screen for glaucoma.

20. Normal range for intraocular pressure is between _____ and _____ mm Hg.

21. List the three areas of assessment during physical examination of the ear:
    a.
    b.
    c.

22. Tophi, deposits of uric acid that form hard nodules in the helix of the ear, are characteristic of:
    1. Meniere's disease
    2. gout
    3. glaucoma
    4. Sjögren's syndrome

23. Identify the purpose of each of the following tests:

Test	Purpose
Weber test	
Rinne test	
Romberg test	

BEST PRACTICES

24. State the procedure that must be performed prior to application of the tonometer.

25. State the instructions the nurse would give to a client after completing an examination of both internal and external structures of the eye.

26. Electrocochleography is used to evaluate the presence of _____, which involves disabling problems with balance.

27. A client reports clear drainage from his ear. Identify the clinical significance of the drainage and state the appropriate nursing action.

KEEPING DRUG SKILLS SHARP

28. Medications that are ototoxic and can cause hearing loss in nontherapeutic levels include: (Select all that apply)
    1. aminoglycosides.
    2. antiprotozoal agents.
    3. aspirin.
    4. chemotherapeutic agents.
    5. salicylates.

29. Prior to beginning an intravenous pyelogram (IVP), the medication _____ may be given prophylactically for possible allergic reactions to the contrast dye.

30. Identify the possible drug interactions that can occur from the use of over-the-counter eye medications.

Management of Clients with Visual Disorders

OBJECTIVES

67.1 Identify common clinical manifestations of clients experiencing glaucoma and cataracts.

67.2 Describe nursing care and medical/surgical management of clients with glaucoma and cataracts.

67.3 Describe nursing care and medical/surgical management of other visual disorders.

67.4 Describe nursing care and medical/surgical management of ocular manifestations of systemic disorders.

UNDERSTANDING PATHOPHYSIOLOGY

1. Manifestations that characterize glaucoma include all of the following except:
   1. increased intraocular pressure.
   2. optic nerve atrophy.
   3. visual field loss.
   4. dry eyes.

2. Compare and contrast between the various types of glaucoma:

Type	Cause	Manifestations
Primary Open Angle		
Angle-Closure		
Normal Tension		
Secondary		

3. List the common causes of primary open-angle glaucoma:
   a.

   b.

   c.

   d.

4. Risk factors for the development of cataracts include: (Select all that apply)
   1. diabetes.
   2. Down syndrome.
   3. living at low altitudes.
   4. retinal detachment.
   5. blunt trauma.
   6. lacerations.
   7. radiation.
   8. chronic use of corticosteroids.
   9. working in dim lighting.
   10. glass-blower or welder without eye protection.

5. True or False

   _____ The leading cause of blindness worldwide is trauma to the eye.

6. Age-related macular degeneration affects _____ vision.

7. Compare and contrast between "dry" and "wet" macular degeneration:

Type	Etiology	Manifestations
Dry		
Wet		

8. Common causes of keratitis include: (Select all that apply)
   1. dry eyes.
   2. ineffective eyelid closure (i.e., comatose client).
   3. retinal detachment.
   4. systemic collagen order (i.e., rheumatoid arthritis).

9. Compare and contrast the follosing common refractive disorders:

Type	Etiology	Manifestations
Myopia		
Hyperopia		
Astigmatism		

APPLYING SKILLS

10. The range for normal intraocular pressure is between _____ and _____ mm Hg.

11. Intraocular pressure is highest upon _____ during a diurnal cycle.

12. True or False

    _____ Clients with cataracts will experience blurred vision, photophobia, and glare.

    _____ Cataracts cause a dull, aching pain, especially at night.

    _____ Secondary glaucoma is a result of the edema caused by removal of a cataract.

    _____ Only serous drainage is expected following eye surgery.

    _____ If the red reflex is absent during opthalmoscopic examination, the nurse should suspect cataracts.

13. A client reports a shadow or "curtain falling across the field of vision." This is a classic manifestation of _____.

14. Identify the common ocular manifestations for each of the following systemic disorders:
    a. Graves' disease:

    b. Rheumatoid arthritis/connective tissue disorder:

c. SLE (lupus):

d. Myasthenia gravis:

e. Multiple sclerosis:

f. Hypertension:

g. AIDS:

h. Lyme disease:

BEST PRACTICES

15. Nursing interventions to assist the client in coping with vision loss due to glaucoma include: (Select all that apply)
    1. Recognizing that the client is experiencing grief over the loss and will be anxious during examinations fearing discovery of more problems.
    2. Counseling the client to prepare to accept further vision loss even with treatment.
    3. Assisting the client in identifying effective coping skills used in the past.
    4. Maintaining professional relationship with the client, using therapeutic communication to express empathy.
    5. Allowing the client to verbalize feelings regarding visual problems/loss.

16. It imperative for the nurse to intervene to calm an anxious client with glaucoma, because increased anxiety raises _____, which further increases intraocular pressure.

17. Nursing interventions for the client with glaucoma should include all of the following except:
    1. Determine the client's level of understanding.
    2. Use diagrams or pictures to help illustrate important points.
    3. Written information should be in colored ink so the client may read it more easily.
    4. Validate the client's ability to administer eye drops through a return demonstration.

18. State the rationale for the nurse instructing a client to promptly report any nausea or vomiting after cataract removal.

19. List two emergency interventions for the client who has developed retinal artery occlusion and state the rationale for each:
    a.

    b.

20. Nursing interventions to promote comfort for the client receiving treatment for keratitis include: (Select all that apply)
    1. cleansing the eyelids of excessive tears and medications.
    2. applying antibiotic ophthalmic ointment to lower lid margin and cheek to reduce irritation.
    3. identifying rest periods when client will not be disturbed except for eye drops.
    4. giving topical analgesics given at regular intervals.
    5. administering mild sleeping medication at bedtime.

21. True or False

    _____ Removal of a cataract and insertion of an intraocular lens (IOL) requires no stitches.

    _____ A scleral buckle is used to hold the new IOL in place until healed.

    _____ An intraocular lens does not provide the same visual acuity as the natural lens of the eye.

    _____ Clients who have had pneumatic retinopexy should avoid air travel.

    _____ A laser beam can burn the edges of a retinal tear to halt its progression

    _____ Scleral buckling uses silicone bands to hold a retinal tear in place.

KEEPING DRUG SKILLS SHARP

22. Compare and contrast common eye medications used to control glaucoma in clients.

Medication	Dosage	Teaching Points for Client
pilocarpine (Pilcar) (cholinergic)		
timolol (Timoptic)		
carbonic anhydrase inhibitor (Diamox) (diuretic)		

23. _____ help to reduce IOP for the client with glaucoma by acting to constrict the pupil, which opens the canal of Schlemm and aids in drainage of aqueous humor.

24. _____ are prescribed for clients with narrow-angle glaucoma because they reduce the production of aqueous humor and thereby reduce IOP.

25. State the rationale for administering Ismotic instead of Osmoglyn to a diabetic client with an emergency situation of IOP.

26. Nursing responsibilities when infusing IV mannitol to a client include: (Select all that apply)
    1. evaluating cardiovascular and renal status due to diuretic effect of medications.
    2. documenting baseline vital signs before and frequently during infusion.
    3. placing bottle of medication in refrigerator unit for 10 minutes before administering.
    4. placing an in-line filter to prevent infusion of crystal particles.

27. True or False

    _____ Use of beta-blockers and steroids will help to correct cataracts.

    _____ Mydriacyl is used preoperatively to dilate the eyes for removal of a cataract.

    _____ To facilitate the removal of a cataract, the physician may order Cyclogyl, a paralyzing agent for the ciliary muscles.

28. Research has shown that all of the following supplements may help to delay macular degeneration except:
    1. high-dose vitamin C.
    2. high-dose vitamin E.
    3. beta carotene.
    4. iron.
    5. zinc.

Management of Clients with Hearing and Balance Disorders

OBJECTIVES

68.1   Identify common clinical manifestations of clients experiencing hearing disorders.

68.2   Describe nursing care and medical/surgical management of clients with hearing disorders.

68.3   Identify common clinical manifestations of clients experiencing balance disorders.

68.4   Describe nursing care and medical/surgical management of balance disorders.

UNDERSTANDING PATHOPHYSIOLOGY

1.   _____ is the nation's primary disability, affecting 1 in 15 Americans.

2.   Compare and contrast the main types of hearing loss:

Type	Cause	Results
Conductive		
Sensorineural		
Mixed hearing loss		

3.   The most common cause of obstruction of the ear is _____
_____.

4. _____ is a common disorder of the middle ear.

5. Causative factors that result in rupture of the tympanic membrane include: (Select all that apply)
   1. hand slap.
   2. falling in water.
   3. allergic reaction.
   4. high doses of vitamin E.
   5. sports injuries.
   6. cleaning ear with sharp instrument.
   7. welding sparks.
   8. elevated blood pressure.

6. _____ is a type of sensorineural hearing loss that affects older people.

7. Causative factors for sudden hearing loss include all of the following except:
   1. excess cerumen.
   2. rapid infectious processes (meningitis).
   3. ototoxic agents.
   4. trauma.
   5. metabolic disturbances.
   6. immunologic disorders.

8. Common manifestations of hearing loss in a client include: (Select all that apply)
   1. failure to respond to oral communication.
   2. inappropriate response to oral communication.
   3. excessively soft speech.
   4. constant need for clarification of conversation.
   5. listening to radio or television at increasing volume.

9. Sources of infection that can result in otalgia include: (Select all that apply)
   1. insertion of unclean articles into ear.
   2. insertion of anything sharp into ear canal.
   3. instilling contaminated solutions into ear.
   4. swimming in polluted water.
   5. recent upper respiratory infection.
   6. allergies.

10. True or False

    _____ Bullous myringitis is an inflammatory disease that forms blisters on the tympanic membrane.

    _____ Serous otitis media is associated with damage to the pinna.

    _____ Drainage from mastoiditis travels through the middle ear and out the tympanic membrane.

    _____ Cholesteatoma, a type of conductive hearing loss, results from large deposits of cholesterol in the middle ear.

    _____ Perichondral hematomas can develop into a hypertrophic scar known as "cauliflower ear."

_____ Pain from disorders of the tympanic membrane is more painful than disorders of the middle ear.

11. Compare and contrast common types of peripheral vestibular disorders:

Disorder	Cause	Manifestations
Benign paroxysmal positional vertigo		
Labyrinthitis		
Meniere's disease		

12. List the four components necessary to maintain balance:
   a.

   b.

   c.

   d.

APPLYING SKILLS

13. A nurse is assessing a client with hearing loss using the Rinne and Weber tests. State the findings the nurse could expect for each test if there is hearing loss:
   a. Rinne test:

   b. Weber test:

14. Identify the method of assessment the nurse uses to determine if pain reported by a client is from external otitis or from otitis media.

15. A client experiencing a middle ear infection may report all of the following sensations except:
    1. bubbling.
    2. popping.
    3. crackling.
    4. sense of fullness.
    5. pain.
    6. total hearing loss.

16. The nurse should be aware that a _____ may appear to be vertigo, because the temporary loss of blood flow to the brain can cause manifestations similar to balance disorders.

BEST PRACTICES

17. Compare and contrast the three levels of prevention for hearing loss:

Level	Focus	Plans	Interventions
Primary			
Secondary			
Tertiary			

18. Identify an outcome and interventions for the nursing diagnosis Impaired verbal communication related to effects of hearing loss:
    OUTCOME:

    INTERVENTIONS:

19. A client may have trouble coping with the loss of hearing. Appropriate nursing interventions to assist the client include all of the following except:
    1. teaching client to inform others of hearing impairment.
    2. instructing client to request that others communicate by using techniques that improve comprehension.
    3. instructing client to limit social contact with others outside of family.
    4. teaching client to avoid noisy areas that impair hearing.

20. Appropriate postoperative instructions for a client who has undergone a stapedectomy include which of the following? (Select all that apply)
    1. lie on non-operative ear with HOB elevated
    2. surgical packing in ear should not be disturbed
    3. exercise regularly
    4. blow nose gently, one nostril at a time
    5. sneeze with mouth closed
    6. no airplane travel for 1 month

21. List two nursing actions to be completed prior to instilling antibiotic solution into the ear:
    a.

    b.

22. A critical teaching point the nurse should stress to the client receiving antibiotics for an ear infection is that the client must _____ the prescription after the manifestations have cleared.

23. A 23-year-old college student has been admitted due to a complicated sinus infection that also involves his ears. He calls to the nurse's station complaining of discomfort that will not allow him to rest. In addition to medications ordered for pain, interventions the nurse can implement at the bedside to relieve ear pain include: (Select all that apply)
    1. application of cool compress to ear.
    2. soft diet.
    3. quiet environment.
    4. positioning client with affected ear down.

KEEPING DRUG SKILLS SHARP

24. Because the cause is usually viral infection of the inner ear, _____ are often administered to clients who experience sudden hearing loss.

25. An ear solution of _____ is often prescribed because it is a drying agent that cleans the ear of debris and infection.

26. Methods used to remove a live insect from the ear canal include: (Select all that apply)
    1. mineral oil.
    2. mineral water.
    3. lidocaine.
    4. ether-soaked cotton ball.

Chapter 69

Assessment of the Neurologic System

OBJECTIVES

69.1 Discuss the important components required when obtaining a neurologic history from a client.

69.2 Describe the process for performing a physical examination of the neurologic system.

69.3 Identify common diagnostic tests used to assess the neurologic system.

69.4 Describe nursing responsibilities when caring for a client undergoing invasive testing of the neurologic system.

ANATOMY & PHYSIOLOGY REVIEW

1. Label the structures of the brain.

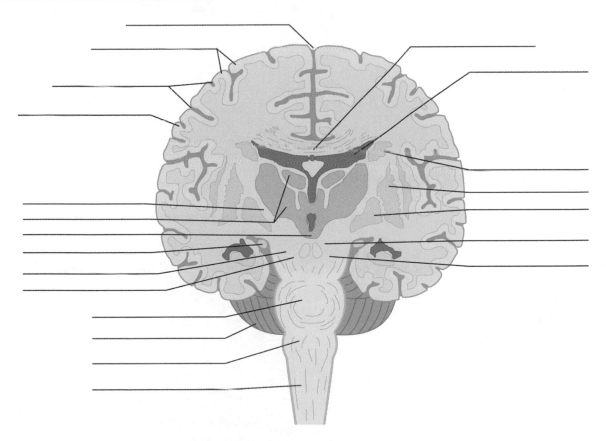

2. Label the parts of a neuron.

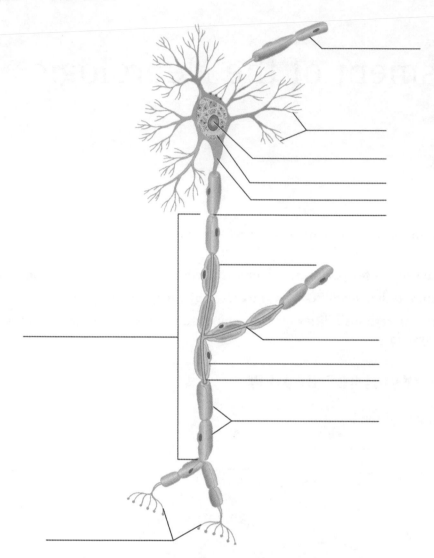

UNDERSTANDING PATHOPHYSIOLOGY

3. The absence of superficial reflexes on one side of the body may be due to the effects of

_____.

4. Childhood diseases that can cause a neurologic sequelae include all of the following except:
   1. rubella.
   2. rubeola.
   3. cytomegalovirus infection.
   4. herpes simplex.
   5. chicken pox.
   6. influenza.
   7. meningitis.

APPLYING SKILLS

5. Identify the clinical significance for each of the areas of the neurologic history.

Area	Clinical significance
Growth and development	
Family health history	
Psychosocial history	

6. _____ is the most sensitive indicator of changes in the neurologic status of a client.

7. An 82-year-old nursing home resident has been admitted to the hospital due to changes in her level of consciousness. As part of her neurologic examination the nurse will assess her orientation to: (Select all that apply)
   1. time.
   2. place.
   3. person.
   4. event/situation.

8. A nurse assess intellectual performance of a client by asking him or her to count by _____ or _____.

9. List the four assessment techniques to examine the head, neck, and spine of a client with a possible neurologic problem.
   a.
   b.
   c.
   d.

10. _____ are dark circles around the eyes caused by periorbital ecchymosis from an anterior basal skull fracture.

11. A 32-year-old computer programmer has come to the clinic with complaints of fatigue, fever, and malaise. When assessing the neurologic system the nurse will ask him to flex his neck, with the chin touching the chest. This technique is used to check for _____ _____, a manifestation of meningitis.

12. Compare and contrast each of the cranial nerves. Identify the function and testing method for each during physical examination of the client.

Cranial Nerve	Function	Testing Method
I		
II		
III, IV, VI		
V		
VII		
VIII		
IX, X		
XI		
XII		

13. A 52-year-old school teacher has come to the clinic with complaints of dizziness. Identify the technique the nurse will use to assess proprioception as part of the physical examination.

14. Compare and contrast testing of the following types of discrimination:

Type	Method of testing
Stereognosis	
Graphesthesia	
Extinction phenomenon	
Two-point simulation	

15. A positive _____ reflex in an adult client indicates significant neurologic problems with transmission of impulses through the spinal cord to higher neuro areas.

16. True or False

_____ Patellar reflex is done by tapping the inside aspect of the arm.

_____ The "snout reflex" is normal in infants but abnormal in adults.

_____ A positive result for testing for the "sucking reflex" is abnormal in adults.

_____ To check for the "chewing reflex" the client is offered a small piece of soft food and observed.

_____ Placing an object in the palm of the hand and curling fingers around it is a positive result of the grasp reflex.

17. Doppler ultrasonography can be used to measure _____.

18. EEG is a measurement of the electrical activity of the cerebral cortex and a defining criteria for _____.

BEST PRACTICES

19. State the rationale for requiring a nurse to accompany a client with a possible neurologic problem to the radiology department for testing.

20. An 18-year-old female client injured in a motor vehicle accident arrives at the hospital via ambulance and is rushed to the radiology department for x-rays. Because it does not require any movement on the part of the client and can help determine whether fractures have occurred, the _____ view x-ray is taken first.

21. Spinal immobilization devices must remain in place on a client with a suspected injury until _____.

22. A client is scheduled for magnetic resonance imaging to assess the cause of frequent headaches. The nurse would instruct the client to remove all _____ objects before the test.

23. A 66-year-old client with diabetes mellitus is scheduled to undergo a PET scan to analyze the effects of a recent stroke. In addition to client education, the nurse should confirm that the client's blood glucose level is below _____ mg/dl prior to the test.

24. List the potential postoperative complications the nurse should assess for in a client who has undergone a lumbar puncture:
    a.

    b.

25. For each nursing action to assist during a lumbar puncture, describe the rationale:
    a. Client on side with back close to edge of bed:

    b. Place pillow under flank:

    c. Place pillow between knees and under head:

    d. Ask client to draw up knees to abdomen:

    e. Nurse places hand on one knee and the other around the neck of client:

26. A 22-year-old college student has just undergone a lumbar puncture. She is resting quietly in her hospital bed and her vital signs are stable. The nurse brings in a large water pitcher and glass, encouraging her to drink large quantities of fluids. State the rationale for administering additional PO fluids to a stable client.

KEEPING DRUG SKILLS SHARP

27. State the rationale for a radiologist asking a client if he or she has an allergy to shellfish prior to administering radiopaque contrast dye.

28. State the rationale for documenting the use of over-the-counter medications and herbal remedies when assessing a client with neurologic problems.

Chapter 70

Management of Comatose or Confused Clients

OBJECTIVES

70.1   Describe etiology and clinical manifestations of disorders of consciousness.

70.2   Discuss various diagnostic tests to evaluate disorders of consciousness.

70.3   Describe nursing care and medical management of the comatose client.

70.4   Discuss nursing care to prevent complications due to altered consciousness of the comatose client.

70.5   Describe etiology and clinical manifestations of common types of confusion, including delirium and dementia.

70.6   Describe nursing care and medical management of the confused client.

UNDERSTANDING PATHOPHYSIOLOGY

1. _____ place pressure on brain stem or structures within the posterior cranial fossa.

2. _____ impair wakefulness by reducing supply of oxygen and glucose, allowing waste products to accumulate in brain.

3. True or False

   _____ Most metabolic comas originate in systems outside the brain.

4. Asterixis is a manifestation of a _____ coma.

5. When muscle groups are not used during periods of immobility, _____ develop.

6. List the three memory impairments that occur with dementia:
   a.

   b.

   c.

7. For each clinical manifestation of confusion, provide an example of a client behavior:

Manifestation	Example
Disorder of attention	
Fluctuations in cognition	
Loss of memory for recent events	
Perceptual errors	

8. State the rationale for using the term "*patient*" when referring to a client who is comatose.

APPLYING SKILLS

9. A client is in a comatose state, receiving enteral feedings. The nurse notes small, frequent liquid stools, which may indicate _____.

10. Conditions a patient must exhibit to be considered "in a coma" include: (Select all that apply)
    1. no response to verbal stimuli.
    2. varying responses to painful stimuli.
    3. no voluntary movements.
    4. altered respiratory patterns.
    5. altered pupillary responses to light.
    6. repeated blinking.

11. The presence of the _____ reflex in the comatose patient indicates that brain stem functioning is preserved.

12. Initial assessment of a comatose patient includes: (Select all that apply)
    1. level of consciousness.
    2. presence/absence of neurologic manifestations.
    3. pupil size and reactivity to light.
    4. deep tendon reflexes.
    5. response to noxious stimuli.
    6. evidence of trauma.
    7. lab values if metabolic coma is suspected.
    8. history from significant other.

13. Absence of pupillary, corneal, or oculovestibular responses in the comatose patient is highly predictive of _____.

14. The _____ Scale is the most common neurologic assessment tool used in clinical practice.

15. Characteristics of *confusion* include all of the following except:
    1. alterations in thought.
    2. attention deficit.
    3. loss of long-term memory.
    4. irritability alternating with drowsiness.

BEST PRACTICES

16. State the appropriate nursing action for prevention of corneal abrasions in the comatose patient.

17. True or False

    _____ Comatose patients may have sips and ice chips in high Fowler's position.

    _____ After suctioning the trachea, the nurse may use the same suction catheter for oral or pharyngeal suctioning but not vice versa.

    _____ If the patient has facial paralysis, position him or her with the affected side up.

    _____ Dried mucous may form, break off, and be aspirated in the comatose patient.

    _____ Suctioning of a comatose patient is limited to no more than 30 seconds of suctioning time to prevent hypoxia.

18. The nurse should place the recovering comatose patient in the _____ position to test the gag reflex.

19. State the appropriate nursing action for switching a client from tube feedings to oral feedings.

20. After checking the residual volume of a tube feeding on a comatose patient, the nurse notes 75 ml residual volume. State the action the nurse should take after making this observation.

21. An 82-year-old client has been admitted to the hospital for treatment. After assisting the patient to her room, the nurse notices her wandering around the hallways. The client is assisted back to her room. Nursing interventions to assist this confused client would include: (Select all that apply)
    1. reorient patient as often as necessary.
    2. placing clocks and calendars in the hospital room.
    3. using familiar objects from home.
    4. reducing unfamiliar noises.
    5. using bright lighting.
    6. allowing restful sleep at night without unnecessary interruptions.
    7. administering sedatives.

22. Compare and contrast management and delegation of tasks for providing an enteral feeding to a comatose patient:

Task	Responsibility	Can RN Delegate?
Verification of MD order		
Verification of placement of feeding tube		
Reconstitution of feeding		
Preparation of feeding		
Priming the feeding pump		
Irrigation of feeding tube		
Tube site care		
Monitoring fluid/nutritional balance		

KEEPING DRUG SKILLS SHARP

23. Seizures from an overdose of cocaine are treated with _____.

24. Identify the nursing action that should be performed prior to administering a diuretic to a comatose patient.

25. Administration of seizure medications be accurately timed in order to maintain high _____.

Chapter 71

Management of Clients with Cerebral Disorders

OBJECTIVES

71.1 Describe etiology and clinical manifestations of various seizure disorders.

71.2 Discuss nursing care and medical/surgical management of the client experiencing seizure disorders.

71.3 Describe etiology and clinical manifestations of brain tumors.

71.4 Discuss nursing care and medical/surgical management of the client experiencing brain tumors.

71.5 Identify etiology and clinical manifestations of other types of cerebral disorders, including aneurysms, hemorrhage, and structural malformations.

71.6 Discuss etiology and clinical manifestations of various types of headaches.

71.7 Describe nursing care and medical management of the client experiencing headaches.

UNDERSTANDING PATHOPHYSIOLOGY

1. A _____ is a sudden, abnormal electrical discharge from the brain.

2. _____ is a chronic disorder of recurrent seizures.

3. Identify the mechanism for development of severe hypoxia and lactic acidosis in brain tissue during seizures.

4. For each area of the brain, identify the clinical manifestations of seizure activity originating in that area.

Area of Brain	Manifestations
Parietal region	
Occipital region	
Posterior temporal area	
Anterior temporal lobe	

5. Tonic-clonic seizures, formerly known as "grand mal" seizures, follow a pattern of manifestations. Place the manifestations in the correct order according to this pattern:

_____ a. tonic phase

_____ b. postictal phase

_____ c. aura

_____ d. sudden loss of consciousness

_____ e. clonic phase

6. True or False

_____ Most primary brain tumors do not metastasize out of the brain to other areas.

_____ Brain tumors are space-occupying lesions and the compression of tissue causes a decrease in intracranial pressure.

_____ Astrocytomas are the most common type of glial cell tumor.

_____ Oligodendrogliomas are slow-growing and calcify, making them recognizable on x-ray studies.

_____ A meningioma is a rapid growing malignant tumor of the spinal cord.

_____ Acoustic neuromas affect the sense of balance and can cause dizziness, tinnitus, and unilateral hearing loss.

7. For each area of the brain, identify the clinical manifestations that would develop due to a brain tumor in that area.

Area of Brain	Manifestations
Frontal lobe	
Temporal lobe	
Parietal lobe	
Occipital lobe	
Cerebellar	
Brain stem	
Pituitary/ hypothalamus	
Ventricle	

8. Conditions that can accelerate development of an intracranial aneurysm include all of the following except:
   1. hypotension.
   2. atherosclerosis.
   3. aging.
   4. stress.

9. Compare and contrast the common types of headaches.

Type	Etiology	Manifestation
Tension		
Cluster		
Migraine		

APPLYING SKILLS

10. A major diagnostic tool for assessment of clients with suspected epilepsy is
_____.

11. A client has been admitted to the hospital with a possible seizure disorder. While he is undergoing diagnostic testing, the nursing staff are instructed to closely observe any clinical manifestations during the seizure. State the rationale for observing a client during a seizure.

12. Explain how the nurse can differentiate between actual seizures and "pseudoseizures" which occur in clients with psychiatric disorders.

13. The "classic triad" of clinical manifestations for ICP consists of: (Select all that apply)
    1. headache.
    2. nausea.
    3. vertigo.
    4. vomiting.

14. The clinical manifestation of sudden, severe headache accompanied by vomiting may indicate that a client is experiencing an _____.

15. The hallmark of a ruptured aneurysm is the presence of
_____ in the CSF.

16. A 22-year-old college student is rushed to the emergency room with suspected meningitis. While completing a full physical exam and neurological assessment, the clinician should be alert to the classic manifestations listed below. Describe what the client would present with clinically if she had developed meningitis:
   a. Nuchal rigidity:

   b. Brudzinski's sign:

   c. Kernig's sign:

BEST PRACTICES

17. List four nursing management goals for clients with seizures:
   a.

   b.

   c.

   d.

18. During an actual seizure, the priorities of care include: (Select all that apply)
   1. maintaining an airway.
   2. protecting the client from injury.
   3. observing the seizure.
   4. restraining the client.
   5. administering anticonvulsant medications.

19. Identify the nursing responsibilities for the preoperative neurosurgery client.

20. A client who is postoperative from removal of a pituitary tumor has a "moustache" dressing in place. The nurse notes clear fluid on the pad. State the action the nurse should perform after making this observation.

21. For a client with a seizure disorder, prior to discharge the nurse should emphasize all of the following client teachings except:
    1. how anticonvulsants prevent seizures.
    2. limiting physical activity.
    3. the importance of taking medications regularly.
    4. care during a seizure.

KEEPING DRUG SKILLS SHARP

22. Explain what modifications should be made for the older adult taking anticonvulsant medications.

23. Anticonvulsant medications should be resumed _____ after surgery to obtain therapeutic levels of the medication.

24. State the rationale for contraindicating alcohol consumption for clients taking anticonvulsant medications.

25. The medication _____ is given to terminate status epilepticus and prevent exhaustion.

26. The medication _____ is administered to treat the decreased secretion of ADH after pituitary surgery.

27. Identify the technique used to facilitate delivery of chemotherapy through the blood brain barrier.

28. _____ are administered to reduce cerebral edema in the treatment of brain abscesses.

29. Drug absorption is impaired during a migraine due to reduced _____.

Chapter 72

Management of Clients with Stroke

OBJECTIVES

72.1 Describe etiology and clinical manifestations of the two major types of stroke.

72.2 Discuss the physical and psychosocial effects of a stroke on the client.

72.3 Describe nursing care and medical/surgical management of the client experiencing a stroke.

72.4 Discuss the etiology and clinical manifestations of transient ischemic attacks (TIAs).

72.5 Describe nursing care and medical/surgical management of TIAs.

UNDERSTANDING PATHOPHYSIOLOGY

1. Identify the causes for the two major types of strokes.
   a. Ischemic:

   b. Hemorrhagic:

2. The _____ type of stroke has a higher incidence.

3. The degree of damage to brain tissue from stroke is determined by the length of time the area was deprived of _____.

4. Identify the mechanism that leads to the development of a thrombus in a blood vessel, which can cause a stroke.

5. Clients with _____ are at greatest risk for development of a thrombotic stroke.

6. Intracerebral hemorrhage results from effects of _____ on blood vessels, causing them to rupture.

7. List the modifiable risk factors for stroke:
   a.

   b.

   c.

   d.

   e.

8. The brain requires a mean arterial pressure of _____ mm Hg to maintain adequate blood flow.

9. The most common site of ischemic stroke is the _____.

10. Explain why *right*-sided hemiplegia affects speech.

11. Differentiate between dysarthria and aphasia.

12. Differentiate between a stroke and a transient ischemia attack (TIA) and explain how they are related.

13. Identify the characteristics of each type of aphasia due to stroke.

Type	Characteristics
Wernicke's	
Broca's	
Global	

APPLYING SKILLS

14. Compare and contrast the early warning manifestations of the major types of strokes:

Type of Stroke	Warning Manifestations
Ischemic	
Thrombotic	
Hemorrhagic	

15. Manifestations of unilateral neglect after a stroke include: (Select all that apply)
    1. attention to only one side of the body.
    2. failure to respond to stimuli on one side of the body.
    3. use of only lower extremities.
    4. orienting the head and eyes to one side.

16. List the pertinent information the nurse should include when completing an *initial* assessment of a client who has suffered a stroke:
    a.

    b.

    c.

    d.

    e.

    f.

    g.

    h.

BEST PRACTICES

17. Identify the difficulties of nurse-client communication for each type of aphasia.
    a.   acoustic aphasia:

    b.   visual aphasia:

18. Appropriate nursing actions to communicate with an aphasic client who has suffered a stroke include: (Select all that apply)
    1.   establishing a yes/no communication method early.
    2.   using verbal communication.
    3.   using written communication.
    4.   using gestures can aid communication.

19. For a client with dysphagia, the nurse would teach all of the following steps to prevent choking or aspiration except:
    1.   opening the mouth properly.
    2.   leaving lips slightly open after food is placed inside mouth.
    3.   using the tongue to move food bolus toward oropharynx.
    4.   contracting the muscles to swallow.

20. Identify the priority action for emergency care of the client with stroke.

21. State the rationale for reducing elevated temperatures in the client who is experiencing a stroke.

22. The nurse is assisting a client with ROM exercises to improve his strength after suffering a stroke. He doesn't understand how having the nurse "do all the work of the muscles really helps." List the benefits of *passive* ROM:
    a.

    b.

    c.

23. Identify an appropriate nursing action to assist a client in the prevention of hip contractures after a stroke.

KEEPING DRUG SKILLS SHARP

24. State the rationale for performing a non-contrast CT scan of the head prior to beginning thrombolytic therapy.

25. Contraindications for beginning thrombolytic therapy include: (Select all that apply)
    1. current use of oral anticoagulants.
    2. use of intravenous dextrose solution.
    3. platelet count less than 100,000.
    4. blood glucose less than 50 mg/dl or greater than 400 mg/dl.
    5. history of myocardial infarction.
    6. diabetes mellitus.
    7. rapidly improving neurologic signs.

26. After a thrombolytic infusion, the nurse should wait _____ hours before beginning administration of anticoagulants and antiplatelet medications.

27. Activated partial thromboplastin time (aPTT) should be at _____ times the control value for anticoagulation to be effective.

Chapter 73

Management of Clients with Peripheral Nervous System Disorders

OBJECTIVES

73.1 Discuss the etiology and clinical manifestations of disorders of the lower back and spine.

73.2 Describe nursing care and medical/surgical management of the client with disorders of the lower back and spine.

73.3 Describe etiology and manifestations of other spinal disorders.

73.4 Discuss nursing care and medical management of spinal disorders.

73.5 Describe etiology and manifestations of other peripheral nervous system disorders.

73.6 Discuss nursing care and medical/surgical management of other peripheral nervous system disorders.

UNDERSTANDING PATHOPHYSIOLOGY

1. Provide examples for each of the three groups of problems leading to the development of low back pain.

Cause	Example
Biomechanical and destructive	
Destructive origins	
Degenerative	

2. Identify the mechanism for increased damage to intervetebral disks due to normal aging.

3. True or False

    _____ Lumbar disks are more likely to rupture than cervical disks.

    _____ Ruptured intervetebral disks may occur at any level of the spine.

    _____ Factors increasing risk of disk injury include extended sitting, aerobic exercise, and high cholesterol.

4. For each spinal disorder, identify the cause and resulting body changes.
   a. Lordosis:

   b. Spondylothesis:

   c. Spondylosis:

   d. Spinal stenosis:

5. Any lesion that destroys the upper motor neuron will result in _____ _____.

6. _____ and _____ are the most common spinal cord tumors. Both are benign and operable.

7. Trigeminal neuralgia, or tic douloureux, is an irritation of the _____ _ cranial nerve and is characterized by intense pain of sudden onset along maxilla and mandible.

8. Bell's palsy affects the motor aspects of the _____ cranial nerve and presents as _____ of the facial muscles of expression.

9. Peripheral neuropathy causes different clinical manifestations, depending on the type of nerves affected. For each type of nerve, identify the ways in which the manifestation will present in the client:

Type	Manifestation
Motor nerves	
Sensory nerves	
Autonomic nerves	

10. Repetitive motion of the wrists can result in _____ syndrome, which occurs when the median nerve is compressed.

11. Pain from sciatic nerve compression begins in the _____ and extends down the _____.

APPLYING SKILLS

12. State the rationale for evaluating occupation and working equipment of a client with low back pain.

13. The nurse should assess both the surgical site of the spine of a spinal fusion client and the _____ site on a postoperative client.

14. A critical nursing assessment for a client who is postoperative from cervical disk surgery is to check the site for excessive _____ that may compromise breathing.

15. Label the assessment techniques for carpal tunnel syndrome.

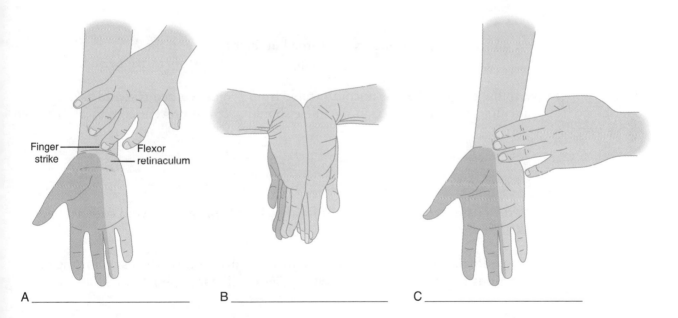

Finger strike — Flexor retinaculum

A _____ B _____ C _____

16. A client returns after surgical correction to relieve pressure from carpal tunnel syndrome. State the rationale for delaying assessment of sensation of the fingers after surgery.

17. Identify the information the nurse should document in the initial assessment if a client's hand is injured.

BEST PRACTICES

18. A client calls for the nurse with complaints of discomfort due to his sciatica. State the appropriate nursing intervention to assist him and reduce the discomfort.

19. Important client teaching points the nurse should discuss to assist in resolving low back pain include: (Select all that apply)
    1. using good body mechanics.
    2. keeping objects close to the body when lifting.
    3. locking knees when lifting.
    4. avoiding twisting when lifting.

20. Identify an effective intervention for preventing future low back injuries.

21. Clients who have undergone spinal surgery are turned in their beds with the
    _____ maneuver in the postoperative period.

22. A postoperative spinal surgery client is uncomfortable from prolonged bed rest and asks for assistance from the nurse. Identify the action the nurse should *avoid* to prevent complications from his immobility.

23. Normal protocol for postoperative voiding calls for the client being able to void sufficiently within _____ hours after spinal surgery.

24. Many clients who undergo cervical disk surgery complain of discomfort when swallowing or talking. Nursing actions to improve comfort include: (Select all that apply)
    1. soft diet.
    2. throat lozenges.
    3. viscous lidocaine solution.
    4. cool, dry air.
    5. minimal talking.

KEEPING DRUG SKILLS SHARP

25. To reduce pain and spasms from low back pain, all of the following medications may be prescribed except:
    1. NSAIDs.
    2. beta blockers.
    3. COX-2 inhibitors.
    4. muscle relaxants.

26. A PCA pump filled with _____ is the best way to control postoperative pain for the spinal surgery client.

27. Why is use of Capsaicin topical cream indicated for the postpolio client?

28. A postpolio syndrome client complains of significant discomfort from overuse, pain, and cramps in her muscles. She doesn't understand why she "must suffer" with these pains and wants to take strong medications to "take all the pain away." Her physician has cautioned against this. State the rationale for the physician's advisory against pain medication.

29. _____ is prescribed for treatment of trigeminal neuralgia because it dampens the reactivity of the neurons within the trigeminal nerve, reducing pain stimuli.

Chapter 74

Management of Clients with Degenerative Neurologic Disorders

OBJECTIVES

74.1 Describe etiology and clinical manifestations of dementia.

74.2 Discuss nursing care and medical/surgical management of the client with Alzheimer's disease.

74.3 Describe etiology and clinical manifestations of other degenerative neurologic diseases.

74.4 Discuss nursing care and medical/surgical management of the client experiencing degenerative neurologic diseases.

UNDERSTANDING PATHOPHYSIOLOGY

1. Compare and contrast the major types of dementia:

Type	Characteristics
Alzheimer's disease	
Multi-infarct disease	
Lewy body dementia	
Pick's disease	

2. Describe the stages of Alzheimer's disease and the manifestations of each stage:

Stage	Manifestations
Preclinical	
Mild Alzheimer's	
Moderate Alzheimer's	
Severe Alzheimer's	

3. A client with Huntington's disease has a _____% chance of passing his disease on to future children.

4. Areas of the body most affected by multiple sclerosis include all of the following except the:
   1. optic nerves.
   2. cerebellum.
   3. cerebrum.
   4. cervical spinal cord.

5. Although clinical manifestations may vary due to the random distribution of the MS plaques on nerves, they can include: (Select all that apply)
   1. bowel and bladder dysfunction.
   2. hair loss.
   3. vision loss from optic neuritis.
   4. weakness.
   5. uncoordination.
   6. constipation.
   7. fatigue.
   8. insomnia.

6. During the recovery phase of GBS, remyelination occurs in a
   _____ pattern.

7. The cause of muscle weakness in MG is loss of _____
   at the neurotransmitter junction.

8. Although Amyotrophic Lateral Sclerosis involves degeneration of both upper and lower motor neurons, it does not affect _____.

9. Progressive muscle weakness from ALS will eventually lead to _____ _____.

10. Compare and contrast between a myasthenic crisis and a cholinergic crisis in the client with myasthenia gravis.
    Myasthenic crisis:

    Cholinergic crisis:

APPLYING SKILLS

11. Assessing pain or discomfort in the client with advanced AD is difficult due to communication problems. Behaviors that would indicate discomfort include: (Select all that apply)
    1. noisy breathing.
    2. negative vocalizations (mutterings).
    3. sad or frightened facial expression.
    4. frowning.
    5. tense body language.
    6. motionlessness.

12. List the *classic triad* of clinical manifestations of Parkinson's disease:
    a.

    b.

    c.

13. Identify a classic feature of myasthenia gravis (MG).

14. A common test for MG is to ask the client to hold an upward gaze for 3 minutes. If the test is positive, a manifestation of _____ of the upper eyelid will be observed.

15. A client suspected of having MG is to undergo a Tensilon test. After injecting Tensilon IV into the client, a positive result would be _____ in muscle strength.

BEST PRACTICES

16. A nursing diagnosis of Risk for injury related to impaired judgment has been developed for a client with AD. List the appropriate interventions to prevent injury to the client:
    a.
    b.
    c.
    d.
    e.

17. A nurse caring for a client with MS develops the nursing diagnosis of Impaired physical mobility related to weakness, contractures, and spasticity. List the appropriate interventions for this client:
    a.
    b.
    c.
    d.
    e.

18. Upon entering the room of a client who has been diagnosed with AD, the nurse notes manifestations of increased frustration. The client is pacing the room and shaking his fist at the air. Interventions the nurse can implement to help the client include all of the following except:
    1. increase environmental stimuli.
    2. approach client calmly.
    3. do not place any demands on client.
    4. gently distract client.
    5. use multiple sensory methods, but not all at the same time.

19. An 84-year-old female client diagnosed with early stages of AD has begun to show manifestations of skin breakdown in the perineal area due to incontinence. Nursing interventions for incontinence appropriate to her age and physical/mental condition include: (Select all that apply)
    1. schedule voiding and defecation times.
    2. monitor client for nonverbal clues of needing to void/defecate.
    3. post bright, clear signs indicating where bathroom is located.
    4. use an indwelling catheter to reduce risk of infection.
    5. use disposable undergarments in later stages of AD.

20. A 79-year-old client diagnosed with Parkinson's disease suddenly stops moving in the middle of walking to the bathroom. This phenomenon called "freezing" can be corrected through which nursing actions? (Select all that apply)
    1. Have client step over an imaginary line to get moving again.
    2. Assist client to rock to get momentum.
    3. Instruct client to lift toe of foot off ground to begin walking.
    4. Gently push client forward.

21. Nursing interventions to assist the client with HD who is experiencing problems eating due to dysphagia include: (Select all that apply)
    1. diets that include easy-to-swallow foods.
    2. two large meals a day.
    3. have the client sit upright.
    4. have the client keep chin down toward the chest while swallowing.
    5. have the client hold his or her breath before swallowing and cough to clear the throat afterward.

KEEPING DRUG SKILLS SHARP

22. Identify the primary indication for prescribing medications such as tacrine, donepezil, and rivastigmine for clients with Alzheimer's disease.

23. Explain how Sinemet (combination of levodopa and carbidopa) works to correct manifestations of Parkinson's disease.

24. The dopamine blocker _____ helps control the abnormal movements that result from HD by altering neurotransmission of signals for movement.

25. The standard therapy to treat an acute exacerbation of MS is administration of _____ to reduce inflammation.

Chapter 75

Management of Clients with Neurologic Trauma

OBJECTIVES

75.1 Describe etiology and clinical manifestations of increased intracranial pressure.

75.2 Discuss nursing care and medical/surgical management of the client experiencing increased intracranial pressure.

75.3 Describe the etiology and clinical manifestations of traumatic brain injury.

75.4 Discuss nursing care and medical/surgical management of the client with traumatic brain injury.

75.5 Describe etiology and clinical manifestations of spinal cord injury.

75.6 Discuss nursing care and medical/surgical management of the client with a spinal cord injury.

UNDERSTANDING PATHOPHYSIOLOGY

1. To maintain a balance between the brain tissue, blood, and cerebrospinal fluid, intracranial pressure should not exceed _____ mm Hg.

2. List the common causes for increased intracranial pressure (ICP):
    a.
    b.
    c.
    d.
    e.
    f.

3. List the three mechanisms that compensate for increased ICP:
    a.
    b.
    c.

4. List the two initial manifestations of increased ICP:
    a.
    b.

5. The leading cause of traumatic head injuries is _____.

6. Identify the characteristics of each type of common brain injury.

Injury	Characteristics
Concussion	
Open head injury	
Closed head injury	
Contusions	
Subdural hematoma	

7. Spinal cord injuries occur most often in _____ between the ages of _____ and _____.

8. _____ are the most common type of spinal cord injury.

9. Clinical manifestations of spinal cord damage *below* the level of injury include loss of: (Select all that apply)
    1. voluntary movement.
    2. sensation of pain, temperature, pressure, proprioception.
    3. bowel and bladder function.
    4. spinal and autonomic reflexes.

10. A spinal cord injury to the cervical area results in _____.

11. Injuries to the thoracic or lumbar spinal segments produce _____.

12. Clinical manifestations of autonomic dysreflexia include: (Select all that apply)
    1. sudden onset of severe hypertension.
    2. throbbing headache.
    3. profuse diaphoresis.
    4. flushing of the skin above level of the lesion.
    5. blurred vision.
    6. nausea.
    7. bradycardia.

13. When the spinal cord is damaged, the immediate response is "spinal shock" with the loss of all of the following except:
    1. skeletal muscle function.
    2. bowel and bladder tone.
    3. vision.
    4. sexual function.
    5. autonomic reflexes.

APPLYING SKILLS

14. A young motorcyclist has arrived in the ICU after being stabilized in the ED. The nurse begins her initial physical assessment, including a thorough neurological exam using the Glasgow Coma Scale. Factors that can cause an invalid scale score include that the: (Select all that apply)
    1. client cannot speak or is intubated.
    2. client's eyes are swollen closed.
    3. client unable to communicate in English.
    4. client has hearing loss/blind.
    5. client is aphasic.
    6. client is paralyzed/hemiplegic.

15. A client arrives in the emergency department from an accident via ambulance. Upon assessment, the nurse notes ecchymosis around the eyes and drainage of clear fluid from the ear. These manifestations are consistent with the injury _____

_____.

16. Explain why the description of the accident causing a head injury is critical to care.

17. A client has been diagnosed with Brown-Séquard syndrome. Upon assessment the nurse would expect to find all of the following clinical manifestations except:
    1. ipsilateral motor paralysis (same side as lesion).
    2. ipsilateral motor paralysis (opposite side of lesion).
    3. loss of vibratory and position sense.
    4. contralateral loss of pain and temperature sensation (opposite side).

18. When completing an assessment of a client with a, SCI, levels of sensation are documented according to _____.

19. Assessment of the major reflexes includes: (Select all that apply)
    1. Achilles.
    2. patellar.
    3. biceps.
    4. triceps.

BEST PRACTICES

20. List the immediate interventions that should be implemented to decrease ICP and state the rationale for each:
    a.

    b.

    c.

21. Open head wounds should be covered and pressure applied except if there is evidence of
_____ or _____
fracture.

22. A client with traumatic brain injury is at risk for ineffective airway and aspiration. Nursing actions to protect the airway include: (Select all that apply)
    1. clearing mouth and oropharynx of foreign bodies.
    2. suctioning oropharynx and trachea to remove secretions.
    3. placing the client in supine position to facilitate drainage of secretions.
    4. using humidified oxygen or intubation as needed to maintain PaO_2 within parameters.

23. List the emergency interventions that should be implemented to correct autonomic dysreflexia:
    a.
    b.
    c.
    d.
    e.

24. When turning a client with a suspected spinal injury, the nurse should use the
_____ maneuver to maintain straight body alignment.

25. Clients with SCI have altered thermoregulation due to loss of hypothalamic control of the sympathetic nervous system. Nursing actions to maintain normothermic status include (Select all that apply)
    1. rectal or core temperature monitoring every 24 hours.
    2. palpation of skin surfaces for areas of warmth or coolness.
    3. control of environmental temperature.
    4. use of bed linens and eliminating drafts in room.

26. For each rehabilitation goal for the client with SCI, identify appropriate nursing interventions:
    a. promote mobility:

    b. reduce spasticity:

    c. improve bladder control:

    d. bowel control:

    e. prevent pressure ulcers:

    f. reduce respiratory dysfunction:

    g. control pain:

    h. promote psychological adjustment:

KEEPING DRUG SKILLS SHARP

27. State the rationale for controlling seizure activity prophylactically with phenytoin or carbamazepine in the client with increased ICP.

28. If a client with increased ICP begins shivering from a fever _____ would be administered to prevent shivering which would increase metabolism.

29. True or False

_____ Clients with severe traumatic brain injury are not candidates for barbiturate therapy (undergo a prophylactic barbiturate coma).

_____ A client undergoing barbiturate therapy should have respirations monitored with pulse oximetry and incentive spirometer every 4 hours.

_____ Barbiturate therapy can cause hypothermia.

_____ Even when a client is in a coma, the pupils dilate if the brain stem is compressed.

30. State the indication for each type of medication used to treat acute SCI:

Medication	Indication for Use
Vasoactive agents	
Steroids	
Thyrotropin releasing hormone	
H_2 receptor blocking agents	

31. _____ is used for neurogenic bladder control to stimulate contractions and _____ to reduce the contractions.

32. Pain control for the client with SCI includes analgesics, which may need to be supplemented with other medications such as _____ to control neuropathic pain.

33. Heterotopic ossification is the formation of bone in abnormal locations. Clients with SCI who develop this complication are treated with _____.

Chapter 76

Assessment of the Hematopoietic System

OBJECTIVES

76.1 Describe the components of the health history specific to the hematopoietic system.

76.2 Discuss the review of systems and common clinical manifestations associated with hematopoietic disorders.

76.3 Describe common diagnostic tests used to diagnose hematopoietic disorders.

76.4 Recognize values for a complete blood count.

ANATOMY & PHYSIOLOGY REVIEW

1. Label the organs of the immune system.

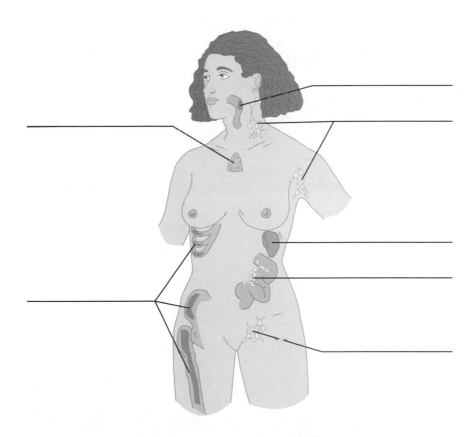

UNDERSTANDING PATHOPHYSIOLOGY

2. List the two groups of individuals that have a diminished immune response:

   a.

   b.

3. Which of the following clinical manifestations is typically found in a client that presents with anemia?

   1. epistaxis
   2. recurrent infections
   3. fatigue
   4. chronic diarrhea

4. List the major types of allergic triggers:

   a.

   b.

   c.

   d.

5. Explain why clients who have had a partial or total gastrectomy may develop anemia.

6. What physiologic response occurs when clients live at altitudes above 10,000 feet?

7. Which of the following clinical manifestations is most likely to occur with severe anemia? (Select all that apply)

   1. weakness
   2. fatigue
   3. exertional dyspnea
   4. ringing in the ears

8. Clients with immunodeficiencies are most likely to present with a history of:

   1. recurrent infections.
   2. pruritis and ruddy skin.
   3. petechiae and purpura.
   4. scleral jaundice.

9. Explain the underlying rationale for the presence of tachycardia in a client with anemia.

10. The hematocrit value is roughly _____ times the hemoglobin concentrations.

11. True or False

_____ The type of allergen and individual sensitivity pattern may vary clinical manifestations.

_____ Strict vegetarians are not at greater risk for deficiency anemia than people who eat regular diets.

_____ Clients who abuse alcohol may be at risk for bleeding disorders.

_____ A glossy, bright red and sore tongue is a clinical manifestation associated with thrombocytopenia.

_____ Clients experiencing sickle cell crisis may complain of severe, excruciating bone pain.

_____ The RBC count varies with age and gender.

APPLYING SKILLS

12. Which of the following responses from a client may alert the nurse to a possible immunodeficiency?
    1. "It takes a long time for me to heal even the smallest wound."
    2. "I have occasional diarrhea."
    3. "I rarely get a cold."
    4. "I haven't had an infection that required an antibiotic for over a year."

13. List the nine areas to assess with regard to family health history when conducting the hematopoietic assessment:
    a.
    b.
    c.
    d.
    e.
    f.
    g.
    h.
    i.

14. List the portions of the lymphatic system that are accessible for a physical examination:
    a.
    b.
    c.

15. List the four specific blood tests that are generally needed to diagnose hematopoietic disorders:
    a.
    b.
    c.
    d.

16. Explain the uses of the Coombs' test.

17. List the four laboratory studies used to pinpoint bleeding disorders:
    a.
    b.
    c.
    d.

18. Identify the following laboratory tests as low, normal, or high.

Laboratory Test	Low, Normal, High
a. RBC woman 3.7	
b. RBC man 4.9	
c. Hemoglobin woman 12.6	
d. Hemoglobin man 12.6	
e. Hematocrit woman 50%	
f. Hematocrit man 40%	
g. WBC 12,000	
h. Neutrophils 60%	
i. Eosinophils 6%	
j. Basophils 0.5%	
k. Lymphocytes 50%	
l. Monocytes 6%	
m. Platelets 200,000	

19. True or False

    _____ Some hematologic tests are age-specific and gender-specific.

    _____ When conducting a symptom analysis it is important to ask about onset and timing.

BEST PRACTICES

20. Explain why it is important to ask a client if he or she has donated blood or blood components recently.

21. Which of the following preoperative nursing interventions are not appropriate for a client having a bone marrow aspiration?
    1. Advise the client the procedure is painless.
    2. Inform the client he or she will sign a consent form.
    3. Explain the procedure and what the client should expect.
    4. Provide sedation that is prescribed.

22. The most important nursing observation for a client who has had a bone marrow aspiration is to
_____.

KEEPING DRUG SKILLS SHARP

23. Over-the-counter medications containing _____ can aggravate bleeding tendencies.

24. List the antibiotics that can cause hemolysis:
    a.

    b.

25. In addition to aspirin, the _____ group of medications can interfere with platelet aggregation and prolong bleeding.

26. Match each herbal preparation and nutritional supplement with the appropriate reason they may be taken.

Herbal Preparation/Nutritional Supplement	Reason for Taking
_____ a. comfrey	1. hay fever
_____ b. echinacea	2. antiviral
_____ c. St. John's wort	3. anticancer
_____ d. licorice	4. pernicious anemia
_____ e. stinging nettle	5. reduce inflammation, fight viruses
_____ f. vitamin e	6. boost the immune system
_____ g. folic acid	7. anti-inflammatory

27. True or False

    _____ Tissue plasminogen activator (t-PA) can cause a decrease in the bleeding time.

    _____ Ephedra might reduce the effect of prednisone.

Chapter 77

Management of Clients with Hematologic Disorders

OBJECTIVES

77.1 Discuss major disorders of the hematologic system.

77.2 Discuss risk factors, clinical manifestations, and outcome management of nursing interventions for clients with hematologic disorders.

77.3 Recognize common laboratory findings for selected hematologic disorders.

UNDERSTANDING PATHOPHYSIOLOGY

1. Which of the following is essential for RBC production?
   1. manganese
   2. Vitamin A
   3. Vitamin C
   4. folic acid

2. Which of the following depicts a compensatory mechanism for tissue hypoxia?
   1. a shift in oxygen-hemoglobin dissociation curve to the left
   2. redistribution of blood from tissues of low O_2 needs to tissues of high O_2 needs
   3. decreased cardiac output
   4. decreased rate of RBC production

3. List the four factors that determine the severity of clinical manifestations associated with anemia:
   a.
   b.
   c.
   d.

4. List the three situations in which the production of erythrocytes is decreased:
   a.
   b.
   c.

5. The most common etiologic factor in men for iron-deficiency anemia is _____ _____ .

6. Thalassemia disrupts the synthesis of _____.

7. Megaloblastic anemias result in defective _____ and are caused by deficiencies of _____ and _____.

8. A common GI symptom associated with pernicious anemia is:
   1. weight gain.
   2. increased appetite.
   3. abdominal distention.
   4. flatulence.

9. A failure of bone marrow results in _____ anemia.

10. Clients with aplastic anemia are at great risk of succumbing to fungal infections caused by _____.

11. The cause of polycythemia vera (PV) is excessive activation of _____.

12. The most common clinical manifestation of hemochromatosis is _____.

13. The means used to rid the body of excess iron in hemochromatosis is _____.

14. Agranulocytosis is characterized by a profound decrease in _____.

15. The most common presenting complaint in multiple myeloma is _____.

16. List the four factors essential for normal clot formation:
   a.
   b.
   c.
   d.

17. The most common thrombocytopenic disorder is _____.

18. Prothrombin synthesis is dependent on _____ to act as a catalyst.

19. List the four primary causative factors of DIC:
   a.
   b.
   c.
   d.

20. List the eight primary manifestations of acute DIC:

a.

b.

c.

d.

e.

f.

g.

h.

21. Hemophilia is most often found in _____.

22. True or False

_____ Anemia is a disease with a number of underlying pathological processes leading to an abnormality in RBC numbers.

_____ Older adults are at increased risk for anemia.

_____ Clients with mild anemia typically present with complaints of exertional dyspnea.

_____ People whose diets lack meat are at greatest risk for iron-deficiency anemia.

_____ Iron-deficiency anemia is the most prevalent hematological disorder worldwide.

_____ Infants, children, and all adolescents are high risk for iron-deficiency anemia.

_____ A lack of interest in food preparation contributes to a higher prevalence of iron-deficiency anemia in older adults.

_____ Iron is used in the bone marrow to form iron compounds called heme that are responsible for synthesis of the molecule responsible for transport of oxygen.

_____ Thalassemia is thought to be a response to endemic malaria.

_____ Due to a diminished sensitivity and nerve damage, clients with pernicious anemia are at high risk for injury.

_____ Folic acid deficiency can occur during pregnancy due an increased demand for folate.

_____ Idiopathic cases of aplastic anemia are most common in infants and older adults.

_____ Sickle cell anemia is a hereditary hemoglobinopathy.

_____ Sickle cell anemia is the most common anemia worldwide.

_____ The peak incidence of PV is in the group 50 to 70 years of age.

_____ Clinical manifestations of PV are related to hypoxia.

_____ The most common cause of agranulocytosis is drug or chemical toxicity or hypersensitivity.

_____ If left untreated, clients with agranulocytosis develop overwhelming infection and septicemia and die.

_____ Multiple myeloma is a malignancy of the plasma B-cell.

_____ The EBV, which causes 85% of infectious mononucleosis, is a herpes virus.

_____ Spleenectomy cures secondary hypersplenism.

_____ Hypoprothrombinemia is a congenital or acquired deficiency of the clotting factor VIII.

_____ Disseminated intravascular coagulation is a loss of balance between the clotting and lysing systems in the body.

APPLYING SKILLS

23. Which of the following statements by a client with anemia indicate that he or she needs further teaching about iron supplement therapy?
    1. "I should take one 325 mg tablet orally 3-4 times a day."
    2. "When possible I should take my pills with milk to increase absorption."
    3. "My stools may look black."
    4. "I may experience constipation when taking this drug."

24. A client has a nursing diagnosis of Activity intolerance related to decreased blood supply or low Hgb levels. A nurse would know that the outcome of activity tolerance has been met when the client:
    1. has difficulty sitting up.
    2. participates in ADLs without dyspnea.
    3. walks short distances with a heart rate of 110.
    4. complains of shortness of breath while bathing.

25. A nurse provides teaching to a client with a nursing diagnosis of imbalanced nutrition: less than body requirements related to disease, treatment, or lack of knowledge of adequate nutrition. Which statement made by the client indicates that teaching has been effective?
    1. "I should eat a diet high in proteins and fats."
    2. "I should eat three regularly scheduled meals daily"
    3. ""I should eat egg whites instead of the yolk."
    4. "Liver is the richest source of iron."

26. Complete the table for the laboratory values for *iron deficiency anemia* and indicate if the value is increased or decreased.

Laboratory Value	Increased or Decreased
1. Hgb	
2. RBC	
3. MCV	
4. MCH	
5. MCHC	
6. Serum iron	
7. Total iron binding capacity	

27. A nurse teaches a client with aplastic anemia measures to prevent infection and bleeding. Which of the following statements made by the client indicate that further teaching is needed?
    1. "I should use a humidifier."
    2. "I need to be meticulous in performing oral hygiene."
    3. "I can use my straight razor for shaving."
    4. "I should avoid crowds when my white count is down."

28. The two primary indications for splenectomy are _____
and _____.

29. True or False

_____ In folic acid deficiency, the Schilling test is abnormal.

_____ African-American parents should be encouraged to have themselves and their children tested for the presence of Hb-S.

BEST PRACTICES

30. List the eight interventions that are used to control the causes of anemia:
    a.
    b.
    c.
    d.
    e.
    f.
    g.
    h.

31. When clients with severe chronic anemia have responded poorly to other forms of therapy, _____ is an appropriate intervention.

32. Explain the procedure that is initiated if the nurse suspects a transfusion reaction.

33. The nurse should instruct a client with aplastic anemia who is neutropenic to avoid eating:
    1. yogurt.
    2. eggs.
    3. well-cooked meats.
    4. bread products.

34. Explain the rationale for encouraging activity, such as walking, for the client with multiple myeloma.

35. A critical nursing intervention for clients with DIC and their families is to provide

_____.

36. True or False

_____ Because most of the care for clients with anemia occurs in an outpatient clinic or the client's home, teaching is critical to effective management.

_____ Blood components that contain a significant volume of plasma or other diluents are infused at a slow rate through a large gauge needle.

_____ Blood components not used can be returned to inventory for up to 3 hours out of monitored storage.

_____ An estimated 40% of transfusion reactions are due to labeling errors.

_____ Blood warmers are used to promote comfort for the client and have no therapeutic value.

_____ Bone marrow transplantation is the treatment of choice for clients with aplastic anemia.

_____ Sickle cell crisis is a medical emergency and requires immediate attention.

_____ Teaching clients with sickle cell disease to avoid dehydration is one way to avoid crisis.

_____ The treatment of choice for multiple myeloma is bone marrow suppression using chemotherapy.

KEEPING DRUG SKILLS SHARP

37. A positive response to iron therapy is evidenced by an increase in

_____ in _____ days.

38. What multidrug combinations are used to treat neurologic complications of pernicious anemia?

39. The drug of choice for acute pain control in sickle cell crisis is

_____.

40. Which of the following drugs is used to treat deep bone pain in clients with sickle cell disease?
    1. morphine elixir
    2. NSAIDs
    3. acetaminophen
    4. tricyclic antidepressant

41. The drug of choice to treat hyperuricemia in clients with PV is

_____.

42. True or False

_____ Clients with a history of a transfusion reaction may receive Benadryl prophylactically.

_____ Recommended daily iron intake for women is 10 mg/daily.

_____ Persons with pernicious anemia require Vitamin B_{12} supplementation for life.

_____ Folic acid deficiency can occur with long-term use of Dilantin.

_____ Hydroxyureas are the drug of choice in the treatment of all clients with sickle cell disease.

_____ Infectious mononucleosis is aggressively treated with antibiotics and steroids.

_____ Clients with hemophilia should be taught to take aspirin to decrease joint pain.

CONCEPT MAP EXERCISE

The following questions are based on the concept map *Understanding DIC and Its Treatment* in your textbook.

43. Which of the following treatments in DIC is instituted first?
    1. administration of platelets.
    2. administration of fresh frozen plasma.
    3. administration of heparin.
    4. treatment of the underlying problem.

44. The pathophysiologic process that leads to tissue necrosis is:
    1. consumption of clotting factors.
    2. endothelial damage.
    3. occlusion of small blood vessels.
    4. inhibition of platelet function.

45. A factor that directly contributes to the intrinsic pathway of coagulation is:
    1. activation of fibrinolytic system.
    2. consumption of clotting factors.
    3. increased tissue thromboplastin.
    4. endothelial damage.

Chapter 78

Management of Clients with Immune Disorders

OBJECTIVES

78.1   Discuss the pathophysiologic process associated with immune disorders.

78.2   Describe common hypersensitivity reactions including common allergens, clinical manifestations, and medical management.

78.3   Describe nursing interventions for clients with common hypersensitivity reactions.

UNDERSTANDING PATHOPHYSIOLOGY

1. Which of the following statements are true regarding allergy?
    1. Allergy involves immunoglobulin E (IgE) formation.
    2. Hypersensitivity and allergy are not synonymous.
    3. Allergy represents a decreased response to an allergen.
    4. Over 50% of the population has allergies.

2. Factors that influence manifestations of allergies include: (Select all that apply)
    1. gender.
    2. exposure to second-hand smoke.
    3. noise pollution.
    4. age.

3. List the four routes by which an allergen can enter the body:
    a.

    b.

    c.

    d.

4. Factors that influence the likelihood of developing an allergy include: (Select all that apply)
    1. exposure later in life rather than earlier.
    2. the type of allergen.
    3. the allergen load.
    4. having January as a birth month.

5. Arrange the following pathophysiologic events in the order in which they occur in an immediate reaction.

_____ a. increased vascular permeability

_____ b. IgE production in response to allergen

_____ c. Degranulation of mast cells and basophils

_____ d. Activation of mast cells and basophils

_____ e. Release of prostaglandins

6. The cells responsible for delaying an inflammatory response after mast cells have been activated are the _____ cells.

7. List the four main types of hypersensitivity reactions:
   a.
   b.
   c.
   d.

8. Which of the following is associated with an anaphylactic hypersensitivity reaction?
   1. chills and fever
   2. hypertension
   3. coughing
   4. hives

9. Arrange the following pathophysiologic events in the order in which they occur in a cytotoxic reaction.

_____ a. tissue injury

_____ b. antibody binding

_____ c. cell destruction of cell where antigen is bound

_____ d. activation of the complement system

10. Clinical manifestations associated with a blood transfusion reaction include (Select all that apply)
    1. hypertension
    2. glucosuria
    3. bradycardia
    4. urticaria

11. A localized area of tissue necrosis that results from immune complex hypersensitivity is called a _____ reaction.

12. A typical clinical manifestation of contact dermatitis reaction is:
    1. hypotension.
    2. hematuria.
    3. vesicular lesions.
    4. pain.

13. List three factors that are considered in the diagnosis of allergic disease:
    a.
    b.
    c.

14. List the two classifications for adverse food reactions:
    a.
    b.

15. Food intolerances:
    1. occur most often in young- and middle-aged adults.
    2. are less prevalent than food allergies.
    3. result in food-induced anaphylaxis.
    4. commonly manifested by diarrhea and vomiting.

16. Match each allergen associated with allergic rhinitis with the appropriate time of occurrence.

	Allergen	**Most Frequent Time of Occurrence**
_____	a. animal dander	1. spring
_____	b. ragweed	2. summer
_____	c. tree pollen	3. fall
_____	d. grasses	4. winter
		5. year-round

17. Arrange the following pathophysiologic events in the order in which they occur in allergic rhinitis.
    _____ a. watery discharge, sneezing, and nasal itching
    _____ b. mediator release
    _____ c. allergen exposure
    _____ d. binding of IgE to receptors on mast cells and basophils
    _____ e. increased production of IgE
    _____ f. nasal swelling

18. True or False
    _____ It is believed that environmental factors acting either before or after birth contribute to the increasing prevalence of allergic disease.
    _____ Due to a direct correlation between higher concentrations of allergens and the intensity of the response, subsequent lower concentrations can induce more severe reactions when reexposure occurs.
    _____ Blood transfusions are associated with anaphylactic hypersensitivity reactions.
    _____ Serum sickness develops 21 to 28 days after injection with a foreign serum.
    _____ A positive skin test reaction indicates antibody response to a previous exposure to an antigen.
    _____ The distinguishing factor between food allergies and food intolerances is a specific IgE mediated response.

APPLYING SKILLS

19. The allergy test used for the diagnosis of asthma is:
    1. blood assays for IgE.
    2. skin testing.
    3. radioallergosorbent test (RAST).
    4. pulmonary function tests.

20. Negative results of a skin test may indicate: (Select all that apply)
    1. the client is immunocompromised.
    2. the client has taken antihistamines within 72-96 hours.
    3. the antigen was likely introduced subcutaneously.
    4. antibodies present did not react to the antigen.

21. A radioallergosorbent test:
    1. is more sensitive than skin testing.
    2. is less time-consuming and costly.
    3. involves blood incubated with a paper disc bound with allergen.
    4. is most widely used due to increased sensitivity and specificity.

BEST PRACTICES

22. List the four nursing interventions to be initiated if the nurse suspects a transfusion reaction:
    a.
    b.
    c.
    d.

23. State the most important nursing intervention to prevent a serum sickness.

24. An indication that a client has understood teaching about skin care measures is that the nurse observes the client:
    1. bathing in hot water.
    2. scratching his or her skin.
    3. applying Alpha Keri after bathing.
    4. bathing with a strong antibacterial soap.

25. List appropriate nursing interventions for itching and discomfort at the injection site for a skin test:
    a.
    b.

26. Explain the rationale for having clients wait 20-30 minutes after receiving immunotherapy injections.

27. The most important component of therapy for the client with allergic rhinitis is
_____.

KEEPING DRUG SKILLS SHARP

28. Which of the following types of medication may be administered to a client with severe serum sickness reaction?
    1. analgesic
    2. antihistamine
    3. steroids
    4. diuretic

29. Explain why newer over-the-counter antihistamines are safer to use than traditional antihistamines such a diphenhydramine (Benadryl).

30. A beta$_2$ agonist used to control bronchospasm in asthma is
    1. fluticasone (Flovent).
    2. cromolyn sodium (Intal).
    3. ipratropium (Atrovent).
    4. albuterol (Ventolin).

31. List the three types of medications commonly used to treat atopic dermatitis:
    a.
    b.
    c.

32. The primary drug for the treatment of urticaria is an _____.

33. True or False

    _____ The administration of penicillin can initiate a serum-sickness–like reaction.

    _____ Oral sympathomimetics such as pseudoephedrine should be used with caution in clients with heart disease and hypertension.

Chapter 79

Management of Clients with Rheumatic Disorders

OBJECTIVES

79.1   Identify the etiology and risk factors for the development of rheumatic disorders.

79.2   Describe clinical manifestations of rheumatoid arthritis.

79.3   Discuss nursing care and medical/surgical management of clients with rheumatoid arthritis.

79.4   Describe etiology and clinical manifestations of other connective tissue disorders.

79.5   Discuss nursing care and medical/surgical management of clients with other connective tissue disorders.

UNDERSTANDING PATHOPHYSIOLOGY

1.   _____ is the primary reason for work-related disability and the leading cause of disability in people 65 years old or older.

2.   Factors that have been identified by researchers as having a role in the development of autoimmune inflammatory disorders include: (Select all that apply)
   1. overuse.
   2. injury.
   3. anorexia.
   4. gene defects.
   5. infection.
   6. immunosuppression.
   7. environmental agents.

3.   In addition to morning stiffness in joints, other systemic manifestations of RA include: (Select all that apply).
   1. obesity.
   2. weight loss.
   3. fatigue.
   4. muscle ache.

4.   List the three types of deformities that can result from chronic inflammation of joints and synovial involvement:
   a.
   b.
   c.

5. Identify the manifestations that develop with CREST syndrome in clients with systemic sclerosis:

   C:

   R:

   E:

   S:

   T:

6. Describe the physiologic changes that occur during Raynaud's phenomenon:
   WHITE:

   BLUE:

   RED:

7. The rheumatic joint disease _____ can result as sequelae to infection from a tick-borne spirochete.

APPLYING SKILLS

8. When evaluating effectiveness of therapy for clients with arthritis, the American College of Rheumatology has set the standard as _____.

9. The areas most affected by RA include: (Select all that apply)
   1. wrists.
   2. metacarpophalangeal (MCP) joints.
   3. proximal interphalangeal (PIP) joints.
   4. knees.
   5. feet.

10. A 28-year-old client who has had arthritis for years has undergone an elbow arthroplasty. Upon returning to the orthopedic unit, the nursing interventions for postoperative care includes elevating the arm above the shoulder and assessing hand strength to check for _____
    _____.

11. A 30-year-old bank teller comes to the clinic complaining of fatigue, painful swollen joints, and fever. Upon physical examination, the nurse notes a reddened rash over the bridge of the nose and cheeks. These symptoms may be indicative of the rheumatic disorder
    _____.

12. Explain why the nurse should evaluate occupation and hobbies when completing a history from a client with complaints of bursitis.

BEST PRACTICES

13. In teaching the client with ankylosing spondylitis (AS) about measures to maintain mobility, the nurse would instruct the client to: (Select all that apply)
    1. maintain good posture.
    2. engage in exercises that promote stretching/extension of the spine (e.g., swimming).
    3. select ergonomic chairs and work station equipment.
    4. sleep on one side.

14. A client who works in a business office has been diagnosed with RA. Nursing interventions for client education should include all of the following except:
    1. use of adaptive equipment to protect joints.
    2. evaluation of work space for ergonomics.
    3. replacement of incandescent lights with fluorescent lights.
    4. medications to reduce inflammation and pain.

15. State the rationale for each type of exercise used to assist the client with RA:
    a. Range-of-motion:

    b. Strengthening:

    c. Endurance:

16. List four interventions which research has shown to be effective in assisting clients with RA who experience joint pain:
    a.
    b.
    c.
    d.

17. Nursing actions to protect skin integrity for clients with scleroderma include: (Select all that apply)
    1. use of pressure-reducing beds or air mattresses.
    2. careful removal of dressing.
    3. dressings secured with stretchable gauze.
    4. IM injections/IV therapy at sites free of fibrosis and sclerosis.
    5. use of large amounts of tape.

18. A client with RA complains of fatigue and disrupted sleep. Nursing interventions to assist this client would include: (Select all that apply)
    1. medication for pain and inflammation.
    2. maintaining a regular sleep schedule.
    3. consumption of one glass of wine before bed.
    4. use of flannel nightwear or sleeping blankets to retain warmth.
    5. engaging in soothing activities.

KEEPING DRUG SKILLS SHARP

19. Common disease modifying anti-rheumatic drugs (DMARDs) used today in the clinical setting include: (Select all that apply)
    1. Methotrexate.
    2. Leflunomide.
    3. Etanercept.
    4. Infliximab.

20. Treatment of SLE involves use of _____ and _____ to suppress inflammation.

21. Use of NSAIDs to control inflammation in SLE should be closely monitored if there is evidence of _____.

22. To control the symptoms of Raynaud's disease, _____ is used as a calcium channel blocker resulting in vasodilation.

23. In the treatment of scleroderma, _____ is used as an immumodulating agent that interferes with the cross-linking of collagen, reducing the deposits.

24. List the three categories of medications used to treat clients with Fibromyalgia and the rationale for each:
    a.

    b.

    c.

CONCEPT MAP EXERCISES

The following questions are based on the concept map *Understanding Rheumatoid Arthritis and Its Treatment* in the textbook.

25. How does administering intravenous Immunoglobulin G treat the manifestations of rheumatoid arthritis?

26. When the synovium of the joint is inflamed, as with RA, how does that result in subsequent destruction of that joint area?

27. What combination of medications is given during the inflammatory phase of RA to decrease pain?

28. During the destruction phase of RA, what mechanism *causes* the tissue damage?

29. What clinical manifestations are treated with direct injection of steroids into the joint space?

30. Which clinical manifestations are permanent without surgical correction?

Chapter 80

Management of Clients with Acquired Immunodeficiency Syndrome

OBJECTIVES

80.1 Discuss the etiology and risk factors for HIV.

80.2 Describe the pathophysiology of HIV.

80.3 Discuss the clinical manifestations and management of clients with HIV.

80.4 Discuss nursing interventions for clients with HIV/AIDS.

UNDERSTANDING PATHOPHYSIOLOGY

1. The genetic subtype of HIV that predominates in North America and Europe is
    _____.

2. List the three primary modes of HIV transmission:
    a.
    b.
    c.

3. The greatest risk of occupational exposure to HIV for the health care worker is through
    _____.

4. Place the following steps in the depletion of T helper cells in the order in which they occur.

    _____ a. The virus is uncoated, and RNA enters the cell.

    _____ b. The cell may function abnormally.

    _____ c. The newly created DNA moves into the nucleus and the DNA of the cell.

    _____ d. The enzyme known as reverse transcriptase is released, and viral RNA is transcribed into DNA.

    _____ e. A provirus is created when the viral DNA integrates itself into the cellular DNA or genome of the cell.

    _____ f. The host cell dies, and viral budding occurs.

    _____ g. When the provirus is in place, its genetic material is no longer pure cell but is part virus.

5. An individual will likely develop an infection at a CD4 cell count below
   _____.

6. Differentiate between a long-term non-progressor and a long-term survivor.

7. Normally antibodies to HIV can be detected _____ weeks after exposure.

8. Which of the following individuals is at risk for having a false-positive test result for HIV?
   1. person with osteoarthritis
   2. person with lung cancer
   3. person with lupus erythematosus
   4. person with anemia

9. List the four main types of opportunistic infections:
   a.
   b.
   c.
   d.

10. A constitutional manifestation of infection is:
    1. chest pain.
    2. joint pain.
    3. skin lesions.
    4. weight loss.

11. List the five methods of contracting salmonella infection:
    a.
    b.
    c.
    d.
    e.

12. List the predisposing factors of recurring bacterial pneumonia:
    a.
    b.
    c.
    d.
    e.

13. Clients with cutaneous infection with *Candida albicans* present with
    _____.

14. The first manifestation of *P. carinii* pneumonia is _____.

15. True or False

_____ HIV ranks third among the leading causes of death worldwide.

_____ The lack of economic resources to treat the disease causes HIV to be a rapidly progressing fatal illness in some parts of the world.

_____ HIV-1 and HIV-2 are two distinct and separate viruses.

_____ The ability of the HIV virus to change its appearance or mutate is called genetic promiscuity.

_____ Sexual preferences versus sexual practices place individuals at greatest risk for HIV.

_____ Most people are infected with *P. carinii* in the early preschool years.

_____ Toxoplasmosis can be acquired through direct handling of contaminated dog feces.

_____ Profuse diarrhea is a common clinical manifestation of cryptosporidial disease.

_____ Cervical intraepithelial neoplasia occurs at a high rate in women infected with HIV.

APPLYING SKILLS

16. List two monitoring parameters that are used to follow a client with HIV:
    a.
    b.

17. Which of the following viral load test results poses a high risk for AIDS?
    1. 10,000 copies/ml
    2. 10,000-100,000 copies/ml
    3. >100,000 copies/ml

18. Prior to initiating teaching for the client with HIV, it is important for the nurse to assess the client's _____.

19. List the two criteria used to determine whether to treat a client for *M. avium* complex infection:
    a.
    b.

20. True or False

_____ Urine tests for detecting HIV infection are as accurate as serologic testing.

_____ During the assessment of clinical manifestations of HIV infected clients, it is important to try to quantify the clinical manifestation.

BEST PRACTICES

21. Explain how the health care worker can decrease his or her risk of occupational exposure to HIV.

22. List the crisis points at which the nurse can anticipate anxiety, fear, or depression in the client with HIV disease:

    a.

    b.

    c.

    d.

    e.

    f.

23. Which of the following should the nurse include in the teaching plan for an HIV-infected person? (Select all that apply)
    1. interpretation of viral load tests
    2. the importance of limiting exercise
    3. eating a high-calorie, low-protein, low-fat diet
    4. routine mouth care
    5. proper hand washing
    6. skin care

24. To help control recurrent infections with Candida, the nurse should instruct the client to eat

    _____.

25. List the nonpharmacologic nursing interventions for a client with fever:

    a.

    b.

    c.

26. Explain the rationale for avoiding tepid sponge baths for the treatment of fever.

27. The nurse should teach the client with fatigue to avoid consumption of all of the following except:
    1. coffee.
    2. tobacco.
    3. sugar.
    4. alcohol.

28. True or False

    _____ Autologous blood programs limit the transmission of HIV through blood product administration.

    _____ When an HIV client's CD4 cell counts fall below 200 mm^3, the client should receive prophylactic therapy for *P. carinii* pneumonia.

    _____ Alternate and complementary therapies provide positive benefits and should be encouraged if the client believes they are helpful.

    _____ Aerobic exercise, which increases endurance, can reduce fatigue.

    _____ Cooking with herbs and spices is an appropriate intervention to counter anorexia secondary to hyperosmia.

    _____ Physical therapy modalities such as massage, TENS, and application of heat and cold can be helpful in reducing pain.

KEEPING DRUG SKILLS SHARP

29. Identify the absolutely, very, and probably safe practices to limit exposure to HIV through injected drug use.
    a. absolutely safe:

    b. very safe:

    c. probably safe:

30. The antiretroviral agents that prevent HIV from entering healthy T-cells in the body are:
    1. NRTIs.
    2. PIs.
    3. NNRTIs.
    4. entry inhibitors.

31. The first NRTI was _____.

32. Match each drug with the appropriate reason for administration:

	Drug	**Reason for Administration**
_____	a. trimethoprim-sulfamethoxazole	1. respiratory infections
_____	b. clarithromycin	2. traveler's diarrhea
_____	c. pyridoxine	3. *P. carinii* pneumonia
_____	d. ciprofloxacin	4. *M. avium*-intracellulare complex
_____	e. pneumococcal vaccine	5. peripheral neuropathy

33. To sustain the durability and efficacy of antiretroviral therapy, clients must maintain compliance _____ of the time.

34. List the three drugs used in combination to treat mycobacterium tuberculosis:
    a.
    b.
    c.

35. True or False

    _____ Most clinicians recommend starting an antiretroviral combination therapy regimen early in the course of the disease.

    _____ A potential benefit of antiretroviral therapy is decreased risk for development of HIV resistance to drugs.

    _____ A potential risk of antiretroviral therapy is unknown long-term toxicity of antiretroviral therapy.

_____ Amphotericin B is used to treat disseminated disease of *Candida albicans*.

_____ It is unusual for clients to sleep for extended periods during the first few days of a pain control regimen.

_____ Pain therapy regimens increase the diarrhea common in clients with HIV.

Management of Clients with Leukemia and Lymphoma

OBJECTIVES

81.1   Discuss the pathophysiology, clinical manifestations, and management of the client with leukemia and lymphoma.

81.2   Describe nursing care for clients undergoing treatment for leukemia and lymphoma.

81.3   Discuss care provided to clients receiving bone marrow transplantation.

UNDERSTANDING PATHOPHYSIOLOGY

1.   Match each term with the appropriate definition.

Term	Definition
_____ a. hemotopoietic cells	1. cancer of the bone marrow
_____ b. lymphoid cells	2. cells that originate in the bone marrow
_____ c. leukemia	3. cancer of the lymphoid tissue
_____ d. lymphoma	4. cells that originate in the lymphoid cells

2.   List the risk factors for leukemia:
  a.
  b.
  c.
  d.
  e.

3.   The leukemia most commonly found in children is _____.

4.   The leukemia most commonly found in adults is _____.

5.   List the three classic symptoms commonly associated with leukemia:
  a.
  b.
  c.

6. A complication associated with the rapid destruction of a large number of WBCs is known as
_____.

7. Characteristic clinical manifestations of NHL include: (Select all that apply)
   1. ascites.
   2. back pain.
   3. abdominal masses.
   4. painful lymphadenopathy.

8. Identify and explain the three sources of bone marrow.

9. GVHD may occur _____ to _____ days after infusion of viable lymphocytes.

10. True or False

_____ The client's risk for acquiring chronic lymphocytic leukemia increases with age.

_____ Non-Hodgkin's Lymphoma (NHL) is 60 times more common in people with AIDS than in the general population of the United States.

_____ Chronic GVHD resembles systemic lupus erythematosus.

APPLYING SKILLS

11. A client with leukemia reports having an increased sensitivity to sour and sweet tastes. The nurses recognizes this is associated with:
    1. facial nerve involvement.
    2. meningeal irritation.
    3. anorexia.
    4. lymphadenopathy.

12. The primary diagnostic tool for leukemia is _____.

13. A nurse is caring for a client experiencing tumor lysis syndrome. The nurse would expect the electrolytes to reveal:
    1. hyponatremia.
    2. hypercalcemia.
    3. hypokalemia.
    4. hyperkalemia.
    5. hypernatremia.

14. List two criteria the nurse should check for before administering blood to a client receiving treatment for leukemia.
    a.
    b.

15. A nurse is assessing a client with chronic lymphocytic leukemia. Which of the following manifestations would the nurse expect due to the reduced production of RBCs?
    1. insomnia
    2. increased appetite
    3. weight gain
    4. decreased attention span

16. A manifestation consistent with a decrease in platelet function is:
    1. hard, brown stool.
    2. diminished menstrual flow.
    3. hematuria.
    4. heat intolerance.

17. A client is experiencing altered tissue perfusion related to anemia. The nurse would expect to find all of the following when assessing the vital signs except:
    1. increase in respirations.
    2. increase in blood pressure.
    3. increase in pulse.
    4. decrease in blood pressure.

18. True or False

    _____ A complete blood count of a patient with leukemia may reveal a white blood cell count (WBC) as normal, low, or high.

Case Study

A client has a nursing diagnosis of Ineffective protection/risk for infection related to neutropenia or leukocytosis secondary to leukemia or treatment.

19. Identify appropriate outcomes for this nursing diagnosis.

20. Calculate the absolute neutrophil count (ANC) for this client with the following values: 1% bands, 42% segs, 1650 WBC.

21. Based on the ANC count of the client described above, would the nurse place the client in protective isolation? Why or why not?

22. The client ordered a fresh fruit salad on the menu but did not receive it when the meal was served. The client noted that the salad had been marked out and was substituted with applesauce. What explanation would the nurse provide to the client?

23. Which of the following orders for this would the nurse question and why?
    1. Notify physician for temperature > 38°
    2. Frequent oral hygiene with soft bristle brush
    3. Pericolace, 1 PO, OD
    4. Tylenol suppository for fever > 37.5°

BEST PRACTICES

24. Explain the rationale for not performing a lumbar puncture during the acute phase of leukemia.

25. What should the nurse teach the client with a nursing diagnosis of Imbalanced nutrition: less than body requirements related to anorexia, pain, or fatigue about his or her diet?

26. A client voices concern about losing his or her hair secondary to chemotherapy. What should the nurse teach the client about this hair loss?

27. Explain the role of the clinical nurse specialist or case manager for the client with a nursing diagnosis of Risk for ineffective therapeutic regimen management and risk for ineffective family therapeutic regimen management.

KEEPING DRUG SKILLS SHARP

28. Which of the following medications is added during stage IV treatment of chronic lymphocytic leukemia?
    1. prednisone
    2. leukeran
    3. fludarabine
    4. potassium chloride

29. Explain why the client with a nursing diagnosis of Ineffective protection/risk for hemorrhage related to thrombocytopenia secondary to either leukemia or treatment should not receive aspirin or medications containing aspirin.

30. List the drugs administered in ABVD therapy for HD and explain why this regimen is preferable to MOPP.
    a.
    b.
    c.
    d.

Chapter 82

Management of Clients Requiring Transplantation

OBJECTIVES

82.1 Identify the major contributing factors to successful organ transplantation.

82.2 Discuss nursing roles and responsibilities related to organ transplantation.

82.3 Discuss the basic criteria used for transplantation.

82.4 Discuss pertinent nursing care for clients having transplantation.

82.5 Describe ethical and family considerations associated with transplantation.

UNDERSTANDING PATHOPHYSIOLOGY

1. There is a significant limitation to organ transplantation due to:
    1. increased use of medications that affect transplant reactions.
    2. shortage of organ donors.
    3. numerous insurance claims which do not cover cost.
    4. clients choosing other options.

2. _____ is the leading cause of morbidity and mortality after transplantation.

3. Acute rejection of organs usually occurs within _____.

4. Chronic rejection of organs usually occurs after _____.

5. Opportunistic infections are very common within the first 6 months after transplantation. These infections include: (Select all that apply)
    1. *Pneumocystis carinii* pneumonia.
    2. candidiasis.
    3. CMV infections.
    4. *Staphylococcus aureus*.

APPLYING SKILLS

6. The nurse's role in organ donation and organ recovery includes: (Select all that apply)
    1. identifying early potential donors.
    2. making referrals to OPO.
    3. assisting in medical management of organ donors.
    4. acting as a liaison with donor families.

BEST PRACTICES

7. The improved success of organ transplantation today is due to: (Select all that apply)
    1. availability of new immunosuppressive therapies.
    2. advancements in organ preservation.
    3. improved surgical techniques.
    4. risk factor recognition that enhances survival.

8. The _____ (amended 1972) covers the cost of dialysis and transplantation for end-stage renal disease.

9. The criteria used by the Uniform Determination of Death Act state that an individual is considered dead if: (Select all that apply)
    1. there is irreversible cessation of circulatory and respiratory functions.
    2. there is irreversible cessation of all functions of the entire brain and brain stem.
    3. only respiratory functions remain.
    4. cardiac functions are maintained only due to medication administration.

10. Which act was passed to prohibit the sale of human organs?
    1. Social Security Act of 1972
    2. United Network of Organ Sharing Act
    3. Uniform Determination of Death Act
    4. National Organ Transplant Act 1984

11. _____ is the transplantation of organs, tissues, or cells from one species to another, and has been proposed as one answer to the organ donor shortage.

12. The primary responsibility of an organ transplant team is to:
    1. transplant organs into clients who have the best chance for a long-term successful outcome.
    2. identify donors and maintain a list for future transplants.
    3. maintain a database of successful transplants for future research.
    4. educate other health professionals regarding organ transplant procedures.

13. Successful transplant recipients will have: (Select all that apply)
    1. improved functional status.
    2. long-term graft function.
    3. improved quality of life.
    4. no need for other medications for life-sustaining purposes.

14. True or False

   _____ The nurse plays an integral role in preoperative education of potential organ recipients.

   _____ Nurses are encouraged to meet with other health professionals to discuss their feelings and difficult cases, as well as to develop plans of care for their clients.

15. The goal of education of a potential organ recipient is to: (Select all that apply)
   1. provide family with factual information regarding waiting time for organs.
   2. explain surgical procedures.
   3. explain post transplantation regimens (diet, exercise, medications).
   4. explain routine skin grafting procedures.

16. The criteria maintained by the United Network of Organ Sharing (UNOS) for listing a client for organ transplantation is based on: (Select all that apply)
   1. urgency.
   2. blood type.
   3. recipient weight and height.
   4. medical condition.

17. During the period when clients are waiting for organ transplants, the nurse will: (Select all that apply)
   1. establish a trusting relationship with the client.
   2. participate in client education.
   3. work with clients so they grasp the realities of life after transplantation.
   4. refer clients to another system of care if needed.

18. Problems that clients with organ transplants may encounter include: (Select all that apply)
   1. medication side effects.
   2. rejection of organs.
   3. financial limitations.
   4. preservation of other organs.

19. Organ transplantation teams consist of: (Select all that apply)
   1. transplant surgeon, psychologist, other physicians.
   2. nurse coordinator, nurse practitioner.
   3. social worker.
   4. pharmacist, nutritionist.
   5. clergy.

KEEPING DRUG SKILLS SHARP

20. The goal of immunosuppressive therapy in organ transplantation is to: (Select all that apply)
   1. suppress immune response to prevent organ rejection.
   2. prolong complications from therapy itself.
   3. give massive doses of medications.
   4. identify graft resources.

21. Excessive immunosuppressive therapy can lead to: (Select all that apply)
    1. increased risk of infection.
    2. liver or kidney insufficiency.
    3. joint necrosis.
    4. cataracts or malignancies.
    5. rejection of transplanted organ.

Chapter 83

Management of Clients with Shock and Multisystem Disorders

OBJECTIVES

83.1 Describe the basic etiologies of shock.

83.2 Identify similarities and differences among the various types of shock.

83.3 Describe generally recognized stages of shock.

83.4 Explain the systemic effects of shock.

83.5 Identify the appropriate interventions for clients with shock.

84.6 Discuss current medications used to treat shock.

UNDERSTANDING PATHOPHYSIOLOGY

1. Shock can be defined as:
    1. failure of the circulatory system to maintain adequate perfusion of vital organs.
    2. decreased oxygenation at the cellular level.
    3. anaerobic cellular metabolism.
    4. accumulated waste products in the system.

2. Shock can be categorized into which of following types? (Select all that apply)
    1. distributive
    2. hypovolemic
    3. cardiogenic
    4. muscle-related

3. A client admitted to the clinic with burns, hemorrhage, or dehydration may develop:
    1. hypovolemic shock.
    2. distributive shock.
    3. cardiogenic shock.
    4. neurologic shock.

4. Cardiogenic shock is caused by: (Select all that apply)
    1. inadequate pumping action of the heart.
    2. primary cardiac muscle dysfunction.
    3. mechanical obstruction of blood flow.
    4. valvular insufficiency resulting from disease or trauma.

5. All clients with spinal cord injuries experience some degree of:
   1. septic shock.
   2. neurogenic shock.
   3. distributive shock.
   4. cardiac shock.

6. The primary events that precipitate hypovolemic shock are: (Select all that apply)
   1. inadequate circulation.
   2. reduction in the circulating blood volume.
   3. metabolic needs of the body not being met.
   4. absence of creatine in the circulation.

7. Clients admitted the clinic with large partial thickness or full thickness burns will be prone to: (Select all that apply)
   1. hypovolemic shock.
   2. distributive shock.
   3. anaphylactic shock.
   4. neurogenic shock.

8. The major pathology behind irreversible or refractory shock is:
   1. renal failure.
   2. intestinal mucosa disturbed.
   3. failure of sympathetic nervous system compensation.
   4. cardiac compromise.

APPLYING SKILLS

9. When mechanical obstructions cause blood flow problems that lead to cardiogenic shock, which of the following may occur? (Select all that apply)
   1. large pulmonary embolism
   2. pericardial tamponade
   3. tension pneumothorax
   4. multiple CVA events

10. Clients admitted to the clinic with anaphylactic reactions may be sensitized to which of the following agents? (Select all that apply)
    1. penicillin
    2. bee stings
    3. chocolate
    4. snake venom

11. The major cause of death in shock is _____.

12. During shock, the nurse can expect a client's pulse rate to:
    1. usually increase due to increased sympathetic stimulation.
    2. decrease due to vascular collapse.
    3. usually increase with resultant drop in cardiovascular collapse.
    4. undergo no changes.

13. Clients who have a declining diastolic blood pressure can be potential candidates for:
    1. neurogenic collapse.
    2. decreasing systemic vascular resistance.
    3. abnormal pulse pressures.
    4. no significant changes.

14. Clinical manifestations that are expected with hypovolemic shock include which of the following lab data? (Select all that apply)
    1. urine osmolarity increases
    2. specific gravity of urine increases
    3. sodium and water reabsorption
    4. no change in urine status

15. Confusion, agitation, and restlessness are clinical signs that a client's level of consciousness has changed due to:
    1. decreased circulation to brain tissue.
    2. abnormal output from urinary status.
    3. elevated cardiac enzymes.
    4. constant change in pH values.

16. Clients who have massive thermal burns and are heading toward irreversible shock will show which of the following laboratory findings?
    1. increased liver enzymes
    2. decreased cardiac enzymes
    3. elevated pH levels
    4. decreased HCO_3 levels

17. When using Ringer's lactate for fluid replacement therapy for clients with shock, the nurse needs to monitor:
    1. serum pH levels.
    2. CPK and LDH levels.
    3. ammonia levels.
    4. serum calcium levels.

18. Arterial blood gas analysis may be done during the shock phase to determine: (Select all that apply)
    1. if metabolic acidosis that occurs with shock is being effectively combated by hyperventilation.
    2. adequate oxygen levels.
    3. if further respiratory assistance is needed.
    4. a baseline for CO_2 replacement.

19. The primary goals in treating shock are to: (Select all that apply)
    1. establish vaso-peripheral circulation.
    2. maintain adequate circulating blood volume.
    3. restore vital potassium circulating levels.
    4. increase demands for oxygenation.

BEST PRACTICES

20. The priority in emergency management of shock is to: (Select all that apply)
    1. provide for emergency intubations.
    2. place client in reverse Trendenlenburg position.
    3. provide fluid resuscitation.
    4. establish intravenous access sites.

21. A _____ is an example of a mechanical device that assists circulation or decreases the workload of the heart.

KEEPING DRUGS SKILLS SHARP

22. The mainstay of hypovolemic shock therapy is: (Select all that apply)
    1. expansion of circulating blood volume.
    2. IV administration of blood or other appropriate fluids.
    3. increased dilation of heart vessels.
    4. establishment of baseline respiratory status.

23. When large volumes of fluid are given, the nurse must be aware of the client's urinary status. Aggressive fluid replacement should be tapered off when: (Select all that apply)
    1. urinary output is at least 60 ml/hr.
    2. blood pressure is greater than 100 mm Hg.
    3. heart rate is 60-100 beats per minute.
    4. the client's ability to tolerate foods has been assessed.

24. IV fluids used in shock management may include: (Select all that apply)
    a. warmed crystalloids.
    b. balanced salt solutions.
    c. colloids.
    d. blood products.

25. When hemorrhage is the primary cause of shock, rapid administration which of the following is indicated? (Select all that apply)
    1. large volumes of packed cells
    2. whole blood
    3. IV fluids of dextrose
    4. rapid rate extenders of fluids

26. The drug of choice for treating of allergic reactions and anaphylaxis is:
    1. epinephrine.
    2. antibiotics.
    3. urinary stimulants.
    4. glucose inhibitors.

27. Medications that improve myocardial contractions are used in treating types of shock that decrease cardiac output. Examples of these medications include: (Select all that apply)
    1. digitalis.
    2. amiodarone.
    3. lidocaine.
    4. atropine

Chapter 84

Management of Clients in the Emergency Department

OBJECTIVES

84.1 Discuss nursing assessment, triage categories, documentation, and discharge teaching in the emergency department.

84.2 Discuss priority nursing interventions for selected emergency situations.

84.3 Identify signs and symptoms associated with selected medical-surgical conditions and emergencies.

84.4 Discuss appropriate medical management and priority discharge teaching of clients with medical-surgical emergencies.

84.5 Discuss relevant terminology unique to the emergency department.

84.6 Explain proper handling of evidentiary specimens obtained in the emergency department.

UNDERSTANDING PATHOPHYSIOLOGY

1. _____ is a procedure that can be used when suspected chest trauma clients have large amounts of blood loss from a hemothorax.

2. Match the following definitions or descriptions with the correct term.

	Definition/Description	Term
_____	a. chest moves opposite of normal respiratory patterns	1. pneumothorax
_____	b. occurs with a sucking chest wound	2. hemopneumothorax
_____	c. blood and air in the pleural space	3. tension pneumothorax
_____	d. fractures of two or more ribs on the same side	4. open pneumothorax
_____	e. blood in the pleural space	5. flail chest
_____	f. contents of the mediastinum are pushed toward the unaffected side	6. mediastinal shift
_____	g. air enters the pleural space and becomes trapped	7. paradoxical motion
_____	h. air in the pleural space	8. hemothorax

APPLYING SKILLS

3. Which of the following types of incidents seen in the emergency department must be reported to federal, state, and local authorities? (Select all that apply)
   1. suspected child abuse
   2. suspected domestic violence
   3. suspected elder abuse
   4. motor vehicle accidents

4. Match the following definitions or descriptions with the correct term.

	Definition/Description	**Term**
_____	a. any sudden illness or injury that is perceived to be a crisis that threatens the physical or psychological well-being of a person or group	1. secondary nursing interventions
_____	b. interventions may be delayed beyond a few hours	2. priority nursing interventions
_____	c. occurs when the emergency department is called for help with a crisis	3. emergent
_____	d. a complete focused assessment	4. emergency
_____	e. requires interventions within a few hours	5. urgent
_____	f. life threatening: the client may die without immediate interventions	6. telephone triage
_____	g. interventions focused on emergency care	7. non-urgent
_____	h. the process of determining priorities	8. triage

5. The _____ obligates emergency department personnel to follow the client's advance directives.

6. If no written information regarding advance directives is available for a client who requires emergency treatment, emergency department personnel must: (Select all that apply)
   1. stabilize the client.
   2. resuscitate any client if necessary.
   3. follow appropriate standard treatment guidelines regardless of a family member's expressed wishes.
   4. not provide any treatment for the client.

7. For any client arriving at the emergency department with a major traumatic injury, primary assessment includes:
   1. determining when the patient ate last.
   2. overall assessment of vital signs.
   3. evaluation of cervical spine area for any potential injury.
   4. location of relatives in the next state.

8. Before clients can be discharged from the emergency department, they must receive: (Select all that apply)
   1. fluid and foods to be eaten at home.
   2. oral and written discharge instructions.
   3. written identification of diagnosed problem.
   4. explanation of treatments, complications, and recheck times.

9. Nursing documentation in the emergency department must include: (Select all that apply)
   1. assessment findings.
   2. diagnostic tests and interventions.
   3. responses to treatment.
   4. client education.

10. The first priority of care with any client in the emergency department is:
    1. maintaining a patent airway.
    2. observing for respiratory distress.
    3. securing medical insurance information.
    4. documenting time of arrival.

11. Unstable clients admitted to the emergency department with suspected abdominal injury or trauma would likely undergo:
    1. diagnostic peritoneal lavage (DPL).
    2. venogram.
    3. AST evaluation.
    4. stress ECG.

BEST PRACTICES

12. The goals of the emergency medical services include:
    1. providing emergency care to a client as quickly as possible.
    2. assuring that the "right client arrives at the right hospital."
    3. maintaining professional relationships with the community.
    4. assisting families in securing appropriate referrals when needed.

13. Minors for whom consent of a parent or legal guardian does not need to be obtained in order to treat them include: (Select all that apply)
    1. emancipated minors.
    2. minors seeking treatment for communicable diseases.
    3. minor-aged females requesting treatment for pregnancy or pregnancy-related concerns.
    4. children with sore throats and fever.

14. Hospital policies and guidelines must comply with which of the following organizations regarding the use of restraints on clients in the emergency department? (Select all that apply)
    1. American Medical Association.
    2. Joint Commission on Hospital Accreditation.
    3. Centers for Medicare and Medicaid Services.
    4. National Alliance of Hospital Organizations.

KEEPING DRUG SKILLS SHARP

15. Clients who have received fibrinolytic medications in the emergency department must be continuously monitored for:
    1. increased intracranial pressure.
    2. active bleeding.
    3. visual disturbances.
    4. beta blocker corrections.

16. When conscious sedation is used in the emergency department, nursing responsibilities include: (Select all that apply)
    1. continually monitoring for airway patency.
    2. maintaining oxygen saturation levels.
    3. monitoring cardiac activity.
    4. determining patient response to physical or verbal stimulation.

17. When a client is admitted to the emergency department for any kind of poisoning, whether accidental or intentional, the nurse must obtain accurate information, including:
    1. amount and time of ingestion.
    2. information about the offending substance.
    3. whether the client has vomited since exposure.
    4. any previous episodes of intentional or accidental poisoning in the past.

18. The drug of choice for clients who presents with a narcotic overdose is:
    1. methylpredinosolone.
    2. Narcan.
    3. Valium.
    4. lisinopril.

Answer Key

CHAPTER 1

1. Health is a state of complete physical, mental, and social well-being and not merely the absence of disease or infirmity.
2. high-level wellness
3. True
4. 1
5. Health promotion is a process of fostering awareness, influencing attitudes, and identifying alternatives so that people can make informed choices and change behavior to achieve an optimal level of physical and mental health and improve their physical and social environments.
6. 3
7. a. genetic or biologic (age, race, family history), b. behavioral (personal health habits such as overeating, smoking, lack of exercise), c. environmental (air pollution, water pollution, noise pollution)
8.

Modifiable Risk Factor	Non-modifiable Risk Factor
• Capable of being changed • Include such things as tobacco use, dietary indiscretion, deficiencies, and over consumption, sedentary lifestyle, alcohol and drug abuse, fatigue and lack of sleep, pollution, unsafe sexual behavior, and misuse of motor vehicles and or firearms	• Are unchangeable • Genetic and biologic characteristics cannot be modified

9. self-efficacy
10. confidence
11. Allostatic load is the resulting deterioration that the body experiences from repeated activation of the stress response.
12. In a recessive disease, one abnormal gene is inherited but the individual doesn't show signs of the disease; however, they pass the abnormal gene to 50% of their offspring. In a dominant disorder, one abnormal gene is inherited and the offspring will likely show signs of the disease.
13. carcinogen
14. Their training is disease focused rather than wellness or prevention oriented.
15. a. physical activity, b. overweight and obesity, c. tobacco use, d. substance abuse, e. responsible sexual behavior, f. mental health, g. injury and violence, h. environmental quality, i. immunization, j. access to health care
16. True
17. a. 2, b. 5, c. 4, d. 3, e. 1
18. In gene therapy a normal copy of DNA fragments are injected into cells of a client with a disease. The fragments find their way to the nucleus and repair enzymes to restore normal function to the cell.
19. 2
20. A broad definition is needed because health can be viewed in many contexts of individual human experience. A broader definition reflects a multi-dimensional, holistic view.
21. 1, 3, 4
22. a. progression toward a higher level of functioning, b. integration of the whole being, c. an open-ended future with the challenge of fuller potential
23. *Healthy People 2010*
24. True, True, False, False, True, False, True, False, True, False, True, True
25. Health risk appraisal
26. 2, 3, 4
27. high fiber, vegetables
28. Moderate alcohol intake raises HDL levels, has anticlotting properties, and reduces the risk of heart disease.
29. autoimmunity
30. a. asthma, b. lung cancer
31. a. 2, b. 3, c. 1
32. 1, 3, 5
33. Social support decreases levels of hormones, provides a sense of meaning or coherence that promotes a healthy lifestyle, and helps clients adhere to medical treatment and seek medical care.
34. Alcoholics Anonymous
35. 4
36. 3
37. 10%
38. 4
39. 1

40. 2
41. Nurses empower clients with the provision of information, skills, services, and support needed to undertake and maintain positive lifestyle changes. The nurse teaches the client self-care.
42. a. performance attainment (successful performance of a desired behavior), b. vicarious experiences (watching others successfully perform a behavior), c. verbal persuasion (convincing a client of the capability to perform a specific behavior), d. physiologic status (interpretation of physiologic states that may occur when a behavior is performed).
43. 2
44. 3
45. The nurse can implement intervention to promote physical safety, to prevent alterations in skin integrity, to promote social interactions, to promote adequate nutrition, and to encourage cancer screening.
46. Relaxation

CHAPTER 2
1. a. 2, b. 1, c. 3, d. 3, e. 1, f. 2, g. 3
2. a. stress resistance, b. cognitive reappraisal, c. effective coping skills
3. The 3-day dietary log not only identifies what types and amounts of food eaten but when, why, and how the client ate the food. This information helps the client and nurse identify patterns and problem behaviors.
4. 1, 2, 4
5. one hour
6. Physical activity improves mental functioning, decreases depression, and increases physical endurance.
7. perception, interpretation
8. a. occupational exposure to blood or blood products
   b. men who have sex with men
   c. injectable drug users and their partners
   d. multiple sexual partners
   e. history of sexually transmitted disease
   f. travel to countries with endemic Hepatitis B.
9. 2, 3, 4
10. a. mode, b. intensity, c. duration, d. frequency
11. a. confident in ability to perform activity, b. finds activity pleasurable, c. have social support
12. True, True, True
13. assessment
14. decrease
15. a. helpful for the worrier. Clients learn to stop obsessive dialogue such as "what if" and replace with positive thought.

b. based on rational emotive therapy and helps clients recognize irrational thought and replace it with rational self-talk.
   c. clients learn how to image a relaxing event or dialogue with self for problem solving.
   d. clients learn how to recognize stressors, determine how significant the stressor is, and use problem solving to cope with the stressor.
16. 2, 3, 4, 6
17. 4
18. 4
19. 1
20. a. assess lifestyle
    b. assess for risk factors
    c. intervene to modify lifestyle
    d. intervene to reduce modifiable risk factors.
21. 4
22. 4
23. 3
24. 1, 2, 3, 4
25. 4
26. 3
27. 1, 2, 3, 5
28. 4
29. 3
30. 1, 2, 4
31. a. regular use of lap and shoulder restraints: protect from injury sustained from forward movement of the body or being thrown from the vehicle during a crash.
    b. avoid drug use: drugs impair judgment and delay motor responses.
    c. avoid alcohol use: alcohol impairs judgment and delays motor responses.
32. 4
33. 2
34. safety
35. 1, 2, 3, 4, 7
36. To identify client readiness to modify physical activity, screen for contraindications, and develop an individualized activity plan.
37. a. not recommended: simple carbohydrates increase energy temporarily but then this is followed by weakness and lethargy.
    b. not recommended: over eating decrease energy and lowers self-esteem.
    c. recommended: eating fruits increases energy and provides increased physical ability to cope.
    d. recommended: adequate sleep and rest are essential for healing and repairing physiological effects of stress.
38. a. Ask the client if he/she wants to quit now.
    b. Determine motivation to change.

c. Identify what is needed to support the cessation efforts.
d. Help the client identify strategies for managing triggers.
e. Refer the client to community resources for additional assistance.
39. Any woman can be abused and any man/partner can be an abuser
40. a. up-to-date immunizations
    b. practicing safe sex
41. a. Frequency: Periodic
       Rationale: detect obesity
    b. Frequency: every 3 years
       Rationale: detect cervical cancer
    c. Frequency: periodic
       Rationale: detect problem drinking
42. a. fecal occult blood or sigmoidoscopy less often
    b. mammogram and clinical breast exam

CHAPTER 3

1. ADLs are basic self-care activities while IADLs include ADLs plus the ability to shop, perform housework, manage money, prepare food, and engage independently in transportation activities such as driving, riding a bus, or taking a taxi.
2. Ageism is the prejudices and stereotypes applied to older people purely because of their age.
3. The ingestion of any compound in quantities that may be harmful to health or well-being.
4. True, True, True
5. Accentuates the positive ability of the individual
6. Ageism limits older person's self-confidence, may force early dependence, influences attitudes of health care providers, influences attitudes of political powers, may contribute to less aggressive treatment of diseases in older individuals, and may contribute to underfunding of social programs.
7. a. low self-esteem, b. no friends or support, c. increased worries, d. high levels of alienation, e. poor self-perception of health, f. depression
8. 1, 2, 3, 4
9. 2
10. 3
11. a. normal changes of aging, b. chronic health conditions, c. autonomy, d. feelings of stress, e. powerlessness
12. a. increased energy, b. improved eating, c. improved sleeping, d. decreased discomfort and stress, e. decreased smoking and alcohol use.
13. a. socioeconomic: seniors live on fixed income and may choose to buy medications and pay rent over buying food. Also, they may be unable to afford fresh fruits and vegetables.

b. social: seniors may lack transportation to get groceries and may be unable to carry heavy grocery bags. They may live alone and lack motivation to prepare and eat balanced meals.
c. psychological: depression and stress can lead to under eating.
d. medication use: some medications can decrease appetite, cause constipation, nausea and vomiting, or alter fluid and electrolyte balance.
e. physiological: decreased energy may alter appetite and altered dentition may affect the ability to chew food.
14. True, True, True, True, False, True, True
15. 1, 2, 3, 4, 5
16. Older adults have more difficulty falling asleep, awaken more easily, spend more time in the drowsiness stage of sleep, and spend less time in deep sleep.
17. Sensory impairments can affect safety, ability to communicate, ability to perform ADLs and IADLs, and increase the risk of medication errors and falls.
18. 40%
19. a. alcohol, b. illicit drugs, c. prescription drug abuse
20. living wills, durable power of attorney for health care
21. Family support helps maintain independence, promotes effective coping with illness, and helps the older adult remain functional.
22. 2
23. abilities, disabilities
24. 3
25. 1, 2, 3, 4
26. 3
27. 2
28. Polypharmacy contributes to increased risk of drug interactions and adverse drug reactions, may duplicate therapy, decrease quality of life, and increase unnecessary financial and societal costs.
29. a. minimize conflict within families, b. alleviate burden of guilt
30. functional
31. Delivery of services is seamless and encompasses a large range of health, community-based, and in-home services.

CHAPTER 4

1. chief complaint
2. a. 6, b. 7, c. 5, d. 2, e. 4, f. 1, g. 3
3. a. 8, b. 5, c. 7, d. 1, e. 12, f. 4, g. 10, h. 11, i. 3, j. 9, k. 2, l. 6

4. a. body temperature greater than normal range, b. body temperature less than the normal range, c. heart rate greater than 100 BPM, d. heart rate less than 50 BPM, e. respiratory depth, f. systolic pressure less than 95 mm Hg or diastolic pressure less than 60 mm Hg, g. systolic pressure greater than 140 mm Hg or diastolic pressure greater than 90 mm Hg, h. difference between the systolic and diastolic pressure reading, i. a period of silence between two levels of systolic pressures.

5. a. 4, b. 1, c. 2, d. 3

6. A genetic risk involves changes in chromosomes which can lead to deformities in future offspring, whereas somatic risk involves changes that occur in body tissues that receive excessive radiation.

7. angiography

8. Endoscopy is the direct visualization of a body system or part by means of a lighted, flexible tube. This examination is more accurate due to the direct visualization.

9. a. 3, b. 7, c. 5, d. 6, e. 4, f. 2, g. 1

10. A computerized health history assessment provides accurate, legible databases. It can be completed by the client or the nurse and tends to be more complete due to branching programs.

11. This approach helps to identify health patterns, deviations from normal, and actual or potential nursing diagnoses.

12. 3, 4, 5

13. False, True, False, False, True, False, True, True, True, True, True, False, True

14. *long*: also known as exhaustive, uses holistic approach, time-consuming, elicits a wealth of data, may be impractical for an acute care setting *short*: also known as episodic, used when client presents with an uncomplicated, short-term health problem, proficiency required to perform this type of assessment

15. a. demographic information, b. review of systems, c. family history, d. psychosocial assessment, e. client's health maintenance and health promotion behaviors

16. 2

17. 1, 2, 3, 4

18. 2

19. a. 2, b. 3, c. 1

20. anatomy, physiology

21. a. Inspection is a systematic, deliberate visual examination of the entire client. This technique provides information about size, shape, color, texture, symmetry, position, and deformities. It is the first examination technique. b. Palpation is generally the second physical assessment and uses touch. Palpation determines information about masses, pulsation, organ size, tenderness or pain, swelling, tissue firmness and elasticity, vibration, crepitation, temperature, texture, and moisture. Palpation uses the most sensitive parts of the hands to palpate. Palpation uses three levels: light, deep, and bimanual. c. Percussion is used to assess tissue density with sound produced from striking the skin and is usually the third technique. Percussion helps to confirm suspected abnormal findings from palpation and auscultation. There are two methods of percussion: direct and indirect. d. Auscultation is listening to internal body sounds to assess normal sounds and detect abnormal sounds, is the final step in the physical examination, and uses a stethoscope to enhance sounds.

22. general survey

23. balance

24. septicemia

25. 1, 2, 4

26. finger tip

27. 3

28. a. establish presence of a mobility or structural problem, b. follow progress, c. evaluate effectiveness of treatment

29. not exposed to ionizing radiation

30. 1

31. 4

32. 2

33. 4

34. 3

35. 1

36. 3

37. a. 2, b. 3, c. 4, d. 1

38. a. 12, b. 10, c. 8, d. 6, e. 4, f. 2, g. 11, h. 9, i. 7, j. 5, k. 3, l. 1

39. 4

40. 1, 3, 4

41. 2

42. 4

43. 1

44. 4

45. 1

46. 3

47. False, True

48. A lavender top tube contains an additive EDTA. Collecting blood in this tube first increases the risk of contaminating blood in the red top tube, thus altering the test results.

CHAPTER 5

1. a group of diverse medical and health care systems, practices, and products that are not presently considered part of conventional medicine

2. Integrative medicine combines mainstream medical therapies and CAM therapies for which there is some high-quality evidence of safety and effectiveness.

3. A placebo effect suggests that the persons being treated with the placebo experienced an improvement in their condition as the result of psychological or other factors, rather than because of the inert substance administered.

4. A redox agent acts in some situations as an antioxidant, whereas in other situations it can act as pro-oxidant.

5. Therapeutic touch is derived from an ancient technique called "laying-on of hands" and is based on a premise that the healing force of the therapist affects the client's recovery. Healing is promoted when the body's energies are in balance. By passing their hands over the client, healers can identify energy imbalances.

6. Complementary medicine is used together with conventional medicine, whereas alternative medicine is used in place of conventional medicine.

7. a. alternative medical systems, b. mind-body interventions, c. biologically based therapies, d. manipulative and body-based methods, e. energy therapies

8. True, False, True, True

9. False

10. The DSHEA ruling of 1994 placed the actual burden of proof on the U. S. federal government to disprove dietary supplement claims.

11. Vitamin C, E, and beta-carotene

12. 1

13. 2

14. Create a respectful and open communication environment, ask about CAM at each interaction with the client, educate the client about possible adverse reactions, provide information from NCCAM, and teach life-style modification behavior.

CHAPTER 6

1. The cost of providing employees with health care benefits contributes to greater cost of consumer goods, decreases competitiveness of American goods in the world market, and stagnates employee salaries.

2. Consumers are more interested today in receiving quality health care at an affordable cost and are looking more positively at health promotion and disease prevention.

3. Department of Health and Human Services

4. a. Medicare – federal
   b. Medicaid – joint
   c. Department of Veteran Affairs – federal
   d. workers compensation – joint
   e. indigent care – state

5. a. Agency for Healthcare Research and Quality (AHRQ)
   b. National Institutes of Health (NIH)

6. Center of Disease Control and Prevention (CDC)

7. American Hospital Association

8. The health care industry shifts costs by increasing charges to individuals and other payers to offset underpayment by Medicare, Medicaid, and other contracted payers.

9. women and children

10. Introduction of insurance has as its goal the provision of a stronger financial base for community hospitals and the spread of risk of economic loss from individuals to larger groups of peoples. The availability of insurance contributed to an increased demand for and utilization of hospital and health care services. Concurrently, due to wage and price controls, American industries used the provision of health care benefits as a means of recruiting and retaining workers. This, in turn, contributed to increased consumption of and rising cost of health care services.

11. Eliminate shortage of hospitals, especially in rural and economically depressed areas

12. Through a pay-back mechanism, facilities had to provide health care to indigent clients equal in value to the dollar amount of money received by the hospital, prorated over time.

13. Johnson's administration War on Poverty

14. a. Medicare – federal
    Medicaid – federal and state
    b. Medicare – payroll tax by workers who pay Social Security and premiums
    Medicaid – matching formula funds between the federal and state governments
    c. Medicare – Part A hospitalization: Part B physician services
    Medicaid – core health care services

15. Allow states to convert Medicaid services to a managed care system without obtaining a federal Medicaid waiver.

16. a. reduce the number of uninsured
    b. provide coverage of pre-existing conditions after 12 months
    c. provide continuation of group health insurance after COBRA ends

17. They are decertified as Medicare providers and thus face the loss of revenue.

18. a. increased deductibles
    b. larger and more frequent co-payments
    c. initiation of managed care programs
    d. mandatory second opinions
    e. increased contracts with HMOs and PPOs
19. a. Introduction of certificate of need requirement aimed at eliminating duplication of services and facilities.
    b. Introduction of prospective-payment system based on diagnostic related groups for Medicare aimed at reducing health care costs.
    c. Development of a restructured payment system by Blue Cross and other insurers to protect them from cost shifting.
    d. HMOs and PPOs sought to contract with employers to provide insurance to their employees
    e. Capitation was introduced which established per-member-per-month fee paid in advance for specified health care services.
    f. Oversight systems were introduced primarily by HMOs to control delivery of services without authorization
20. To address health care cost, access, and quality.

CHAPTER 7

1. Primary health care focuses on the right to basic health care while primary care focuses on the coordinated care by one primary provider.
2. Telehealth nursing practice is practice using the nursing process to provide care for individual clients or client populations through telecommunications media.
3. 2
4. a. changes in technology, b. emphasis on demonstrated outcomes, c. aging of population, d. reduced revenue to health care organizations, e. large number of uninsured people, f. growing shortage of nurses
5. True, False, True, True, True, True, True
6. Because encounters are of short duration, nursing assessment must be clearly focused. Due to the time factor important assessments may be missed or important questions not asked.
7. physician's offices, hospital outpatient departments, hospital emergency departments.
8. Clients are classified by their health status such as acutely ill, chronically ill, or chronically ill with an acute episode. Another classification is by a major illness or body system such as heart failure, diabetes, or ear, nose, and throat. The last type of classification is by the source of reimbursement such as private insurance, Medicaid, worker's compensation, or self-pays.
9. During telephone triage, the nurse sorts encounters based on the immediacy of need and type of problem, addresses how the problem should be resolved, and advises the client on whether or not the client should be seen in person.
10. cardiac, high-risk obstetric
11. Every encounter should be documented and include assessment data, nursing analysis, recommendations made, client level of understanding of instructions, and requirement for follow-up.
12. Accreditation offers the setting an opportunity to be evaluated by an external group for quality, demonstrates that the setting complies with a uniform set of standards, and allows the organization to be compared with others, thus enhancing a competitive edge.
13. a. Joint Commission of Accreditation of Healthcare Organizations (JCAHO), b. National Committee for Quality Assurance, c. Accreditation Association for Ambulatory Health Care.
14. 2, 3, 4
15. Because the client's family or significant other is responsible for managing the client's care between visits, it is important to understand and respect the client's culture, traditions, and perspectives on health and illness so that care can be provided within this value system.
16. 1, 2, 3, 4
17. 2
18. 1
19. 3

CHAPTER 8

1. a. 3, b. 1, c. 2
2. This is a physician who specializes in the care of hospitalized clients.
3. Swing beds are hospital beds that can be utilized for acute care or postacute care depending on need.
4. a. 2, b. 3, c. 1
5. One-level-of-care means that the same care is provided throughout an institution for the same given situation.
6. Culturally competent care is knowing, explaining, interpreting, and predicting nursing care within the knowledge of the client's cultural and ethnic beliefs and practices.
7. Risk management is a planned program of loss prevention and liability control.
8. True
9. to determine if the hospital has complied with specific rules and regulations.

10. 3
11. Diagnosis-related groups (DRGs)
12. client-driven, payer-driven
13. True, True, False, True, False, True, True, False, False, False, False
14. a. government, b. voluntary/not-for-profit, c. for-profit
15. a. promoting self-care, b. upgrading quality of life, c. using resources efficiently
16. To determine if and how a specific job function can be performed more efficiently.
17. Quality care is delivered while controlling costs.
18. per diem
19. cross-training
20. a. Occupational and Safety and Health Act (OSHA), b. Civil Rights Act of 1964, c. Rehabilitation Act of 1973, d. Age Discrimination and Employment Act (ADEA), e. Americans with Disabilities Act
21. a. medication errors, b. complications from diagnostic or treatment procedures, c. falls, d. client or family dissatisfaction, e. refusal of treatment or refusal to sign consent for treatment
22. 1, 2
23. 3
24. Informal education is continuous and includes explanations to clients and/or family members about medications, what to expect during a treatment, or the importance of particular assessments. Informal education is invaluable to client outcomes. Formal education may be provided to individuals or groups of clients and families. More formal methods of teaching are used, including videotapes. The content provided in formal education is consistent among clients.
25. 4
26. 2
27. a. provide excellent nursing care, b. have good medical outcomes, c. provide medical services for complex clients requiring a team of health care providers, d. high retention rate of staff, e. high staff morale, f. good payment systems
28. False, True, True
29. a. budgeting process, b. strategic planning, c. performance improvement plan, d. risk management input, e. utilization review data, f. client satisfaction, g. physician input, h. census data, i. changes in client population.
30. the client's opinion

CHAPTER 9
1. 1, 3, 4
2. True, True, True, True, False

3. a. These clients often require ventilators to assist with respiration. The equipment requires intensive monitoring and skilled nurses to evaluate the client's response. b. These clients are hemodynamically unstable and require cardiac monitoring, monitoring of the pressures within the heart. These clients require skilled nurses to assess for potential changes and further instability. c. These clients require constant monitoring to assess for changes in the brain's perfusion. d. These clients require constant monitoring to control blood pressure, maintain perfusion of the heart, brain, kidneys, and lungs. In addition, these clients require intensive medication and fluid management. e. These clients require intensive monitoring and medication administration to control and treat the underlying metabolic problems. f. These clients are potentially unstable due to the trauma and loss of blood from major surgery and require intensive hemodynamic monitoring. g. These clients are at risk for cardiac and pulmonary complications due to their previous history and require intensive monitoring to detect any potential change in status.
4. ICU psychosis
5. a. ICU, b. PACU, c. ER
6. the bedside nurse
7. A critical care nurse specialist is a Master's prepared nurse with advanced level of knowledge of critical care, pharmacology, and pathophysiology. This nurse may act in an educator role, consultant, manger, researcher, or practitioner. The acute care nurse practitioner is a Master's prepared nurse with advanced knowledge of acute care nursing. This nurse may practice in ICUs, ERs, and step-down units and may plan and coordinate care for clients in these settings.
8. a. American Association of Critical Care Nurses, b. Society of Critical Care Medicine
9. 4
10. The nurse can provide open visitation as much as possible to decrease separation from family, provide appropriate day and night cycles to promote improved quantity and quality of sleep, minimize noise, and conversation to promote a restful environment, provide privacy to promote the client's dignity and worth, explain all equipment, noise and activities to decrease the client's fear of the unknown, provide a means of communication for clients on mechanical ventilators to promote control and communication, and monitor the client frequently for manifestations of pain or anxiety and provide appropriate medication if ordered.

11. a. massage, b. prayer, c. music therapy, d. therapeutic energy provision
12. As demands on the family increase, their ability to adapt and cope effectively is diminished. This can manifest itself as fear, guilt, anger, and hostility. These negative emotions can have an adverse effect on the client and contribute to his or her stress.
13. Visitor assistants can help family members meet physical and emotional needs which improves their ability to cope. By using visitor assistants for the family, the nurse has more time to concentrate on the client.
14. Nurses have an ethical and moral obligation to act in the client's best interest. Because hospitalization in an ICU is an emotional and potentially traumatic event for the client and family, coping mechanisms are diminished and they may experience hopelessness. By advocating for the client and family, the nurse ensures that interventions are taken which best support the client's basic values, rights, and beliefs. This support can provide hope for the client and family.
15. Due to the ever-increasing changes in technology and treatments, the ICU nurse must engage in continuing education to maintain a level of knowledge and skill to meet the ongoing needs of clients in the ICU.

CHAPTER 10
1. The skilled services needed to treat an individual's disease and disability in collaboration with his or her family and designated caregivers.
2. 1
3. a. introduce a prospective payment system, b. initiate a per client service limit, c. change billing procedures, d. mandate the use of Outcome and Assessment Information Set (OASIS)
4. The primary role is to coordinate the delivery and payment of services that target individual client needs.
5. Be Prepared. This is important because nurses visiting clients in their home are on their own. They don't have colleagues readily available for consultation and they don't have an endless amount of supplies down the hall. Therefore, careful preparation and planning is essential to make the home visit successful.
6. education, experience, common sense
7. a positive nurse-client relationship
8. a. domains are four areas that represent groupings of client problems including environmental, psychosocial, physiologic, and health-related behaviors, b. problems is a list of 40 nursing

diagnoses that represent matters of concern that adversely affect the client's health status and well-being, c. modifiers are terms used to identify ownership of the problem and degree of severity, d. clinical manifestations are objective and subjective evidence of the client's problem
9. The Problem Rating Scare for Outcomes provides a framework for measuring a client's problem specific knowledge, behavior, and status. The scale can be used throughout the time of service to the client and provides a mechanism for documentation. In addition, the scale is used to measure the client's progress and to determine the effectiveness of interventions.
10. True, True, True, True, True, True
11. 1, 2, 4
12. The intervention scheme is an arrangement of nursing actions and activities designed to help the user identify and document plans and interventions. It includes four categories of care such as health teaching, guidance and counseling, targets for nursing intervention, or activities such as dressing change/wound care, and a separate area for identifying client-specific information.
13. The Nightingale Tracker is a computerized communication system designed to be used by students having clinical experiences in home health settings. The system facilitates student completion of clinical activities.
14. Multiple disciplines may be involved in the care of a client at home. It is essential that staff communicate effectively so that services provided by each discipline can be coordinated.
15. Core values include the use and importance of the multidisciplinary team, the provision of care within a seamless health care environment, conducting of disease prevention and health promotion activities, respect for the client's rights and responsibilities, recognition that clients must be knowledgeable about their own health and involved in the decision-making process, recognition of the power of the client in that when nurses are in the client's home, it is the client who is in charge, and recognition of the value and contribution of family and other caregivers to the client's health and well being.
16. The nurse needs to recognize that she is a guest in the client's home; she needs to respect the client's culture, religious, and ethnic beliefs, develop and implement interpersonal skills, enlist the support of the client's family or caregiver, recognize that the nurse's role is to help clients solve their health care problems and to become independent as soon as possible, practice effec-

tive communication and collaboration with peer professionals, and maintain a sense of humor.

CHAPTER 11

1. 3, 4, 5, 6
2. True, True
3. Hill-Burton Hospital Survey and Construction Act of 1946
4. Omnibus Budget Reconciliation Act of 1987
5. a. an RN must be on duty at least 8 consecutive hours per day, 7 days a week, b. a full-time director of nursing must be on staff if the facility has more than 60 beds
6. 14, annually, change in their status
7. Minimum Data Set (MDS)
8. a. assertiveness, b. coaching, c. counseling, d. accurate documentation, e. organizational ability, f. time management, g. effective communication
9. True, True, True, True, False, True, True, True
10. 4
11. 2, 4, 6
12. The MDS does not provide a means of assessing self-concept, spirituality, sense of power, knowledge of health condition and self-care practices, sexuality, patterns of solitude, sense of purpose, immunity, stress management, use of alternative therapies, and attitudes regarding health status and death.
13. a. must be written within 7 days after completion of the assessment, b. the plan is inter-disciplinary and nurses coordinate writing of the plan, c. the resident and family should be actively involved in the development, d. the care plan is a working guide to nursing actions, e. nursing assistants must be familiar with the care plan, f. it is the nurse's responsibility to review the care plan with unlicensed caregivers.
14. Because of daily contact, nursing assistants may be the first to detect a change in health status; this change must be communicated to the nurse who then performs a further assessment to determine the resident's condition. The nurse must document changes in resident status and communicate these to physicians.
15. a. provide the physician with complete information, b. report symptoms and observations, c. take the order directly from the physician and not office staff, d. repeat the order and when possible ask the physician to fax a copy, e. have the order signed within 24 hours, f. ask the physician for clarification of anything that seems inappropriate and report any continuing concerns to the facility medical director and director of nursing.

CHAPTER 12

1. a. advances in science and technology have contributed to populations living longer with more chronic illnesses, b. changes in health policy and financing have contributed to decreased length of stay in acute hospitals.
2. altered functional ability and lifestyle.
3. a. 4, b. 6, c. 7, d. 5, e. 2, f. 3, g. 1
4. a. outpatient, b. home, c. day treatment program, d. sub-acute, e. acute
5. client's needs and medical stability, services offered in a particular setting, intensity and skill level of needed nursing services, the gap between the client's current functional ability and the realistic achievable goal of rehabilitation, and the location of the setting
6. True, True, False, False
7. three, two, nursing, medicine
8. a. client centered: the client and his unique needs are the focus of care, not the underlying medical diagnosis. Nurses and other team members identify the focus and build a plan of care based on that. In this process, the client's right to make decisions is respected and nurses work to support the client's decisions and desired outcomes. The assessment process includes an assessment of the family and the role they will play in the client's rehabilitation. b. goal-oriented: individual goals are determined with the client. Nurses and other team members complete assessments to determine reasonable goals that can be accomplished. c. focus on functional ability: rehabilitation individualizes an approach to maximize functional ability through training and retraining. Nurses and other team members assess functional ability using the Functional Independence Measures tool and determine areas for improvement. d. team approach: the rehabilitation team is comprised of multiple health care disciplines with the client a key member. Team members collaborate and cooperate with one another to help the client reach rehabilitation goals. e. quality of life: successful rehabilitation is dependent upon caregivers understanding what an acceptable quality of life for the client is. Nurses and other team members complete an assessment to determine factors which influence an individual's quality of life that need to be facilitated, maintained, or restored. f. wellness: achieving the highest level of wellness for the individual client is the focus. Nurses and other team members maintain, restore, and promote healthy lifestyles for the client within the context of the client's health. g. adaptation to change: coping with change is an innate

characteristic of living with a chronic illness or disability. Nurses and other team members help clients recognize the anticipation of change and assist them to learn effective means of coping with change. h. coping and adjusting: clients with a disability or chronic illness will have a psychological reaction to the change in their lives. Nurses are instrumental in helping clients and their families understand their reactions and providing interventions that will help them cope effectively. i. culture: the rehabilitation experience is influenced by the client's culture. Rehabilitation nursing requires cultural competence that will enhance the client's achievement of rehabilitation goals. j. client and family education: is a collaborative process between the client, family, and other team members. Nurses and other team members work together to provide client and family teaching in ways that are accessible and meaningful to the client and family.

9. 1
10. True
11. Because these settings may look physically similar it may be difficult for clients and family members to understand the differences. By explaining these differences and emphasizing the rehabilitation principles and concepts, the client and family member can make a successful transition from one setting to the other.

CHAPTER 13

1. See Figure U3-1 in the textbook.
2. dehydrated
3. hyperosmolarity
4. a. vascular, b. interstitial
5. 1
6. a. hypertonic, b. isotonic, c. hypotonic
7. decreased fluids
8. 1, 2, 3
9. sugar, caffeine
10. 2
11. 1, 2, 3, 4
12. 1, 2, 3, 4
13. 1, 2, 3
14. 1, 2, 3
15. 1, 2, 3
16. 240 cc
17. pulmonary overload, cerebral edema
18. 1
19. 1, 2, 3, 4, 5, 6
20. 1, 2, 3, 4
21. 1, 2, 3
22. 1, 2, 3, 4, 5
23. 2, 3, 4

24. 1, 2, 3, 4
25. D_5W
26. lactated Ringer's
27. fluid loss, myocardial contractility
28. 1, 2
29. False, True, False, True
30. 2
31. 4

CHAPTER 14

1. electrolyte deficiency
2. a. Risk for injury
   b. Risk for activity intolerance
   c. Risk for decreased cardiac output
   d. Altered mucous membranes
3. decreased sodium
4. increased sodium
5. 1, 2, 3, 4
6. water loss or sodium gain
7. a. heart disease, b. liver disease, c. renal disease
8. Dysrhythmias
9. 3.5 mEq/L
10. 1, 2, 3, 4
11. excessive excitability of the myocardial cells
12. decreased
13. occurrence of carpal spasm when a blood pressure cuff is inflated on the arm for 5 minutes
14. occurrence of spasms of facial muscles elicited by lightly tapping the facial nerve below the temple region in front of the ear
15. 1, 2, 3
16. Hyponatremia, extreme perspiration
17. 1, 2, 3, 4
18. Hyponatremia
19. 1, 2, 3
20. 1, 2, 3
21. Intravenous therapy of hypertonic saline
22. 1, 2, 3
23. 1, 2, 4
24. 2
25. 2
26. 2
27. sodium
28. 1, 2, 3, 4
29. 1, 2

CHAPTER 15

1. 7.35 – 7.45
2. 7.0
3. 7.0
4. urine
5. True
6. 2

7. 20:1 ratio, pH.
8. acidosis
9. acidemia
10. alkalosis
11. alkalemia
12. 1, 2, 3
13. 1, 2
14. increased
15. decreased
16. decreased
17. elevated
18. a. 1, b. 3, c. 2, d. 4
19. a. 1, b. 2, c. 3, d. 2, e. 3, f. 4
20. 1, 2, 3, 4, 5, 6
21. oxygen
22. 1
23. 1
24. 3

CHAPTER 16
1. hypotension
2. increased risk for thrombus formation due to hypercoagulability secondary to nicotine use, decreased oxygen delivery capacity due to decreased hemoglobin levels, decreased blood flow to surgical wound site to vasoconstriction action of nicotine
3. poor wound healing, wound infection
4. 3
5. a. inadequate ventilation, b. side effects of anesthetic agents, c. side effects of preoperative medications, d. rapid position change, e. pain, f. fluid or blood loss, g. peripheral pooling of blood after regional anesthesia
6. liver, kidney
7. 2, 4
8. abdominal
9. a. extremity pain, b. unilateral edema, c. warmth of calf
10. anesthetic agents are fat-soluble, and much of the drug dose is deposited from the blood into fatty tissue; therefore, excretion of these agents is slower
11. True, False, True
12. a: assess client for allergies, report allergies to surgical personnel and anesthesia, and place an allergy band on the client. b: assess the client's use of any medications or herbal remedies that might contribute to an increased risk for bleeding. c: assess the client for cortisone or steroid use. d: assess the client for a history of diabetes mellitus. e: assess the client for previous embolic events.
13. 3

14. a. chest x-ray is completed to detect any abnormalities, b. pulse oximetry is completed to determine gross levels of tissue oxygenation.
15. a. BUN, b. creatinine, and c. urinalysis
16. a. serum albumin, b. hemoglobin and hematocrit, c. BUN, and d. creatinine clearance
17. 2
18. 1
19. a. heads surgical team and makes decisions about surgical procedures, b. alleviates pain, provides relaxation, maintains the airway, ensures adequate gas exchange, monitors vital signs, estimates fluid and blood loss, administers blood or fluids, administers medications to maintain homodynamic stability, c. coordinates all team members, advocates for the client, d. organize surgical equipment, hand surgeon instruments
20. 1, 2, 5
21. a. recovery from anesthesia, b. discharge from PACU to first day or so after surgery, c. time of healing which may be several weeks
22. 4
23. 96.8° F or 36° C
24. a. color, b. type, c. amount of drainage
25. coughing and deep breathing
26. 3
27. 4
28. 1, 2, 3, 4
29. 3
30. the bed is placed in the lowest position, siderails are up, the client is instructed not to get up without assistance
31. 3
32. a. site of operation, b. age and size of client, c. type of anesthesia used, d. pain normally experienced by the client
33. 4
34. 2, 3, 4, 5
35. airway patency, lateral Sims'
36. 4
37. ventilation with a face mask and ambu bag
38. 2
39. ask another nurse to assess the wound and compare observations
40. return the client to bed if necessary, cover the wound with sterile dressings moistened with normal saline, monitor the vital signs, keep the client calm, notify the surgeon immediately, and prepare the client for emergency surgery
41. instructions on medications, wound care, postoperative appointment, names and telephone numbers in case of emergency, and copies of drug prescriptions

42. True, True, False
43. 2, 4, 5
44. a. 4, b. 3, c. 2, d. 4
45. 4
46. a. spinal, b. epidural, c. caudal, d. topical, e. local infiltration, f. field block, g. peripheral nerve block, h. IV regional block
47. 4
48. 3

CHAPTER 17

1. genes
2. 23
3. autosomes
4. two x, x and y chromosomes
5. nucleotides
6. RNA
7. dementia
8. autosomal dominant
9. random mutations
10. 1, 2, 3
11. 1
12. True, True
13. 1, 2, 3, 4
14. 1, 2, 3, 4
15 1, 2, 3, 4, 5
16. To provide at-risk families with information so that they can make informed choices during pregnancy.

CHAPTER 18

1. lump
2. mass of tissue
3. spread of cancer to distant organs
4. 1
5. Medical Oncologist
6. Epidemiology
7. a. 2, b. 1, c. 3
8. a. 2, b. 1, c. 5, d. 3, e. 4, f. 6, g. 7, h. 8
9. carcinogenesis
10. Stage 1- the progressive alteration of malignant cells with additional genetic changes results in a heterogeneous population of malignant cells with varying degrees of metastatic potential.
    Stage 2- Cancer cell migrate via the lymph or blood circulation or by direct extension.
    Stage 3- Cancer cells are established at the secondary site.
11. immune system
12. True
13. Smoking
14. True

15. 1, 2, 3, 4
16. 1
17. 1, 2, 3, 4

CHAPTER 19

1. 1, 2, 3
2. 20
3. True, True, True, True, False
4. destroy malignant tumor cells without excessive destruction of normal cells
5. 1, 2, 3, 4, 5
6. 1, 2, 3, 4
7. True
8. 1, 2, 3, 4, 5
9. Pain
10. True, True
11. 1, 2, 3
12. time, distance, shielding
13. erythropoietin
14. early aggressive interventions usually offer the best hope of cure
15. from tumors that tend to shed cells from their surface
16. chemotherapy or RT to shrink the tumor mass and decrease the likelihood of micrometastasis
17. 1, 2, 3, 4, 5
18. 1, 2, 3, 4
19. 1, 2, 3, 4
20. infection, catheter occlusion
21. 1, 2, 3, 4
22. surgery
23. 1, 2, 3
24. Extravasation
25. True

CHAPTER 20

1. 1
2.

Phase	Activity
Vascular	Blood vessels constrict
	Clotting process begins
	Platelets release factors to stimulate healing
	Capillaries dilate: wound area is red and warm
Inflammation	Occurs whenever cells are injured
	Limits harmful effects of bacteria
	Inflammatory response: destroy organism
	"Walling Off" effect: fibrin clot blocks lymph
	WBCs clean up wound and initiate further healing

Proliferative	Collagen deposition
	Angiogenesis (new vessels)
	Granulation tissue development
	Wound contraction
Maturation	Remodeling of scar: collagen synthesis and lysis
	Capillaries disappear
	Scar regains 2/3 original strength

3. 2, 4
4. bands
5. matrix mealloproteases
6. True, False, True, False, True, True, True, False, True, False, False, False, True, True, True, True
7. a. tertiary, b. primary, c. secondary (See Figure 20-3 in the textbook.)
8.

Factor	Effect
Diabetes mellitus	Accelerated atherosclerosis: Impairs blood supply to wound
Lack of vitamin C	Impaired collagen synthesis
Neuropathy	Unregulated blood flow to wound
	Possible unintentional injury to area
Foreign bodies	Increases risk of infection
Protein malnutrition	Reduced collagen deposits
	Decreased WBC function
Smoking	Reduces blood flow; vasoconstriction
	CO reduces tissue oxygen levels

9. dilutes toxins released by bacteria, brings nutrients to wound, and carries phagocytes to wound for defense
10. pre-albumin level
11. infection
12. Mark the area to be measured on the client's leg with a pen and a matching area on the non-injured leg.
13. pain level
14. True, True, False, True, True, True, False
15.

Appearance	Clinical Significance
Edges approximated	normal healing with collagen synthesis
Open wound, edges apart	possible infection in wound, opening to drain non-healing wound
Healing ridge under skin	normal finding 5-7 days
Serous exudate	normal finding
Purulent exudate	infection, infiltration by WBC, macrophages

Eschar	necrotic tissue, needs to be removed
Granuloma	chronic infection, "walled off" area

16. Cold compresses cause vasoconstriction to reduce the effects of edema. Application of heat will vasodilate the blood vessels, increase blood flow and removal of waste products.
17. 3
18.

Method	Procedure
Sharp debridement	Surgical removal of eschar
	Used for large wounds with thick eschar
	Eschar removed down to level of bleeding tissues
	Done under sterile conditions
	May need anesthesia or sedation
	Pain medications needed after
Mechanical	Use of irrigation or dressings
	Removes debris, bacteria, necrotic tissue
	Wet-to-dry dressings
	"Non-selective" debridement
	Used only until wound is clean and has granulating tissue
Enzymatic	Proteolytic enzymes applied to necrotic tissue
	Used when client cannot tolerate surgical excision
	Slow process
	Should not be used with infected wounds
	Medicate prior to use: burning pain
	Wound needs to be moist not dry
	Do not place on viable tissue
Autolytic	Use of body's own digestive enzymes to break down necrotic tissue
	Occlusive dressing over wound
	Slow process
	For clients who cannot tolerate other types of procedures
	Contraindicated for infected wounds

19. normal saline
20. The eschar can be scored with small cuts to enhance penetration.
21. Steroids cause a depression of the immune system by blocking prostaglandin production and decreasing the inflammatory response.
22. True, False, True, False, True
23. The increased capillary permeability and blood flow causes edema. Rest, ice, compression and elevation reduce that edema.

24. by blocking the production of prostaglandins which cause inflammation
25. histamine

CHAPTER 21

1. 1, 2, 3, 5
2. 1, 2, 3
3. a. person, b. plant, c. soil, d. food, e. other organic substance, f. combination of substances
4. A carrier may be asymptomatic and can be shedding organisms, spreading the infection unknowingly.
5. 1, 3, 4, 5
6. Cultural practices involving food or hygiene may increase the risk exposure (bathing in contaminated water, eating uncooked foods).
7. 2
8. colonization
9. latent period
10. incubation period
11. 1, 2, 4
12. False, True
13. 1, 2, 3, 4, 5, 6
14.

Category	Etiology
Postoperative	immobility, decreased cough, pain with deep-breathing
Diminished consciousness	high risk for aspiration
Impaired gag reflex	high risk for aspiration
Intubation	high risk for aspiration
Tracheostomy	high risk for aspiration
Old age	decreased immune response, poor nutritional status, decreased activity level
Chronic lung disease	reduced defenses, fatigue
Cardiac disease	reduced defenses, respiratory congestion
Renal insufficiency	decreased immune response
Malignancies	decreased immune response, medications, malnutrition

15. Clients are asymptomatic but can still transmit pathogens to health care workers or other clients.
16. It damages the epithelium and impairs the skin's defense mechanism; increases risk of infection.
17. semi-permeable
18. Handwashing, alcohol-based
19. a. gloves, b. gowns, c. masks, d. protective eyewear
20. a. contact precautions, b. droplet precautions, c. airborne precautions
21. 3
22. 1, 2, 3, 4, 5
23. True, False, True, True, False, True, True, True

CHAPTER 22

1. Pain serves as a warning about potential physical harm and alerts us to problems.
2. Pain causes increased muscle wall tension and spasms, reducing chest wall expansion and making the client reluctant to do deep breathing and coughing postoperatively. The client takes short, shallow, frequent breaths resulting in hypoventilation and atelectasis, which can lead to pneumonia and other pulmonary complications.
3.

Type	Characteristics
Acute Pain	Short duration: less than 6 months
	Identifiable, immediate onset
	Limited and predictable duration
	Described as shooting, stabbing, sharp
	Motivates the person to obtain relief
	Person can return to pre-pain state
Chronic Pain	Lasts months and years
	Constant, continuous
	Not readily treatable
	May have originally been acute pain
	Defined in vague terms
	Many causes remain unknown

4. a. nonmalignant: low back pain, pain from burns
   b. intermittent: migraine headaches, sickle cell crisis
   c. malignant: due to cancerous growths
5. a. superficial/cutaneous: skin and subcutaneous tissues
   b. somatic: muscle, bone, ligaments, joints, blood vessels and nerves
   c. visceral: organs and their capsules
6. False, True, True, True, True
7. Kaposi's sarcoma
8. a. situation (crowded public place, exam room, hospital room), b. age of client (coping mechanisms, previous experiences), c. gender (cultural expectations of gender), d. degree of anxiety, e. past experiences (positive or negative), f. meaning of pain (childbirth pain vs. surgical pain)
9. Pain threshold is the lowest intensity of painful stimulus perceived as pain. Tolerance is the amount of pain a person is willing to endure.
10. 1, 3, 4

11. Transcutaneous electrical nerve stimulation (TENS) unit
12. All pain is real even if the nurse cannot ascertain it or its cause.
13. 1, 2, 3, 4, 5
14. 1, 2, 3, 6, 7
15. a.   recognize and treat pain promptly
    b.   make information about analgesics readily available to clients
    c.   promise attentive analgesic care
    d.   define explicit policies
    e.   examine processes and outcomes with goal of continuous improvement
16. the client's report
17. Wong-Baker
18. 1, 2, 3, 4
19. Nurses are the primary advocates for the client, assessing pain and providing pain relief measures.
20. a. educate clients about pain and pain control measures, b. obtain accurate pain history and assessment
21. False, True, True, True
22. a.   facilitating expression of feelings
    b.   providing support, reassurance and understanding
    c.   teach client self-management strategies
23. chronic intractable
24. application of heat and cold to areas of discomfort
25. a.   Step 1: non-opioids, such as NSAIDs or acetaminophen
    b.   Step 2: mild opioids, such as codeine PLUS non-opioids
    c.   Step 3: strong opioids, such as morphine with/without non-opioids
26. True, False, True, False, True, True, True, False
27. NSAIDs
28. none (there is no ceiling dosage for morphine)
29.

Agent	Characteristics
Lidocaine	Local anesthetic
	Acts within 5-10 minutes
	Lasts 2 hours
Bupivacaine	Local anesthetic
	Long acting 4-8 hours
	4 times more potent than lidocaine
	4-6 times more toxic
	Blocks sensory nerves over motor nerves

30. EMLA cream
31. sulfa drug
32. a. Colace, b. Peri-colace, c. Senokot-S

33. IV: 15 minutes
    IM: 30 minutes
    SC: 90 minutes
    Epidural: 4-12 hours
34.

Medication	Category	Indication
Tegretol	antidepressant	neuropathic pain
Dilantin	anticonvulsant	neuropathic pain
Neurontin	anticonvulsant	muscle spasms from pain
Decadron	corticosteroid	bone pain
Lioresal	muscle relaxant	muscle spasms from pain

35. a. transdermal patch, b. "lollipop"
36. PCAs deliver medication intravenously and are controlled by the client at a pre-set rate ordered by the doctor. The client receives pain medication without delay, reducing anxiety and increasing the client's independence and control over situation.
37. 2

CHAPTER 23
1.   a. denial, b. anger, c. bargaining, d. depression, e. acceptance
2.   Relief of suffering and maximizing quality of life. Palliative care does not emphasize cure.
3.   1, 2, 3, 4, 5
4.   a. socioeconomic status, b. physical health, c. relationships with friends and family, d. satisfaction with self
5.   1, 2, 3, 4, 5, 6, 7
6.

Problem	Example
Disease/treatment-related	Surgery
	Radiation
	Chemotherapy
	Infection/ Anemia
	Malnutrition/cachexia
Physiologic	Overexertion
	Immobility
	Poor sleep
	Pain/discomfort
Psycho-emotional	Stress
	Anxiety
	Grief/depression
Spiritual	Fear
	Distress

7. disease trajectory
8. Mini-Mental Status Exam (MMSE)
9. 1, 2, 3, 4, 5, 6, 7
10. hearing
11. Assessment of sleep disturbances includes review of sleep schedule and the intake of stimulants that interfere with proper rest, evaluation of activity level and daytime napping. Once treatable causes of sleep disturbance are addressed, the client will have proper rest and can be medicated for pain relief without increasing drowsiness.
12. disturbed thought processes including acute confusion or delirium, decreased urinary elimination, reduced peripheral tissue perfusion with mottling of the skin, ineffective breathing patterns [Cheyne Stokes respirations], congested breathing, periods of apnea
13. 1, 2, 3, 4, 7, 8
14. 3
15. a. non-judgmental and non-threatening attitude, b. listening skills that encourage client to talk, c. use of therapeutic silence, paraphrases, reflections, d. offering structure to conversation
16. a. accepting the reality of the loss, b. experiencing the pain of loss, c. adjusting to the environment where deceased is missing, d. finding a way to remember the deceased while moving forward with life
17. 1, 3, 4
18. none (No ceiling amount; titrate to effect to relieve discomfort and achieve satisfactory analgesia)
19.

Medication	Action	Indication
NSAIDs	anti-inflammatory	When inflammation causing pain (i.e.: metastatic bone disease)
Tricyclic antidepressants Anticonvulsants	analgesic effect	Pain syndromes with neurologic component (i.e.: pain described as "burning," "shooting pains," or "shock-like")
Anticholinergics	relieve smooth muscle spasm	"Colicky pain"
Benzodiazepines	relieve anxiety	Physical, emotional and spiritual concerns with terminal illness

20. True, True, False, True, True, False, True
21. haloperidol (Haldol)

22. 4
23. anticholinergics
24. tricyclic antidepressant
25. corticosteroids

CHAPTER 24
1. True, True, False, True, False
2. 2, 3
3. 2
4. 3
5. a. 1, b. 2, c. 1, d. 2, e. 1
6. stress
7. 4
8. a. obesity, b. large adenoids, c. tonsils
9. a. Time-zone-change syndrome is experienced by individuals who cross several time zones. b. Shift-work sleep disorder may be experienced who have a history of long-time shift work where the usual sleep-wake cycle is altered to accommodate work schedules. c. Irregular sleep-wake patterns are seen in the elderly and chronically ill. Erratic schedules or ignoring external cues contributes to erratic periods of sleeping and wakefulness.
10. a. In Parkinson's, 70% of those diagnosed report sleep disorders and is characterized by insomnia initially followed by disturbances in the sleep-wake schedule and visual hallucinations. b. 90% of people with depression suffer from a sleep disturbance. It is most often characterized by sleep-onset insomnia. c. Alzheimer's and other dementias are often accompanied by frequent awakenings, with agitation that progresses to loss of sleep-wake consolidation.
11. a. 4, b. 5, c. 2, d. 1, e. 6, f. 3
12. 3
13. noise level, 24-hour lighting, frequency of care giving interruptions
14. 1, 2, 5
15. True
16. 4
17. The nurse needs to be aware that older adults take longer to fall asleep and are more easily awakened, that REM sleep decreases, and that it takes longer for the older adult to get back to sleep once wakened.
18. depression
19. polysomnography
20. circles under the eyes, lack of coordination, drowsiness, irritability
21. obesity; large adenoids, tonsils; weight; gender; history of snoring; short, thick neck
22. feeling tired upon waking, erectile dysfunction, snoring getting progressively worse

23. taking benzodiazepine. This is a hypnotic sedative which can increase clinical manifestations because of its selective effect in relaxing muscles of the upper airway and depression of arousal.
24. Alcohol is a depressant and can contribute to relaxation of muscles in the upper airway.
25. Teach the client that this is the treatment of choice. CPAP stands for continuous positive airway pressure, which is applied through a face mask. The increased pressure keeps the airway open. The CPAP mask should be applied over the nose and secured in place and should be worn when the client is ready to go to sleep. Inform the client that the machine is portable and can be battery operated. Inform the client he may experience nasal congestion, air leaks, and pressure marks on the face and that if these occur to call the nurse for assistance or referral.
26. 90
27. 4
28. 1, 4, 5
29. The nurse should explain that conventional indoor lighting is not strong enough to have a therapeutic effect. The light being prescribed is very intense and should only be applied for the specific amount of time. During light application, the client should protect her eyes from overexposure.
30. If a male client with an indwelling catheter has REM-associated erections, the nurse must use caution when securing the indwelling catheter. A sufficient amount of slack in the tubing must be present to accommodate the erection.
31. a. reduce noise, b. reduce interruptions, c. provide relaxation measures such as a back rub, d. if prescribed, administer a hypnotic agent.
32. 4
33. These clients are at risk for having symptoms worsen or for having a prolonged relapse with overexertion.
34. 3
35. evening
36. Narcolepsy causes significant disruptions to social and occupational roles and subsequently may affect a client's self-esteem. Decreased self-esteem contributes to depression as does the impaired release of neurotransmitters such as dopamine.
37. Clonazepam and baclofen are skeletal muscle relaxants. They often diminish the limb movements associated with this disorder and thus decrease the frequency of sleep arousals.
38. 3

CHAPTER 25

1. 1, 2, 3, 4
2. a. Anxiety, b. stress, c. coping mechanisms, d. self-esteem. Related factors include culture and family background, exposure to similar stressors, and repeated exposure to stressors.
3. 1
4. Emotion-focused coping behaviors alter a client's response to stress through actions to make him or her feel better such as talking or crying. On the other hand, problem-focused coping behaviors are aimed at altering the stressor such as getting more information or making a plan to relieve the stress.
5. a. 2, b. 1
6. One cause is biology. There is some evidence of a genetic influence as well as evidence of abnormalities in brain structure and neurotransmitters. Additionally, the limbic system is altered with mood disorders and the frontal, temporal lobes and brain stem are altered with anxiety disorders. The second cause is psychological. Alterations in defenses, thinking, and learning processes can distort a person's view of reality.
7. 3
8. a. 1, b. 2, c. 1, d. 1, e. 2, f. 1, g. 2, h. 2
9. 4
10. 1, 3, 4
11. False, False, True, True
12. Denial
13. 3
14. False
15. 4
16. a. definition of the illness, b. medications options, c. treatment options, d. relapse prevention
17. family member
18. 4
19. True
20. a. 3, b. 1, c. 2, d. 3, e. 2, f. 1

CHAPTER 26

1. 1
2. psychoanalytic: person is fixed at the oral stage of development, seeking gratification of needs through drinking; psychodynamic: person experiences interpersonal and intrapersonal difficulties that provide foundation for addiction; behavioral: addiction is a learned behavior that can be unlearned; family systems: emphasizes that relationships and roles and unhealthy communication patterns among family members contribute to addiction

3. a. 4, b. 6, c. 5, d. 7, e. 8, f. 1, g. 3, h. 2
4. 1, 3, 4
5. acute intoxication
6. 1, 3, 4
7. 3
8. cardiovascular, central nervous system
9. 1, 3, 4
10. endorphin
11. 3
12. 1, 4, 6
13. headache
14. marijuana (cannabis)
15. False, True, False, True, True, True, False, True, False
16. 1, 3, 4
17. Respiratory depression places the client at risk for respiratory arrest.
18. brain, 0.10
19. 4
20. 4, 6
21. 1, 4, 5, 6
22. False
23. self-awareness
24. 2
25. methadone therapy
26. a. maintain adequate respiratory status, b. maintain adequate circulatory status, c. provide hydration
27. 2
28. a. education, b. outpatient services, c. impaction or outpatient detoxification and rehabilitation
29. 1, 3, 4, 5
30. True, True, True
31. These drugs cause less respiratory depression and hypertension, and they help prevent delirium tremens (DTs).
32. 1, 2
33. a. providing rest, b. orienting the client as necessary, c. intervening to prevent complications.
34. 2, 3, 4

CHAPTER 27

1. See Figure U6-1 in the textbook.
2. See Figure U6-3 in the textbook.
3. 1, 2
4. a. abnormally increased roundness of the thoracic curve or hump back
    b. lateral deformity of the spine
    c. abnormal increase in the lumbar curve or sway back
    d. bowleg
    e. knock knee
5. See Figure 27-2 in the textbook.
6. 1, 2, 3, 4

7. 1, 2, 3, 4, 5, 6
8. a. 9, b. 8, c. 6, d. 7, e. 4, f. 5, g. 2, h. 3, i. 1
9. 2
10. Review neurovascular assessment sheet
11. 1, 2, 3, 4, 5, 6, 7
12. 4
13. circulatory compromise
14. 2
15. 3
16. a. Tomography
    b. Fluoroscopy
    c. Dual energy x-rays
    d. DEXA scans
    e. Computed tomography
    f. MRI
17. 3
18. 1

CHAPTER 28

1. True, True
2. large weight-bearing joints
3. knee
4. a. 4, b. 1, c. 7, d. 1, e. 7, f. 2, g. 6, h. 2, i. 5, j. 3, k. 3, l. 2, m. 2, n. 4, o. 5, p. 6
5. 1, 3, 4
6. 1, 2, 3, 4
7. 1
8. 2
9. 2
10. 1, 3, 4
11. 3
12. 3
13. 2
14. 1, 2, 3, 4
15. True
16. 1, 2, 3, 4
17. 2
18. 2, 3
19. 1
20. 3

CHAPTER 29

1. 1
2. 1, 2, 3, 4
3. a. 6, b. 1, c. 3, d. 2, e. 5, f. 7, g. 4, h. 10, i. 9, j. 8, k. 11, l. 14, m. 15, n. 12, o. 13, p. 16
4. 1
5. fat embolus
6   False, True, True, True, False
7. 24-48 hours
8. Paralysis
9. 1

10. 2
11. 1
12. 1, 2, 3, 4, 5
13. 1
14. 1, 2, 3, 4
15. higher than the client's heart
16. 2
17. 1, 2,
18. 1, 2, 3, 4, 5

CHAPTER 30

1. See Figure U7-2 in the textbook.
2. cellular
3. a. Increase caloric requirement by 7% for each degree Fahrenheit of temperature increase
   b. reduced protein requirements to reduce workload of kidneys
   c. restriction of dietary fats due to reduction of pancreatic enzymes
   d. restriction of carbohydrates due to loss of insulin release
4. a. increased caloric intake
   b. sedentary lifestyle
5. Primary: adequate nutrition is not delivered to the upper GI tract over an extended period of time (famine, anorexia)

Secondary: when the upper GI tract fails to absorb, metabolize, or use the nutrients (ischemic bowel or Crohn's disease)
6. 1, 2, 3, 4, 5, 6
7. Many diseases, such as ulcerative colitis and Crohn's disease, have a familial component. Other problems such as cancer, ulcers, diabetes, alcoholism or hepatitis also run in families.
8.

Etiology	Characteristics of Pain
Bowel Obstruction	Intermittent, colicky
	Pain near umbilicus=small bowel
	Pain near lumbar area=colon
	Distended abdomen, no flatus
Peritoneal inflammation	Steady, aching
	Directly over area of inflammation
	Gastric acid may produce more pain
	May be associated with s/sx shock
Vascular catastrophe (aortic aneurysm)	May be preceded with 2-3 days mild to moderate pain; hyperperistalsis followed by severe pain and shock
	Back and flank pain=aortic aneurysm

9. 24-hour recall of typical daily intake
10. 3

11.

	Protein Intake	Calorie Intake	Appearance
Marasmus	Inadequate	Inadequate	Thin, cachectic
Kwashiorkor	Inadequate	Adequate	Body weight normal range

12. Albumin has a long half-life and is a more generalized indicator of nutritional status. Prealbumin has a shorter half-life and reflects acute change in nutritional status.
13. a. height, b. weight, c. body mass index, d. frame size. e. circumferential measurements
14. Body Mass Index (BMI)
15. False, True, False, True, True
16. Refer the client for further evaluation. Pre-cancerous lesions can be pain-free and asymptomatic.
17. McBurney's point
18. True, False, True, True, True
19. bruit
20. The action assesses for dysphagia. Clients who have difficulty swallowing are at high risk for aspiration.
21. This test measures absorption in the small intestines of xylose, a monosaccharide. The patient is NPO and a known quantity of d-xylose in water is administered. Blood samples are drawn 2 hours later and compared with normal lab values.
22. This test evaluates the swallowing ability and risk for aspiration. The client should remain NPO until the results of the test have been evaluated by the radiologist, speech therapist, or physician.
23. left lateral decubitus
24. Many elderly clients are prescribed multiple medications for various chronic illnesses. These medications can have drug-nutrient interactions and interfere with normal absorption, metabolic processing, and excretion of nutrients.

25. a. aspirin/aspirin compounds, b. NSAIDs, c. antacids, d. laxatives/stool softeners
26. Because of the wide variation in nutritional content of these products, it is difficult to assess composition and their effect on the nutritional status of the client. There are also potential side effects or drug interactions with prescribed medications of which the client may not be aware.
27. 1, 2, 4
28. Anticholinergic

CHAPTER 31

1. Malnutrition: describes undernutrition OR overnutrition, related to deficient or excess energy or nitrogen stores, possibly due to altered dietary intake. Protein-energy malnutrition: results when the body's needs for protein or energy are not adequately supplied.
2. a. infants: increased nutritional needs for growth and development
   b. pregnant/lactating women: increased nutritional needs for pregnancy and milk production
   c. elderly: medical or socioeconomic status may limit their ability to obtain and ingest nutritionally adequate diets
3. 4
4. 1, 2, 3, 4, 5
5. True, False, True, False
6. a. Environmental: energy expenditure vs. energy intake
   b. Genetic tendency: may be less important than environment
   c. Socioeconomic: lower status has higher obesity rates
   d. Ethnic disparity: higher in Hispanic/African American; etiology not clear
7. 1
8. First-level
9. Nurses are there as clients enter the health care system, have constant contact during hospitalization, and are the last contact as the client leaves the hospital. Early identification of nutritional problems and constant monitoring of progress can help prevent further problems.
10. a. Parkinson's disease
    b. Alzheimer's disease
    c. cataracts or CVA
    d. side effects of medications/nausea
11. Young infants who are breast-fed are receiving adequate levels of protein and calories from the breast milk, but the older children are suffering from kwashiorkor malnutrition due to a lack of protein in their diet. There is muscle wasting

of the extremities, and loss of protein causes changes in colloidal pressure resulting in edema, noted in the abdomens of the children.
12. 1, 3, 4, 5, 6
13. a. Health promotion: activities to support client's knowledge of normal nutrition; example: diet information related to decreasing risk of cancer
    b. Health maintenance: targeting specialized diet therapy for a client with illness; example: Crohn's disease
    c. Health restoration: activities to assist the client to return to normal nutritional behaviors; example: retraining a client to swallow after a stroke or administering TPN to a client with severe inflammatory bowel disease
14. 1, 2, 4
15. 1, 2, 3, 4, 5
16. 2, 3, 4
17. Emergency suction
18. False
19. a. Head of the bed must be elevated at 45 degrees for 1 hour before, during, and 1 hour after feeding: prevent aspiration.
    b. Continuous feedings required HOB elevated at all times: prevent aspiration
    c. Check gastric residuals every 4 hours: assess gastric emptying
    d. Avoid adding blue dye to formula: prevent absorption of dye in critically ill clients
20. 1/2 hour
21. 2
22. Orlistat (Xenical)
23.

Classification	Sample Product
Low-residue	
Standard protein	Isocal, Osmolite, Resource
Fiber supplemented	Jevity, Ultracal, Fibersource
Intermediate	
High protein	Isosource HN, Osmolite HN
Concentrated	Isocal HN, Nutren 2.0
Pulmonary	Pulmocare, Respalor
Renal failure	Nepro

CHAPTER 32

1. The buildup of plaque and bacteria around the tooth causes inflammation of the tissue. The supporting structures of the tooth are damaged, causing the tooth to fall out or to require extraction due to severity of the periodontal disease.

2. a. Mechanical trauma: injury from jagged teeth, cheek biting
   b. Chemical trauma: drugs from chemotherapy, chemicals in mouthwashes
3.

Classification	Etiology	Examples
Primary	direct infection of tissues	Canker sore Herpes simplex Vincent's angina
Secondary	opportunistic infection [immuno-suppression]	Candidiasis

4. 1, 2 ,3, 4
5. biopsy
6. odynophagia
7. The pain from heartburn usually means substernal, midline burning that radiates in waves upward toward the neck. Angina tends to be a heavy, crushing, or tightening sensation in the chest that tends to radiate toward the left arm.
8. Achalasia

9.

Name	Procedure	Result
Nissen fundoplication	suturing fundus around esophagus	creates valve-like sphincter; prevents reflux
Hill operation	narrows esophageal opening	reinforces sphincter anchors stomach and distal esophagus recreates gastroesophageal valve
Belsey (Mark IV) repair	suturing the stomach onto the distal esophagus	creates esophagogastric angle without opening esophagus or diaphragm

10. The extensive lymphatic supply to the mucosa allows the cancer to spread widely and quickly. By the time the client develops swallowing problems, the cancer has invaded the esophagus and spread to other adjacent structures.
11. Hiatal hernia: client experiences heartburn 30-60 minutes after a meal; may have substernal pain
    Rolling hernia: client may complain of fullness after a meal or complain of difficulty breathing; may experience chest pain similar to angina; pain is worse when client lies down
12. Venous drainage causes the darker coloring of the skin.
13. True
14. a. instruct client to bite down gently on gauze pad: maintain pressure over extraction site; reduce bleeding
    b. apply ice over jaw: decrease blood flow to area of extraction and reduce edema
    c. monitoring bleeding from site: small amount expected; call physician if bleeding lasts more than 1 hour
    d. avoid hot/cold foods for several days: extraction site is sensitive to temperature extremes

    e. gentle mouth rinses/avoid tooth brushing: prevent recurrence of bleeding at extraction site
    f. medicate for pain: patient comfort; encourage oral intake
    g. maintain fluid intake: prevent dehydration
15. 1, 3, 5
16. 1, 3, 4, 5
17. False, False, False
18. antimicrobial
19. 1, 2, 3
20. 4
21.

Medication	Category	Action
Biaxin or Amoxicillin	anti-infective	kill bacteria
Flagyl	anti-fungal	kill fungal organisms
Prevacid	proton-pump inhibitor	reduce acid secretions
Protonix	proton-pump inhibitor	reduce acid secretions
Prilosec	proton-pump inhibitor	reduce acid secretions

22. Sucralfate (Carafate)
23. They inhibit the action of histamine on the H_2 receptors that trigger release of gastric secretions.

CHAPTER 33

1. a. chemical irritation of nerve endings from stomach acid
    b. stretching/contracting of stomach caused by muscle tension as in obstructions
2. Esophageal varices
3. potassium
4. 1, 2, 4, 5
5. gastric cancer
6. pernicious anemia
7. High gastric acid secretion and rapid emptying of food from the stomach into the duodenum characterize duodenal ulcers. Gastric ulcers are caused by a break in the mucosal barrier, exposing the stomach to hydrochloric acid.
8. upper GI tract hemorrhage
9.

Procedure	Indication
Vagotomy	eliminate acid-secreting stimulus to gastric cells
Vagotomy with Pyloroplasty	cutting left and right vagus nerves and widening the exit of the stomach at the pylorus; prevents stasis and enhances emptying
Gastroenterostomy	drain made at bottom of stomach, connected to jejunum; drains acid away from ulcerative area and aids in healing
Antrectomy	reduce acid-producing portions of the stomach
Subtotal gastrectomy	partial removal of the stomach; treatment of duodenal ulcers because of recurrent ulceration
Total gastrectomy	total resection of the stomach due to extensive gastric cancer

10. Alkalosis
11. 1, 3, 4, 6, 7
12. 1, 2, 3, 4, 5, 6, 7, 8
13. It is a manifestation of GI tract bleeding; acid digestion of the blood results in dark, granular emesis.
14. Measure NG tube output each shift and monitor serum electrolyte levels from laboratory reports. Notify physician of abnormal lab values promptly.
15. True, False, True, True
16. 3
17. Manifestations can appear 5 to 30 minutes after eating and involve vasomotor disturbances of vertigo, tachycardia, syncope, sweating, palpitations, diarrhea, and nausea.

18. 1, 3, 4
19. right
20. False
21. Report observation to physician promptly. Melena is the result of lower GI tract bleeding and is characterized as black, tarry stools.
22. No, it is not added to the intake. If the irrigation solution is aspirated, it is not intake.
23. Room temperature saline is cooler than body temperature and will create mild vasoconstriction. It is also used to remove blood from the stomach.
24. Maintaining adequate perfusion to the kidneys is vital to client stability; urine output should be monitored hourly with a Foley catheter in place.
25. The tube may be positioned directly over the suture line and repositioning could cause trauma.
26. Compazine
27. The defensive resistance of the mucosa to hydrochloric acid secretion depends on numerous factors, including the presence of adequate gastromucosal prostaglandins. The action of NSAIDs is to inhibit prostaglandin production, which reduces inflammation and pain, but loss of prostaglandins exposes the gastric mucosa to acid secretions, resulting in ulcers.
28. False
29. Many of the OTC preparations contain aspirin (acetylsalicylic acid) and NSAIDs, which can cause ulcers.
30.

Medication	Indication for Use
Enteric-coated aspirin	protects against irritation with loss of mucosa from NSAIDs
Cytotec	protects against irritation with loss of mucosa from NSAIDs
Histamine receptor antagonists	decreases gastric acidity
Proton pump inhibitors	blocks gastric acid production

CHAPTER 34

1. See Figure U8-2 in the textbook.
2. See Figure U8-3 in the textbook.
3. 2, 3, 4, 5, 6

4.

	Urine Output	Associated Conditions
Anuria	less than 100 ml per 24 hours	Acute or chronic renal failure with secondary to systemic events Shock Reduced cardiac output Renal injury or obstruction
Oliguria	100–600 ml per 24 hours	Acute or chronic renal failure
Polyuria	unusually large daily amounts	Systemic diseases such as diabetes mellitus, diabetes insipidus, diuretic medications, chronic renal disease

5. a. Etiology: postoperatively or postpartum, use of certain medications
   b. Manifestations: sudden inability to void, severe suprapubic pain and urgency
   c. Treatment: medical emergency; requires immediate urethral or suprapubic catheterization
6. a. 2, b. 5, c. 1, d. 3, e. 4
7. Pneumaturia
8. True, False, True, True, True, True, False, True, True
9. glomerular
10. a. timing: when problem first noticed, onset abrupt or insidious, where was client when problem began
    b. quality and quantity: describe the problem in detail, aids in diagnosis, pain from referred areas
    c. location: define and locate, aids in identifying possible organ involvement
    d. precipitating factor: events that occur in relation to problem, change in client's diet/location/travel
    e. aggravating/relieving factors: what has client already tried to alleviate problem; did it work?
    f. associated manifestations: problems in GI tract can cause symptoms in other areas; assists in diagnosis
11. False, True, True, True
12. prostate gland
13. cervix of the uterus
14. 1, 2, 3, 4, 5
15. 2, 3, 4, 7, 8
16. 1, 3, 4, 5, 6
17. 2
18. a. Computed Tomography: useful alternative for clients who cannot retain barium; can identify masses

    b. Ultrasonography: used to identify pathology in pancreas, liver, gallbladder, spleen, and retroperitoneal tissue; abdominal gas can interfere with ultrasound waves
    c. Proctosigmoidoscopy: examination of distal sigmoid colon, rectum, and anal canal; not as thorough as colonoscopy but safer
    d. Colonoscopy: visual exam of entire colon with flexible fiberoptic endoscope; used to screen clients at high risk for colon cancer
19. 1, 2, 3, 4
20. a. Instruct client to maintain a low-residue or clear liquid diet 2 days before the test: to reduce feces volume
    b. Teach client to administer a potent laxative and oral bowel prep the night before the test: to cleanse bowel area for examination
    c. Instruct client to maintain NPO after midnight: prevent additional fecal material in bowel
    d. Administer a cleansing enema or suppository the morning of the exam: final preparation for the procedure
21. 1, 2, 4
22.

	Proctosigmoid-oscopy	Colonoscopy
Preparation	bowel cleansing NPO in a.m.	bowel cleansing NPO after midnight
Obtain consent	Yes	Yes
Positioning	left lateral	left lateral
Instrument	rigid sigmoidscope	flexible fiberoptic endoscope
Sedation	No	Yes
Post-procedure	monitor for bowel perforation	monitor for bowel perforation
	monitor for pain	monitor for pain
	monitor for vasovagal response	monitor for vasovagal response
	client is NPO	client is NPO
	monitor vital signs q 30 min until alert	monitor vital signs q 30 min until alert

23. To promote greater concentration of the contrast medium in the kidneys
24. Direct pressure to the site with a sterile dressing for at least 20 minutes to prevent bleeding.
25. 6
26. These medications are often used to treat urinary tract infections.
27. Methylprednisolone
28. Belladonna, opium suppositories

CHAPTER 35

1.

Disorder	Etiology
Hemorrhage	trauma, ulcerations or inflammation
Pain	
Visceral	mechanical factors causing stretching/distending
Somatic	inflammation of specific area, more intense
Referred	pain felt at a distance from affected organ
Nausea/Vomiting	distention of the duodenum
Distention	excessive gas in the intestines; blockage
Diarrhea	infections, malabsorption syndromes, medications
Constipation:	inadequate fluid or bulk, mechanical blockage

2. 3
3. True, False, True, True, True, True, False, True, False, False
4. 1, 2, 3, 5
5. 1, 3, 4, 5

6.

	Crohn's Disease	Ulcerative Colitis
Area affected	entire GI tract	entire colon
	All layers of bowel	mucosa/ submucosa
Age of client	10- 30 yrs of age	15-35 yrs. of age
Amount of diarrhea	5-6 liq. stools/ day	10-20 stools/day
Appearance of stool	liquid, no blood	bloody, mucus
Systemic symptoms	fever, fatigue, wt. loss, malaise	fatigue, wt. loss
Nutritional deficiencies	malabsorption	malabsorption
Medical treatment		
Medications	antidiarrheals	antidiarrheals
	corticosteroids	corticosteroids
	salicylates	salicylates
	Mesalamine	
	Flagyl/antibiotics	
Surgical intervention	Not curative	Remove colon: cure
Prognosis	Chronic; reoccur	Chronic; reoccur

7. Polyps
8. Diverticulosis is the presence of non-inflamed diverticula. Diverticulitis is inflammation of the diverticula.
9. 5

10.

	Cause	Injuries	Treatment
Blunt trauma:	steering wheel pedestrian accidents	shearing crushing compressing rupture of bowel	observation
Penetrating Injury:	gunshot wounds stabbings	damage all structures perforations peritonitis/sepsis	surgery IV antibiotics

11. 1, 2, 3, 4
12. False
13. a. Temperature: increases signify complications
    b. Blood pressure: decrease can signify shock
    c. Respiratory rate: monitor for adult respiratory distress syndrome
    d. Bowel sounds: monitor return of normal functioning
    e. Urine output: evaluate fluid status of client
    f. Skin turgor/mucous membranes: assess hydration status
    g. Laboratory tests (CBC, electrolytes); prevent complications, return levels to baseline
14. 4
15. a. Rest: reduce energy demands on patient
    b. NPO status: rest the bowel, reduce diarrhea
    c. Fluids: replace losses from diarrhea and vomiting
    d. Electrolytes in fluids/IV: return balance to vascular system
    e. Perineal/skin care: remove irritating fluids; prevent breakdown
16. 2, 4

17. a. Acute pain related to inflammation
       OUTCOME: The client describes decreased postoperative pain
       INTERVENTION #1: medicate as ordered and evaluate effectiveness
       INTERVENTION #2: teach client body mechanics to reduce tension on abdominal incision
    b. Risk for infection related to rupture of appendix
       OUTCOME: Infection will not develop/rupture will be diagnosed early
       INTERVENTION #1: monitor vital signs closely
       INTERVENTION #2: teach patient proper wound care
18. a. Diet high in calories, protein and carbohydrates: To provide the nutrients necessary to assist patient cope with stress of surgery and ensure proper wound healing postoperatively
    b. Diet low in residue/liquid diet: to reduce peristalsis, rest bowel
    c. Cathartics, such as GoLYTELY or Fleet Prep Kit: clean out the bowel and minimize bacterial growth in the bowel
    d. Administration of antibiotics: reduce bacterial growth and prevent postop infections
    e. Administration of Enemas: to clean the lumen (inside) of the bowel; remove bacteria
    f. Blood transfusions (if needed): correct severe anemia and enhance wound healing
    g. Enterostomal nurse consult: provide emotional support and information before the surgery
19. a. Insertion of a nasogastric tube: Decompress; remove fluids/gas
    b. NPO status: rest the bowel
    c. IV fluids with electrolytes: replace losses; maintain balance
    d. Monitor vital signs frequently: signifies complications; infection
20. gastroenteritis
21. it has been shown to cause spasms of the colon

22.

Medication	Indication for Use	Action
5-ASA Azulfidine Asacol/Rowasa Dipentum	Ulcerative Colitis and Crohn's	block production of prostaglandins/leukotrienes decrease inflammatory process
Steroids	UC and Crohn's IBD fails to respond to salicylates	reduce inflammation
Antacids/antihistamines	steroid use for UC/Crohn's	prevent gastric ulceration
Budesenide	Crohn's	new, non-systemic steroid
Purinethol	UC and Crohn's	immunosuppression
Methotrexate Imuran Sandimmune	IBD fails to respond to salicylates/steroids	immunoregulatory
Remicade	Crohn's	block action of tumor necrosis factor
Antegren	IBD	immune modulator attach to immune cells and prevent them from leaving blood stream to go to site of inflammation
Anticholinergic	UC and Crohn's	relieve abdominal cramps
Antidiarrheals	UC and Crohns's	relieve diarrhea
Antispasmodic	UC and Crohn's	reduce spasms, rest the colon
Flagyl	UC and Crohn's	prevent/control infection
Cipro		treat anal fistulas/perianal disease

CHAPTER 36
1. microorganisms, 100,000
2. a. length of the male urethra
   b. antibacterial properties of prostatic fluid
3. 1, 2, 3, 5, 6, 7
4. urine culture
5. pyelonephritis
6. Urethritis
7. a. urinary stasis, b. supersaturation of the urine with poorly soluble crystals

8.

Type of Calculi	Etiology
Calcium	Paget's disease
	hyperparathyroidism
	impaired renal absorption
	increased intestinal absorption
Oxalate	inflammatory bowel disease
	postileal resection of bowel
	overdose of ascorbic acid
	concurrent fat malabsorption
Struvite	certain bacteria, Proteus "urea-splitter"
Uric Acid	increased urate excretion
	fluid depletion
	low urinary pH
	increased uric acid production
Cystine	congenital metabolic error
Xanthine	rare, hereditary condition
	xanthine oxidase deficiency

9. True, True
10. benign prostatic hypertrophy (BPH)
11. 6
12. 1, 2, 4, 6, 7, 10
13. 1, 2, 3, 4, 5
14. A change of color from moist red to pale, dark, dusky, gray or cyanotic coloring indicates loss of vascular supply and must be corrected immediately.
15. 1, 2, 4
16. False, True, True, True, True, True
17. 4
18. a. Encourage fluid intake at least 3 liters per day: flush bladder
    b. Avoid caffeinated beverages/alcohol: irritates lining of bladder
    c. Learn risks associated with spermicides: alters pH, irritates
    d. Remind client to void every 2-3 hours: mechanical clearing
    e. Instruct female clients to void before and after coitus: prevent bacterial infection
19. OUTCOME: Client will have return of normal voiding habits within 3 days of starting antibiotic treatment

INTERVENTION: provide instructions about antibiotic therapy
INTERVENTION: instruct on dietary changes/fluid intake
20. OUTCOME: Complications will not develop or will be minimized
INTERVENTION: Administer antispasmodics
INTERVENTION: Increase fluid intake
INTERVENTION: Administer urinary tract antiseptics/analgesics
21. karaya
22. 1, 2, 3, 4, 6
23. Phenazopyridine (Pyridium)
24. a. Renal and hepatic function: ability to clear medications
    b. Cardiovascular status: ability to handle fluid intake
25. Heparin
26. BCG is instilled into the bladder through a urethral catheter, the catheter is clamped or removed, client retains the fluid for 2 hours moving side to side or supine to prone changes in position. After 2 hours, the client voids in a sitting position or catheter is unclamped.
27.

Urge incontinence	Ditropan	increases volume of bladder
	Detrol	before involuntary bladder contractions occur
	Tofranil	bladder wall relaxation
		increases capacity
Stress incontinence	Pseudofed	increases closure mechanism of urethra
Urinary incontinence	Vaginal estrogen	Improved functioning increases circulation to area

CHAPTER 37

1. 1, 2, 3, 4, 5, 6, 7
2. hypertension

3.

	Acute	Chronic
Etiology	bacterial contamination of urethra	chronic obstruction from instrument with reflux
Manifestations	enlarged kidneys	hypertension
	abscesses	azotemia
	high fever/chills	pyuria
	flank pain at CVA	anemia
	cloudy urine, foul smelling	proteinuria
Testing	U/A with C & S	UA with C & S
	KUB x-ray	Blood pressure
	Cystourethrogram	
	MRI/CT scan	
Medical treatment	Antibiotic: Sulfonamides	Control hypertension
	10 days to 2 weeks	High fluid intake
	Analgesic	Antibiotics

4. Removing the obstruction causes sudden release of pressure and diuresis, which can lead to dehydration.
5. True, True, False, False, True, False, True, True, True, True
6. a. hematuria
   b. flank pain
   c. palpable abdominal or flank mass
7.

	Acute	Chronic
Cause	allergic reaction	progressive fibrosis
Onset	rapid onset	chronic inflammatory cell infiltration with atrophy
Manifestations	fever	interstitial edema
	skin rash	altered renal vasculature
	oliguric renal failure	interstitial fibrosis
	gross hematuria	
Prognosis	complete recovery	similar to chronic pyelonephritis
	rapid progression to renal failure and death	
	change to chronic form	

8.

	Acute	Chronic
Onset	suddenly/insidiously	extended period; years
Manifestations	hematuria	malaise/weight loss
	proteinuria	edema
	fever/chills	irritability/mental cloudiness
	weakness/pallor	metallic taste in mouth
	generalized edema	polyuria/nocturia
	ascites	headache/dizziness
	pleural effusion	digestive disturbances
	heart failure	respiratory difficulty/angina

9. a. Contusion
   b. minor laceration
   c. major laceration
   d. "fractured" kidney (shattered)
   e. vascular injury
10. Hematuria
11. a. renal agenesis*: absence of one or more kidneys, *bilateral agenesis is fatal
    b. supernumerary kidney: more than two kidneys
    c. ectopic kidney: kidneys located in thoracic region
    d. aplasia: small and contracted, no functioning renal tissue
    e. hyploplastic: miniature kidney with some functioning tissue
    f. horseshoe kidney: two kidneys are joined in a single organ
12. 1, 2, 4
13. Spontaneous pneumothorax
14. Damage caused by poststreptococcal infections leads to glomerulonephritis
15. Rhabdomyolysis: IV fluids and bed rest
    Rationale: maintain adequate perfusion through kidneys; reduce muscle metabolism; prevent further damage
    Hypertension: medication and diet changes
    Rationale: reduce blood pressure to stop damage to arterioles/arteries
16. 3
17. OUTCOME: The client will have balanced intake and output, maintenance of adequate hydration and absence of signs/symptoms of dehydration
    INTERVENTION #1: Prepare client for diagnostic tests
    INTERVENTION #2: Maintain IV hydration
18. OUTCOME: The client will report no pain or report that pain is controlled.
    INTERVENTION #1: Administer analgesics per orders and evaluate effectiveness
    INTERVENTION #2: Fluid intake of 3-4 liters per day
19. a. relieve pain to allow client to perform deep breathing and coughing exercises
    b. reduce pain during movement, deep breathing/coughing
    c. identify problems with renal function early
    d. paralytic ileus is a common problem

20.

Plan	Intervention(s)
A. Maintain fluid and electrolyte balance	monitor daily weight and intake/output
	loop diuretics [Lasix]
	plasma volume expanders
	dietary restriction of sodium/potassium
B. Reduce inflammation	steroid therapy
C. Prevent thrombosis	long-term anticoagulation
	teach client to monitor for hemorrhage
D. Minimize protein loss	increase protein intake 1-1.5g/kg/day
	24-hr urine to monitor protein loss
	treat inflammation to reduce losses

21. decrease
22. 2, 3, 4
23. Through loss of excessive fluids, the client can experience hypovolemia which reduces kidney perfusion.
24. a. Client may vary in sensitivity and response to medications
    b. Decreased renal perfusion reduces ability to excrete drug
25. 1, 3, 4, 5, 7, 8

CHAPTER 38
1. 1, 3, 4
2. a. Prerenal
   b. Intrarenal
   c. Postrenal
3. a. deposition of heme pigments or myoglobin/hemoglobin in the tubules
      EX: Rhabdomyolysis, surgery, crush injury or electric shock
   b. non-traumatic conditions
      EX: diabetes mellitus, infectious diseases, hypokalemia, heat stroke or rejection of transplanted kidney
4. True, False, True, False, True, True, True

5.

	Nonoliguric Renal Failure	Oliguric Renal Failure
Urine output	2000 ml/day	less than 400 ml/day–600 ml
Urine	dilute	concentrated
	low specific gravity	high specific gravity
		proteinuria
Clinical signs	hypertension	*precipitating event:
	tachypnea	hemorrhage/cardiac insult
	dry mucous membranes	edema/weight gain
	poor skin turgor	hemoptysis
	orthostatic hypotension	weakness from anemia
		hypertension
Prognosis	less morbidity/mortality	mortality as high as 50%
		*when due to trauma/surgery

6. 1
7. a. Reduced renal reserve: BUN is high-normal; no clinical manifestations
   b. Renal insufficiency: more advanced pathology; impaired urine concentration, nocturia, mild anemia; renal function easily impaired by stress
   c. Renal failure: severe azotemia, acidosis, impaired urine dilution, severe anemia, electrolyte imbalances
   d. End-stage renal disease (ESRD): totally impaired excretory and regulatory mechanisms; clinical manifestations in ALL body systems—GI, CV,
   e. Neuromuscular, hematologic, skin, skeletal and hormonal: Kidneys can no longer maintain homeostasis
8. ammonia
9. Ultrafiltration is the removal of fluid from the blood; it uses either osmotic or hydrostatic pressure. Diffusion is the passage of particles from an area of higher concentration to an area of lower concentration.
10. Rapid solute removal from the blood changes the osmotic pressure gradient; the cerebral tissues now absorb more fluids which leads to cerebral edema and increased intracranial pressure. Client will complain of headache and mental confusion and can have a change in level of consciousness.
11. a. Increasing BUN level: decreases seizure threshold; increase in number of seizures
    b. Low RBC, Hct, Hgb: anemia due to decrease erythropoietin production in kidneys decreasing RBC production
    c. Low platelets: elevated BUN levels interfere with platelet aggregation

12. **Electrolyte Imbalances:**
    impaired excretion and utilization by kidneys
    hyponatremia
    hyperkalemia
    hypocalcemia
    elevated magnesium levels
    Metabolic Changes:
    BUN and serum creatinine increase
    proteinuria
    carbohydrate intolerance
    metabolic acidosis
    Hematologic Changes:
    anemia
    bleeding tendencies
    platelet abnormalities
    Gastrointestinal Changes:
    anorexia
    nausea/vomiting
    bitter, metallic taste in mouth
    ammonia-like breath
    stomatitis
    esophagitis/gastritis/colitis
    GI bleeding/ diarrhea
    constipation
    Immunologic Changes:
    depression of humoral antibody formation
    suppression of delayed hypersensitivity
    decreased chemotactic function of leukocytes
    Changes to Medication Metabolism:
    high risk for medication toxicity
    Changes in:
    absorption
    distribution
    metabolism
    excretion
    Cardiovascular Changes:
    hypertension
    left ventricular hypertrophy

congestive heart failure
dysrhythmias
atherosclerosis; accelerated deposition of
plaques
Respiratory Changes:
pulmonary edema
"uremic lung" (pneumonitis)
tachypnea from metabolic acidosis
Musculoskeletal Changes:
osteodystrophy
osteomalacia
osteoporosis
osteosclerosis
impaired conversion of vitamin D to active form
reduced absorption of calcium from intestines
increased phosphate retention
Integumentary Changes:
dry skin due to atrophy of sweat glands
intractable pruritus
petechiae due to bleeding tendency
bruising
anemia; pallor
brittle hair; falls out
thin brittle nails; "half and half nails"
Neurologic Changes:
peripheral neuropathy
sensations: burning feet
restless leg syndrome
gait changes/foot drop/paraplegia
slow nerve conduction
decreased deep tendon reflexes
CNS:
    forgetfulness
    inability to concentrate
    short attention span
    irritability
    nystagmus
    twitching
    seizures
    CNS depression/coma
Reproductive Changes:
menstrual irregularities/amenorrhea
infertility
male impotence
oligospermia/reduced sperm motility
both sexes: decreased libido
Endocrine Changes:
altered insulin utilization
altered parathyroid function
TSH normal but lessened response
Psychosocial Changes:
powerlessness
lack of control over illness/treatment
intrusive therapies
restrictions imposed by regimens

changes to body image
changes in sexuality
role reversal
loss of work/financial strain
scheduling dialysis

13. 1, 3, 4, 5
14. The nurse must palpate for a "thrill" and auscultate for a "bruit" with the stethoscope over the graft site. A positive finding demonstrates adequate blood flow through the graft site.
15. a. Careful replacement of fluids: prevent fluid overload; based on percentage of output; reduce workload of kidneys
    b. Replacement of other fluid losses: must account for insensible losses, vomiting, diarrhea to balance overall fluid level
    c. Cautious use of diuretics to reduce fluid overload: kidneys not functioning properly; avoid dehydration
    d. Electrolyte replacement based on lab data: kidneys' inability to excrete potassium and regulate other electrolytes impaired; prevent hyperkalemia, which may lead to cardiac arrhythmias or arrest.
    e. Electrocardiograph monitors: check for effects of hyperkalemia or hyponatremia
    f. Dietary restrictions: avoid dark green vegetables, seeds, nuts, antacids which contain magnesium; cannot be excreted with renal failure
16. a. High calorie: reverse process of gluconeogenesis
    b. Low protein: reduce workload of kidneys; nitrogenous waste products
    c. Low sodium/magnesium/phosphate/ potassium: impaired excretion
    d. TPN: if oral intake is not sufficient to meet requirements
    e. Adequate/balanced fluids: impaired renal excretion
17. OUTCOME: The client will regain/maintain balanced intake and output
INTERVENTIONS: accurate intake and output
Fluid restrictions
Careful monitoring of fluids each shift
Monitor vital signs
Check skin turgor/mucous membranes
Careful weight measurements
Obtain urine specific gravity
18. OUTCOME: Client will maintain adequate nutrition as evidenced by sufficient intake to prevent protein catabolism and lab values within safe levels
INTERVENTIONS: work with client to establish preferences

pleasant environment at mealtime
medications to alleviate discomfort of
stomatitis/nausea
enteral or parenteral feedings
19. magnesium
20. a. Remove end products of protein metabolism
[urea and creatinine] from the blood.
b. Maintain a safe concentration of serum
electrolytes.
c. Correct acidosis and restore bicarbonate
level.
d. Remove excess fluid from the blood.
21. potassium chloride
22. furosemide (Lasix)
23. heparin
24. Due to decreased kidney function, they are at
higher risk for damage due to possible nephrotoxic effects.
25. 2
26. 1, 2, 5, 7, 8
27. erythropoietin
28. Increased blood urea nitrogen (BUN) and increased serum creatinine levels.
29. The urine will be very dilute, with large quantities produced. In addition, there will be a loss of
sodium in the urine resulting in hyponatremia.
30. Immune disturbances result in ineffective protection against invasion from bacteria, etc.
31. Edema, hypertension and (congestive) heart failure
32. Potassium binding agents and potassium restriction (in the diet)
33. Decreased excretion of nitrogenous waste accu-
mulates in the CNS causing changes in function.
The increased waste products can also cause the
pruritus of the skin.

CHAPTER 39
1. See Figure U9-1 in the textbook.
2. See Figure U9-2 in the textbook.
3. See Figure U9-4 in the textbook.
4. 4
5. 1
6. Pap tests, pelvic examinations
7. is a soft tissue radiographic breast exam, small
invasive and noninvasive tumors and benign lesions
8. 1
9. 3
10. a. 2, b. 1, c. 4, d. 5, e. 3
11. 1, 2, 3, 4, 5, 6, 7
12. 2
13. 1, 2, 4
14. 3

15. 1, 2
16. gynecomastia
17. Bimanual exam
18. rectocele
19. tail of Spence
20. inframammary ridge
21. 1, 2, 3, 4, 5
22. 1, 2, 3, 4
23. 1, 2, 3, 4
24. True
25. 1, 2
26. 1, 2, 3, 4

CHAPTER 40
1. 2
2. 3
3. a. 1, b. 2, c. 9, d. 10, e. 7, f. 8, g. 6, h. 4, i. 5, j. 3
4. 3, 4
5. 1
6. 1, 2, 3, 4, 5
7. 1, 2, 3, 4
8. 3
9. 4
10. 2
11. 3
12. 1, 2, 3, 4
13. bladder
14. True, True

CHAPTER 41
1. 3
2. a. 1, b. 3, c. 6, d. 8, e. 4, f. 7, g. 5, h. 2
3. 2
4. 3
5. uterus, cervix
6. tube, ovaries
7. 1, 3, 4
8. 1
9. a. hot flashes, b. night sweats, c. palpitations, d.
dizziness
10. 1, 2, 3, 4
11. 1, 2, 3
12. 1, 2, 3, 4
13. 4
14. 2
15. 1, 2, 3, 4, 5
16. 2
17. 1, 2
18. 1, 2, 3
19. 1
20. 2
21. 4
22. 1, 2, 3, 4

23. 1, 2, 3
24. caffeine, vitamin B$_6$

CHAPTER 42
1. age
2. 1
3. 4
4. 4
5. 1, 2, 3, 4
6. 1
7. 2
8. a. 3, b. 2, c. 4, d. 5, e. 1
9. 1, 2, 3
10. 3
11. cyst
12. nonpalpable lesions
13. modified radical mastectomy
14. 1, 2, 3
15. True
16. 2
17. 1, 2, 3

CHAPTER 43
1. 1, 2, 3, 4, 5
2. chancroid
3. *C. trachomatis*
4. 1, 2, 3
5. 2
6. 4
7. 3
8. 1
9. 3
10. 1
11. 1, 3, 4
12. 1, 2
13. 1
14. 4
15. 2, 3
16. 2
17. 3, 4

CHAPTER 44
1. See Figure U10-2 in the textbook.
2. True, True
3. a. 12, b. 11, c. 10, d. 9, e. 4, f. 7, g. 8, h. 1, i. 3, j. 2, k. 6, l. 5
4. 1, 2, 3, 4
5. 1, 2
6. 4
7. 4
8. True, True

9. Biopsy
10. Paracentesis
11. Hypovolemia
12. 1, 2, 3, 4
13. 1, 2, 3, 4
14. True, True

CHAPTER 45
1. Euthyroid
2. 1, 2, 3, 4
3. 1, 2, 3, 4
4. 1
5. 2
6. 1, 2, 3
7. myxedema
8. 1
9. 2, 3, 4
10. Graves' disease
11. 2
12. 1, 2
13. 1, 3, 4, 5
14. 1, 4
15. 1, 3, 4
16. 1, 2
17. 1, 2, 3, 4, 5
18. 1, 2, 3, 4, 5
19. 1, 2
20. 1, 2, 3, 4, 5
21. 1, 2
22. thyroid cancer
23. hyperthyroidism
24. 1, 2, 3, 4
25. 3
26. 3
27. 1, 2
28. 1, 2, 3
29. 1
30. 1, 2, 3, 4
31. potassium iodine
32. 1, 2, 3
33. Hypothyroidism
34. 1, 2, 3, 4
35. 4

CHAPTER 46
1. 1, 2, 3, 4
2. Autoimmunity
3. 1, 2
4. 1, 2, 3, 4
5. 1, 2
6. Primary aldosteronism
7. Secondary hyperaldosteronism

8. Hyperpituitarism
9. Hypopituitarism
10. 3
11. True
12. 1, 2, 3
13. 3
14. 2
15. 1
16. 3
17. 3
18. 1, 2, 3
19. 1
20. 1, 2
21. osteoporosis
22. 1
23. True

CHAPTER 47

1. 1, 3
2. 1, 2
3. Type II
4. 2
5. IDDM
6. 1, 2, 3
7. glycosuria
8. ketones
9. 4
10. 1
11. 1
12. 1, 2, 3
13. 1
14. 2 hours after meals
15. 3
16. 2
17. 4
18. 2
19. 3
20. 1
21. 2
22. 4
23. 1
24. 1
25. 1
26. 1, 2
27. Lantus
28. 3
29. 3
30. 2

CHAPTER 48

1. digestion, utilization of glucose
2. True, True

3. 1, 2, 3
4. a. cholecystitis, b. cholelithiasis, c. hyperlipidemia, d. hypercalcemia, e. pancreatic tumor, f. pancreatic ischemia, g. certain medications and alcohol abuse
5. removal of the gallbladder
6. jaundice
7. bluish discoloration of the left flank
8. bluish discoloration of the periumbilical area
9. 1, 2
10. 2
11. 4
12. 4
13. 4
14. 1, 2, 3
15. 1, 2, 3, 4
16. 1
17. 1, 2, 3, 4
18. Morphine
19. 2
20. calcium gluconate
21. 2

CHAPTER 49

1. 1
2. 1, 2
3. 1, 2, 3, 4
4. 1, 2
5. a. 2, 5, 9; b. 2, 3, 6, 8; c. 2; d. 1; e. 10; f. 7
6. hepatic encephalopathy
7. 1, 2, 3, 4
8. 1, 2, 3, 4
9. 1
10. 1, 2
11. 1, 2, 3
12. 1
13. 2
14. 1
15. 1, 2, 3

CHAPTER 50

1. See Figure U11-1 in the textbook.
2. persistent itching or pruritus
3. An allergy is an immunologic response that happens consistently with exposure, while irritation can occur unpredictably.
4. a. alopecia, b. ichthyosis, c. atopic dermatitis, d. psoriasis
5. scabies
6. hirsutism
7. nutrition, respiratory
8. anemia

9. A callus is a flat, painless thickening of a circumscribed area of skin. A corn is a horny induration and thickening of the skin caused by friction and pressure; it is often painful.

10. Linear lesions appear in a straight line whereas satellite lesions appear as small peripheral lesions around a central larger lesion.

11. False, False, False, False

12. A=asymmetry (one half is unlike the other half)
B=border (irregular, scalloped, or poorly circumscribed)
C=color (varied from one area to another, shades of two colors, or changing color)
D=diameter (larger than 6 mm as a rule)

13. Previous experiences may explain unusual lesions or their location.

14. A large number of skin problems are caused or worsened by exposure to irritants and chemicals in the home and work environment.

15. a. 6, b. 7, c. 8, d. 11, e. 1, f. 4, g. 9, h. 10, i. 5, j. 2, k. 3

16. Excessive warmth can produce changes in skin color by causing vasodilation. Colored walls can affect normal skin hue. Privacy is needed so that the client will feel comfortable undressing and putting on a gown.

17. a. buccal mucosa, b. nail beds, lips, and palms, c. white of sclera, d. hard palate

18. dorsum of the hand

19. location, distribution, size, arrangement, color, configuration, secondary changes, and presence of drainage

20. palpate

21. True

22. See Table 50-3 in the textbook.

23. Skin culture is indicated in clients with skin infections that have been unresponsive to routine care.

24. A patch test is done to identify substances that produce allergic skin responses.

25. A patch test is contraindicated when acute dermatitis is present, if the client is taking oral steroids, and if the allergen may worsen the dermatitis.

26. Aspirin can cause prolonged bleeding after the biopsy is completed.

27. A small amount of antibiotic ointment and a clean, dry dressing is applied. The client is instructed about follow-up appointments and told when biopsy results will be available.

28. cutaneous

29. a sunburn-like rash in areas of sun exposure

30. a. 2, b. 3, c. 4, d. 1

CHAPTER 51

1. a. 3, b. 5, c. 2, d. 1, e. 6, f. 4

2. pruritus

3. Irritant contact dermatitis is most common and is from exposure to anything that produces a chemical or physical irritant response. Allergic contact dermatitis is a delayed hypersensitivity reaction resulting from contact with an allergen.

4. body fluids such as in cases of urinary incontinence

5. one month, 3-4 days

6. a. scalp, b. elbows, c. knees, d. genital and sacral region

7. 30, 50, Women, men

8. First-degree sunburn produces mild, tender erythema followed by desquamation that heals without scarring. Second-degree sunburn causes more extreme erythema and edema; blistering results from damage to the epidermal cells.

9. a. basal cell carcinoma, b. squamous cell carcinoma, c. malignant melanoma

10. 3

11. a. fair complexion, b. excessive childhood sun exposure and blistering childhood sunburns, c. increased number of common acquired and dysplastic moles, d. family history of melanoma, e. presence of a changing mole on the skin

12. a. asymmetry, b. border notching, c. color variegation with black, brown, red, or white hue, d. diameter > 6 mm.

13. depth

14. cutaneous T cell lymphoma

15. residual pain called postherpetic neuralgia, itching

16. aesthetic, reconstructive

17. thrombosis

18. False, False, True, True, True, True, True, False, False, True, True, False, True, False, False, True

19. All pressure ulcers are colonized with surface bacteria. A swab culture grows only organisms that colonize the surface.

20. 12

21. excessive swallowing

22. False

23. Application of moisturizers is more frequent if frequent bathing and showering is not possible. Assistive personnel may be needed to help with topical applications. Oral antihistamines are administered in small doses due to possible low tolerance.

24. causative agent

25. a. 2, b. 5, c. 6, d. 1, e. 3, f. 4

26. This measure limits skin destruction, prevents edema, and potentially reduces blisters.

27. 1

28. a. 3, b. 4, c. 5, d. 1, e. 2
29. protect the blood supply of the flap
30. control of hemorrhage through application of direct pressure
31. True, False, False, False, False, True
32. a. client age, b. size of the affected regions, c. condition of stratum corneum, d. cutaneous blood supply, e. molecular weight of the drug, f. medication vehicle.
33. 2, 4
34. 4
35. a. tacrolimus ointment (Protopic), b. pimecrolimus cream (Elidel)
36. taper the dosage as the drug is discontinued
37. 4
38. 1
39. True, True

CHAPTER 52
1. a. 3, b. 1, c. 2
2. a. ability to maintain normal body temperature, b. risk of infection increases due to a loss of the barrier, c. evaporative water loss increases
3. a. 3, b. 4, c. 5, d. 6, e. 1, f. 2
4. 15%
5. higher
6. wound contracture, hypertrophic scarring
7. True, True, True, False, False
8. Thermal burns are caused by exposure to or contact with a flame, hot liquid or semiliquid, or hot objects. Chemical burns are caused by tissue contact with strong acids, alkalis, or organic compounds. Electrical burn injuries are caused by heat that is generated by the electrical energy as it passes through the body. Radiation burns are caused by exposure to a radioactive source.
9. $197 \div 2.2 = 89.55$ kg $\times 0.5 = 4.48$ ml
10. 3
11. 24, 48
12. 2
13. 4
14. Background pain is experienced when the client is at rest or engages in non-procedure-related activities. It is described as continuous in nature and low in intensity. Procedural pain is experienced during the performance of therapeutic measures and is described as acute and high intensity.
15. 1, 2
16. a. pulses, b. capillary refill, c. color, d. movement, e. sensation
17. $146 \div 2.2 = 66.36$ kg $\times 25$ kcal $= 1659 + (40$ kcal $\times 36 = 1440) = 3099$ kcal
18. $212 \div 2.2 = 96.36$ Kg $\times 2 = 192.72 \times 45 = 8672.4$ ml / 24 hours

19. 7% partial-thickness burn for the face, 4% partial-thickness burn for each upper arm, 3% partial-thickness burn for each lower arm, and 2½% full-thickness burn for each hand
20. elevate the head of the bed
21. 75, 100
22. This tissue serves as a medium for bacterial growth.
23. strict handwashing
24. 3
25. a. therapeutic positioning, b. ROM exercises, c. splinting, d. client and family education
26. hip extension
27. 3
28. calories, protein
29. Debridement cases are considered contaminated in the operating room. They are therefore scheduled at the end of the day to decrease the risk to other surgical clients. The OR suite can be terminally cleaned following the last case.
30. False
31. morphine sulfate
32. gastric ulceration
33. False

CHAPTER 53
1. See Figure U12-2 in the textbook.
2. a. predictable: when the client walks, he or she will have pain in the calf
   b. reproducible: the client can walk same distance each time before the pain occurs.
3. 1, 3, 4
4. Lipodermatosclerosis
5. True, False
6. Teleangiectasis
7. It is caused by bleeding outside the vessel wall but within the contained area near the artery. The bleeding can become a site for infection or a source of emboli or may cause a thrombosis.
8. Age: incidence of atherosclerosis increases with age
   Occupation: type of work requiring heavy physical labor, long standing, sedentary work, factors increasing risk of vascular disease
9. baseline
10. True, True
11. contralateral
12. Allen's test
13. Doppler
14. a. elevation of legs, b. exercise
15. a. allows assessment of subtle changes in skin color
    b. prevent vasoconstriction
    c. helpful when auscultating low-pitched sounds in blood vessels

16. 1, 2, 3, 5

CHAPTER 54

1. 2
2. heart attack
3. increase in peripheral arterial resistance
4.

Type	Characteristics
Primary (essential)	90% of all adult cases of HTN Unknown etiology Appears between age 30-50
Secondary	due to identifiable cause: chronic glomerulonephritis renal failure

5. a. Renin is an enzyme produced by the kidney
   b. Converts angiotensin I to form angiotensin II
   c. Angiotensin II causes vasoconstriction and stimulates release of aldosterone
   d. Aldosterone causes sodium and water retention
   e. Increase in volume and vasoconstriction increase blood pressure
6. cortisol
7. 4
8. 140 mm Hg, 90 mm Hg
9. a. the desired "control" of blood pressure is reached, b. treatment choices are tolerated and safe, c. client is willing to commit to regimen over the long term
10. True, False, True, True, True
11.

Risk Factor	Action
Stress	identify coping mechanisms relaxation techniques
Obesity	reduce weight exercise
Nutrients	reduce sodium intake calcium, magnesium, potassium reduce blood pressure adequate water intake
Substance abuse	quit smoking moderate use of alcohol

12. Allow the client to sit quietly and rest for at least 5 minutes prior to taking a blood pressure reading.
13. a. weight reduction, body mass index less than 27
    b. moderate intake less than 2.3 – 6 grams of sodium
    c. decrease saturated fat, increase polyunsaturated fat intake
    d. moderate intensity physical activity most days of the week
    e. no more than 1 ounce/day
    f. not necessary
    g. include if feasible
    h. quit, no use of tobacco products with nicotine
    i. natural food sources not supplements
14. Weight reduction, sodium restriction.
15. compliance
16. a. have clients move slowly when changing positions from lying down to standing, b. instruct the client to breathe deeply and keep both eyes open.
17. a. diuretics, b. beta blockers
18. 1 year
19. Client will demonstrate knowledge of hypertension and its risk factors. Client will list all prescribed medications, including dosage, possible side effects, and indications for use. Client will demonstrate proper technique for measuring BP with home BP machine.
20. Older adults are more likely to experience adverse reactions to antihypertensives medications. Too rapid a reduction in blood pressure can affect cerebral perfusion and result in changes in mental status, dizziness, or weakness. Medications are started at low doses and changes made over longer amounts of time.
21. By blocking the increased aldosterone secretion which causes fluid retention. The reduced fluid

volume will result in a decreased cardiac volume and lower blood pressure.

22. Calcium channel blockers relax the blood vessels and decrease heart rate which will cause a decrease in blood pressure.
23. stimulation of the sympathetic nervous system which increases heart rate and blood pressure.
24. After identification of hypertensive blood pressure readings; to prevent complications from the hypertension.

CHAPTER 55

1. atherosclerosis
2. a. diabetes; b. smoking; c. elevated blood lipid levels
3. 2, 3, 5, 6, 7, 8
4. the client's own saphenous vein
5. infection
6. a. Pain, b. Pulselessness, c. Poilkilothermia, d. Pallor, e. Parasthesias, f. Paralysis
7. a. atherosclerosis; b. hypertension
8. 6 cm
9.

Stage	Physiologic changes
Pallor (white) color in hands	stimuli leads to spasm of digital arteries
	blood flow is decreased
Cyanotic (blue) color in hands	resulting tissue hypoxia venous congestion
Rubor (red) color in hands	spasm resolves, blood flow returns

10. a. venous stasis: immobilization or lack of use of calf muscle pump; b. hypercoagulability: dehydration or blood dyscrasias; c. injury to the venous wall: IV injections, fractures, dislocations
11. True, False, True, True, False, True, True, True, True, False
12. a. constant; b. reproducible; c. not positional
13. Pain at rest indicates limb-threatening disease with a very poor prognosis.
14. Doppler ultrasound
15. a. dorsalis pedis, b. posterior tibial, c. popliteal, d. femoral
16. 1, 2, 3, 4

17. a. documenting character of peripheral pulses, b. comparing one side with the other, c. marking the pulses with ink pen
18. compartment syndrome
19. True
20.

Goal	Specific Teaching Area
A. Reduce risk	stop smoking
	meticulous skin care
	moderate program of exercise
	reduce body weight
	low-fat, low-cholesterol diet
B. promote arterial flow	medications: Trental and Cilostazol, Aspirin, Clopidogrel
	reverse Trendelenburg
	fleece boots to keep feet warm/ protected
C. save the limb of clients with intermittent claudication	arterial bypass surgery to restore blood flow

21. reverse Trendelenburg
22. Preventing injury to the extremities, particularly the feet.
23. 1, 2, 3, 4
24. 2, 3
25. 24 hours
26. A traumatic amputation can usually be reimplanted as the client and the limb were healthy up to the time of the injury, depending on the severity of the injury; but, the client has not had time prior to surgery to grieve the loss of the limb and adjust perceived alterations in body image. Clients with PVD have been chronically ill for some time and have other medical conditions, which would affect the outcome.
27. a. ambulate as tolerated, including stairs and outdoors; b. no heavy lifting of objects more than 15 pounds for 6-12 weeks; c. no activities requiring pushing, pulling or straining; d. driving is restricted due to post operative weakness
28. True, False, True, True, False, False

29.

Medication	Indication	Route	Nursing Considerations
Coumadin	thrombus DVT	PO	given after acute DVT has been treated with injectable heparin
			long half-life: must be stopped 3 days before any invasive procedure
			prescribed based on INR [2.0-2.5]
			hospitalized client: administer in evening
			effects can be reversed with vitamin K
			teaching: avoid other anticoagulants, dark green, leafy vegetables
			safety: bleeding precautions
			teaching: electric vs. standard razor
			gentle tooth brushing
			monitor for bruising/bleeding
heparin	acute DVT	IV	continuous IV infusion
			dosage according to PTT level
			therapeutic: at or above 60 seconds
			therapeutic PTT: 1.5-2.5 times normal
			infused in the range of 700-1400 units/hr
			bleeding precautions
			short half-life of 4 hours
			reversed with protamine injection
			increased effects when given with other anticoagulants
low-molecular-weight heparin	prophylactic for DVT	sub Q	longer acting
			reliable dosing
			no monitoring of lab values
			much more expensive than heparin
			action similar to heparin
			given in the abdomen: bruising at site
			bleeding precautions
			client teaching for safety
			do not massage injection site
heparin	prophylactic for DVT	sub Q	*standard* heparin
			average dose is 5000 units sub Q
			given in abdomen twice daily
			bruising at injection site
			bleeding precautions
			client teaching for safety
			do *not* massage injection site

30. Nifedipine
31. True, True

CHAPTER 56
1. See Figure U13-2 in the textbook.
2. True, True, True
3. coronary artery disease, hypertension
4. 1, 2, 3
5. 1, 2, 3, 4, 5

6. 1, 2
7. 1, 2, 3, 4, 5
8. True, True, True, True, True, True, True, True, True
9. 1, 2
10. 20
11. 1, 2, 3
12. 3, 4
13. influenza
14. thrombophlebitis
15. 1, 2, 3, 4

16. dysrhythmias
17. a. angelica, b. astragalus, c. canola, d. ginkgo, e. motherwort, f. khella, g. cinchome

CHAPTER 57
1. 1, 2, 3, 4
2. rheumatic fever
3. 1, 2
4. 1
5. 2
6. 1, 2, 3
7. 1, 2, 3
8. Acute pericarditis
9. murmur
10. 2
11. 1, 2, 3, 4
12. True
13. 1, 2, 3
14. Aschoff's bodies
15. 3
16. 1, 2, 3
17. 1, 2, 3, 4
18. 1, 2, 3, 4
19. 1, 2, 3, 4
20. 1, 2, 3, 4
21. 1, 2, 3, 4
22. periocardiocentesis
23. 1
24. 2
25. atrial fibrillation
26. Anticoagulants
27. 1, 2, 3
28. Aspirin
29. infection

CHAPTER 58
1. True, True, True, True, True
2. a. smoking, b. hypertension, c. elevated serum cholesterol, d. physical inactivity, e. obesity, f. diabetes mellitus
3. 1, 2, 3
4. menopause
5. intima, arterial wall
6. Collateral circulation
7. True, True
8. 1, 2, 3, 4
9. True, True
10. 1, 2, 3, 4
11. 1, 2, 3, 4
12. 1, 2, 3
13. 1, 2, 3, 4
14. sympathetic nervous system

15. 1, 2, 3
16. True
17. 1, 2, 3, 4

CHAPTER 59
1. 1, 2
2. 1, 2
3. 1
4. sudden death
5. 1, 2, 3
6. 1
7. accelerated
8. Reentry
9. sinus exit block
10. 1, 2, 3, 4, 5
11. 1, 2, 3, 4
12. First degree AV block
13. 1, 2, 3
14. 1, 2, 3, 4
15. 1, 2, 3, 4
16. 1, 2, 3, 4
17. coarse, fine
18. 1, 2, 3, 4
19. 1, 2, 3
20. atrial flutter, saw tooth
21. 1, 2, 3
22. 1, 2, 3
23. 1, 2
24. 1
25. 1, 2, 3, 4
26. 1, 2
27. normal sinus rhythm
28. ventricular tachycardia
29. atrial fibrillation
30. sinus rhythm with premature atrial contractions
31. sinus rhythm with premature ventricular contraction
32. atrial flutter
33. sinus tachycardia
34. sinus bradycardia
35. 1, 2, 3, 4
36. 1

CHAPTER 60
1. atherosclerotic lesions
2. 1, 2
3. Stable angina
4. Unstable angina
5. Variant angina
6. Anterior wall of the left ventricle near the apex
7. 1, 2, 3
8. 1, 2, 3, 4

9. chest pain
10. 1, 2, 3, 4
11. 1, 2, 3, 4
12. 1, 2, 3, 4
13. True
14. dysrhythmias
15. 1, 2, 3
16. 1, 2, 3
17. 1
18. 1, 2, 3
19. 1, 2, 3
20. 1
21. 1, 2, 3, 4

CHAPTER 61
1. See Figure U14-1 in the textbook.
2. See Figure U14-2 in the textbook.
3. Pleuritic pain is described as sharp, stabbing pain on one side of the chest wall that increases with chest wall movement. Angina pectoris is usually described as aching, heavy, squeezing sensation in substernal area.
4. 6
5. 1:2
6. a. Crackles: sudden opening of small airways that contain fluid heard during inspiration; do not clear with cough
   b. Rhonchi: air passing though fluid-filled, narrow passages caused by excess mucus production (pneumonia, bronchitis); heard on expiration; may clear with cough
   c. Wheezes: continuous musical or hissing noise; passage of air through narrow airway; heard during inspiration or expiration; associated with asthma but may be foreign body blocking airway
   d. Pleural friction rub: pleural inflammation; creaking, grating noise heard on inspiration and expiration over area of inflammation
7. sinusitis
8. Visual Analog scale
9. stridor
10.

Factor	Area to be assessed
Occupation	exposure to respiratory irritants hobbies may involve chemicals, dust, airborne particles
Geographic location	recent travel to areas where respiratory diseases are prevalent air pollution
Environment	living conditions crowded household air conditioning climb stairs at home?
Habits	smoking smokeless tobacco drug use alcohol use
Exercise	onset of wheezing with exercise change in activities due to respiratory problems typical activities during the day
Nutrition	decreased nutrition due to fatigue

11. emphysema
12. chronic hypoxia
13. consolidation
14. See Figure 61-4 in the textbook.
15. True, False, True, True, False
16. See Figure 61-3 in the textbook.
17. pulse oximetry reading
18. 1, 2, 3, 4, 5
19. Assess the client, check placement of the probe, ask the client to take some deep breaths and re-assess reading.
20. lifelong, annually
21. smoke, use a bronchodilator for at least 6 hours
22. 5 minutes, anticoagulant
23. Pulmonary embolism
24. gonads
25. Inspiration causes the diaphragm to move downward, allowing better visualization of the lungs.
26. unaffected

CHAPTER 62
1. a. use of sedatives or anesthetic agents, b. deteriorating level of consciousness, c. any other condition potentially affecting ventilatory efficiency
2. cigarette smoking
3. 1, 2, 4
4. 1, 2, 4
5. disruption of normal air flow, swallowing
6. 2
7. beta-hemolytic streptococci
8. 4
9. 2
10. sore throat
11. acute tonsillitis
12. topical nasal decongestant sprays, intranasal cocaine
13. gastric acid
14. 1, 2, 3
15. Tonsillar diphtheria is not life threatening, although it can progress to a fatal form. It is characterized by a low-grade fever, fatigue, headache, and sore throat. Pharyngeal diphtheria is more serious: the client is gravely ill and pres-

ents with a weak pulse, restlessness, and confusion. Fever may or may not be present. Because of the membrane, the airway can be obstructed.
16. hoarseness
17. 2, 3, 4
18. True, False, False, False, False, False, True, True, False, True, False, True, True, True, True, True
19. 1, 2
20. 2
21. a. abnormal respiratory rate and pattern, b. use of accessory muscles to assist breathing, c. abnormal pulse and blood pressure, d. abnormal skin and mucous membrane color, e. abnormal ABG levels or oxygen saturation
22. 1
23. Mild bleeding
24. 3
25. a. presence of bowel sounds, b. passage of flatus, c. complaints of hunger
26. a. coughing upon swallowing, b. ineffective cough, c. decreased breath sounds, d. crackles, rhonchi, or wheezes
27. False, False
28. a. 4, b. 3, c. 5, d. 1, e. 2
29. ability to speak, ability to eat
30. semi-Fowler, high Fowler
31. lateral decubitus
32. a. topical anesthetic throat sprays, b. analgesic agents, c. hot saline throat irrigations, d. saline or alkaline mouthwashes or gargles, e. ice collars
33. a. humidification, b. frequent mouth care, c. increasing oral fluids
34. ice
35. True, True, False, False, True, True, True
36. anaphylaxis, epinephrine
37. epinephrine 1:1000

CHAPTER 63
1. 4
2. 1, 3, 4, 5
3. 3
4. 1, 2
5. 1, 2, 4, 6
6. 2
7. 4
8. ventilation-perfusion mismatch
9. 2, 3, 4, 5
10. 25 mm Hg, 30 mm Hg
11. pulmonary vasoconstriction
12. 1, 2, 3, 4, 5
13. False
14. 4
15. spiral CT scan
16. 1

17. An indication of approaching acute respiratory failure is an inability to auscultate wheezing during exhalation. The airways are too narrow to allow airflow.
18. 1
19. 3
20. 2
21. 2
22. 3
23. 1, 2, 3, 4, 6
24. Peak flow values are known to decrease 24 hours before symptoms of an asthma attack occur. Clients should be instructed to increase routine medications to prevent symptoms.
25. pursed-lip breathing
26. a. Severity of dyspnea is one measure to determine effectiveness of therapy.
   b. Spirometry is an effective tool to determine effectiveness of therapy and to anticipate exacerbations. Accuracy of assessment is important if it is to be used to plan therapy.
   c. Medication delivery is dependent on accuracy of use.
   d. Allergens may be a trigger for asthma attacks.
   e. Some clients may be taking medications which can cause bronchospasms, such as Inderal.
   f. History of triggers is needed to prepare a plan for prevention and control.
   g. Need to know abilities so that guidance can be provided to the client on disease management.
   h. Chronic disease management may be overwhelming. Family support helps decrease anxiety and the burden of self-care. Unsupportive family can increase stress.
   i. This assessment helps identify the presence of possible environmental triggers which can be modified.
27. 3
28. a. early ambulation, b. leg exercises, c. sequential compression stockings, d. low-dose heparin prophylaxis
29. When elevating the legs, flexure of the hips occurs which can contribute to stasis of the lower extremities and thus increase the risk for further clot formation.
30. 4
31. a. 2, i; b. 1, ii; c. 2, ii; d. 1, iv; e. 1, iv; f. 2, vi; g. 2, v
32. 1
33. 4
34. 4
35. 2, 3, 5, 6

36. 2
37. 1
38. 2
39. 1, 3, 4, 5
40. 3

CHAPTER 64

1. a. fever, b. myalgias, c. cough
2. a. advanced age, b. history of smoking, c. upper respiratory infection, d. tracheal intubation, e. prolonged immobility, f. immunosuppressive therapy, g. nonfunctional immune system, h. malnutrition, i. dehydration, j. chronic disease states
3. 1
4. a. 6, b. 1, c. 5, d. 3, e. 2, f. 4
5. Ghon tubercles
6. a. advanced age, b. HIV infection, c. immunosuppression, d. prolonged corticosteroid therapy, e. malabsorption syndromes, f. low body weight, g. substance abuse, h. presence of other diseases, i. genetic predisposition
7. granuloma in the choroids of the retina
8. 2, 7
9. a. small cell carcinoma, b. squamous cell carcinoma, c. adenocarcinoma, d. large cell carcinoma
10. cigarette smoking
11. a. small cell cancers, b. non-small cell lung cancers
12. a. 3, b. 4, c. 1, d. 2
13. interstitial
14. ventilation-perfusion mismatch
15. Transudates are substances that have passed through a membrane or tissue surface. They occur primarily in conditions of protein loss and low protein content or increased hydrostatic pressure. Exudates are substances that have escaped from blood vessels. They contain an accumulation of cells, have a high specific gravity and a high lactate dehydrogenase level, and occur when there is an increase in capillary permeability.
16. empyema
17. a. gastrointestinal perforation, b. surgery of the upper gastrointestinal system, liver, or biliary tract, c. abdominal trauma, d. other intra-abdominal surgery
18. True, False, False, False, True, True, True, True, True, True, True, False, True
19. areas of consolidation
20. a. assess rate and character of respirations, b. auscultate the breath sounds, c. assess skin and nail beds to determine the severity of hypoxia
21. Induration
22. AFB smear, culture
23. if the pulse rate becomes rapid and the blood pressure drops
24. Intermittent bubbling is normal and indicates that the system is accomplishing one of its functions. Continuous bubbling during inspiration and expiration indicates that air is leaking into the drainage system or pleural cavity.
25. Rapid bubbling in the absence of an air leak indicates considerable loss of air from an incision or tear in the pulmonary pleura.
26. False
27. side-lying
28. a. washing hands frequently, b. using gloves appropriately, c. encouraging fluid intake, d. turning clients every 2 hours, e. controlling the client's pain so he or she may breathe deeply and cough effectively
29. Coughing and deep breathing promote lung expansion and the expulsion of air and fluid from the pleural space by increasing intrapulmonary and intrapleural pressures.
30. a. promote adequate oxygenation, b. maintain a patent airway, c. achieve the highest possible functional level
31. a. adequate hydration, b. bronchodilators and mucolytic aerosols, c. effective coughing techniques
32. False, True, False, False, True, True, True
33. 24 hours
34. two
35. amphotericin B
36. Corticosteroids

CHAPTER 65

1. oxygen, carbon dioxide
2.

| • Severe arterial hypoxemia
• Minimally responsive to oxygen
• Caused by diffuse problems such as pulmonary edema, near drowning, ARDS, localized problems | • Client unable to support adequate gas exchange
• Results from CNS depression, inadequate neuromuscular ability to sustain breathing, respiratory system overload |

3. a. decreased minute ventilation with normal dead space ventilation, b. normal or increased minute ventilation with increased dead space ventilation
4. 3
5. carbon dioxide
6. pulsus paradoxus
7. decreased cardiac output
8. 4
9. 2, 3, 4

10. 1, 2, 3, 4
11. inflammatory response, permeability of the alveolar membrane, interstitial, alveolar, noncardiogenic, lung compliance, oxygen transport
12. alveolar, surfactant
13. fibrin
14. increased respiratory rate, profound dyspnea
15. internal bleeding, punctured organs
16. a. atelectasis, b. hemopneumothorax, c flail chest, d. aspiration, e. pulmonary contusion
17. 3
18. air, pleural
19. spontaneous, traumatic
20. 4
21. 2
22. 1
23. 3
24. 1
25. True, True, True, False, True, False, True
26. 3, 4
27. 20
28. 1
29. a. airway patency, b. adequacy of breathing, c. circulatory sufficiency
30. absent, decreased
31. 2
32. 3
33. Raising edematous legs increases venous return and will stress the overtaxed left ventricle. Keeping the legs dependent decreases preload.
34. a. 4, b. 3, c. 1, d. 2
35. a. 4, b. 3, c. 2, d. 1
36. CPAP is applied to a client with spontaneous respirations whereas PEEP is applied during mechanical ventilation. Both are used to apply positive pressure to keep the alveoli open and reduce shunting.
37.

Rapid	Gradual
- used when ventilation has been brief - start in the morning - reduce ventilator rate to half of original rate - obtain ABGs in 30 minutes - if ABGs at or near normal, place client on T-piece at same FiO_2 - obtain ABGs in 30 minutes - if ABGs at or near normal and respiratory rate below 25-30, extubate the client - apply face tent to deliver oxygen and humidity	- used after prolonged ventilation or if neuromuscular disorder is present - determine if spontaneous breathing is present - if spontaneous breathing present, slowly reduce the amount of ventilatory support until the client can accept full responsibility for own ventilatory requirements - may use T-piece for longer periods or decrease the rate of IMV - process may take weeks or months

38. Placing the client in a prone position creates a change in the dependent portions of the lung resulting in increased perfusion to the less damaged portions of the lungs and decreases pulmonary shunting.
39. clear communication, frequent updates
40. a. decreased, b. decreased, c. decreased, d. decreased
41. False, True, True, False
42. 4
43. vecuronium (Norcuron), pancuronium (Pavulon)
44. 1, 3
45. 1
46. 4
47. False, False
48. 2
49. 3
50. 4

CHAPTER 66
1. See Figure U15-2 in the textbook.
2. See Figure U15-4 in the textbook.
3. 2, 4, 5, 7
4. False, False, True, False, True
5.

Manifestation	Cause
Glare/halo	Uncorrected refractive error
	Scratches on glasses
	Dilated pupils
	Corneal edema
	Cataract
Flashing/flickering lights	Retinal traction
	Migraine
Floating spots	Normal vitreous body strands
	Pathologic blood or pigment
Diplopia	Refractive correction
	Muscle imbalance
	Neurological disorders

6.

Complaint	Possible Cause
Hearing loss	Conductive
	Sensorineural
	CNS disorder
	Excess cerumen
Pain	Excessive noise
	Trauma
	Related problems with nose, sinuses
	Oral cavity, pharynx, or TMJ

Ear drainage	Bleeding
	Infection
Tinnitus	Excessive noise
	High doses of aspirin
Loss of balance	Disorder of inner ear
	Excess fluid in inner ear
	Medications

7. 85-90 decibels (dB)
8. Conductive hearing loss
9. sensorineural hearing loss
10. 80%
11. asymptomatic
12. HTN: can affect blood flow to eyes; retinopathy
   MS: diplopia, changes in vision due to nerve damage
   MG: weakness of the eye muscles
   Thyroid: exophthalmos
   RA: Sjögren's syndrome (dry eyes)
   DM: diabetic retinopathy
13. normal (The position properly protects the sclera of the eye.)
14. corneal reflex
15. normal
16. clear, transparent
17. dilate, constrict
18. alignment
19. Applantation tonometry
20. 8, 21
21. a. hearing acuity, b. balance, c. equilibrium
22. 2
23.

Test	Purpose
Weber test	to assess conduction of sound through bone
Rinne test	compares air conduction to bone conduction
Romberg test	assess the inner ear for balance

24. The cornea of the eye must be anesthetized with topical anesthetic drops.
25. Wear dark glasses for several hours until the dilating medication wears off and the pupils can constrict again in the presence of light.
26. Meniere's disease
27. Presence of clear drainage may be due to infection, fistulas, or leakage of CSF. The physician should be notified and a specimen collected for analysis.
28. 1, 2, 3, 4, 5
29. diphenhydramine (Benadryl)
30. Over-the-counter preparations may contain antihistamines and decongestants which can interact with blood pressure and heart medications.

CHAPTER 67

1. 4
2.

Type	Cause	Manifestations
Primary Open Angle	aqueous humor flow is obstructed by trabecular meshwork	no early signs later: increased intraocular pressure (IOP) bilateral
Angle Closure	anatomically narrow anterior chamber angle	unilateral develops suddenly severe pain, blurred vision/vision loss
	sudden blockage of anterior angle by base of iris	
Normal Tension	normal-high IOP	optic nerve is damaged
		IOP not high
		resembles primary open-angle
Secondary	edema, eye injury, inflammation, tumor, cataracts, diabetes blocks outflow of aqueous humor	unilateral/bilateral

3. a. hypertension, b. diabetes, c. cardiovascular disease, d. obesity
4. 1, 2, 4, 5, 6, 7, 8, 9
5. False
6. central
7.

Type	Etiology	Manifestations
Dry	atrophy and degeneration of retina	thinning of macula deposits into retina
Wet	bleeding within and beneath the retina	"metamorphopsia" distorted lines in vision
		opaque deposits
		central vision more distorted
		scar tissue formation
		dark, blurry area in center of vision or "white out"
		color perception changes

8. 1, 2, 4

9.

Type	Etiology	Manifestation
Myopia	light rays focus in front of the retina	difficulty seeing things far away (nearsighted)
Hyperopia	eye is deficient in focusing light rays	difficulty seeing things near (farsighted)
	image that falls on the retina is blurred	
Astigmatism	rays of light are not equally bent in all directions	poor vision for both distant and near objects

10. 12, 22
11. awakening
12. True, False, True, True, True
13. retinal detachment
14. a. Graves' disease: exophthalmos
    b. Rheumatoid arthritis/connective tissue disorder: Sjögren's Syndrome
    c. SLE (Lupus): retinopathy of SLE-cotton wool spots, optic neuropathy, discoid lesions of eyelids
    d. Myasthenia gravis: ptosis of eyelids, diplopia, nystagmus, ocular myopathy, cranial nerve palsy
    e. Multiple sclerosis: optic neuritis
    f. Hypertension: vasoconstriction, leakage, arteriosclerosis of ocular vessels, hypertensive retinopathy, retinal vein occlusion
    g. AIDS: cytomegalovirus retinitis, bacterial corneal ulcers, fungal corneal ulcers, protozoan/viral infections, HIV retinopathy, Kaposi's sarcoma, non-Hodgkins' lymphoma
    h. Lyme disease: optic neuropathy, keratitis, choroiditis, exudative retinal detachment
15. 1, 3, 4, 5
16. blood pressure
17. 3
18. Prolonged vomiting can result in increased IOP and wound dehiscence.
19. a. intermittent massage by a physician: to move the embolus from the central artery into a branch, b. administer 95% oxygen for 10 minutes: maintain oxygen supply to ocular tissues to prevent damage
20. 1, 2, 3, 5
21. True, False, True, True, True, True

22.

Medication	Dosage	Teaching Points for Client
Pilocarpine "Pilocar" (cholinergic)	3-4 times/ day	Causes pupillary constriction (opens canal of Schlemm to increase of aqueous humor)
		May cause blurred vision after instillation of drops
		Space out administration during day
		May cause "brow ache"
Timolol "Timoptic" (beta blocker)	every 12 hours	Decrease production of aqueous humor Space out administration
		Contraindicated with asthma/COPD
		Assess for bradycardia BEFORE administration
Carbonic anhydrase inhibitor "Diamox" (diuretic)	varies	inhibits production of aqueous humor
		Tablets or sustained-release capsules
		Side effects: anorexia, tinnitus

23. Miotics
24. Topical beta-blockers
25. Ismotic is a synthetic glycerin diuretic and will not raise the serum blood glucose level like Osmoglyn, which is glycerin.
26. 1, 2, 4
27. False, True, True
28. 4

CHAPTER 68

1. Hearing impairment
2.

Type	Cause	Results
Conductive	anything that blocks external ear thickening, scarring, retraction, or perforation of tympanic membrane	interference with sound transmission through external and middle ear
	any pathophysiologic change in middle ear that affects the ossicles	
Sensorineural	congenital/ hereditary noise injury aging Meniere's disease ototoxicity	impairment of the function of the inner ear, eighth cranial nerve or brain
Mixed hearing loss	combined	both components present (sensorineural and conductive)

3. cerumen
4. Otitis media
5. 1, 2, 5, 6, 7
6. Presbycusis
7. 1
8. 1, 2, 4, 5
9. 1, 2, 3, 4, 5, 6
10. True, False, True, False, True, True

11.

Disorder	Cause	Manifestations
Benign paroxysmal positional vertigo	Follows head injury or viral infection of inner ear	Slow responses to head movement Brief attacks of vertigo
	Calcium crystals deposited on otoliths	Rapid head tilt to affected ear Self-limited, resolves over weeks to months
Labyrinthitis	Infection or inflammation of cochlear or vestibular portion of inner ear Syndrome occurs in spring or early summer Preceded by URI	Vertigo Nausea Vomiting No hearing changes Resolves in 1-2 weeks
Meniere's disease	Excess endolymph in vestibular and semicircular canals	Hearing changes episodic; waxes and wanes Paroxysmal whirling vertigo Fluctuating hearing loss Tinnitus Aural fullness

12. a. vestibular system (labyrinth or inner ear), b. visual system, c. proprioceptive system (joints and muscles), d. cerebellar system
13. a. Rinne's test: hearing loss results in greater conduction by bone
    b. Weber test: sound will lateralize to the more affected ear
14. Gently pulling on the pinna causes pain when the infection is in the outer ear, because the area is inflamed. Touching the ear does not cause pain when the infection is in the middle ear.
15. 6
16. transient ischemic attack

17.

Level	Focus	Plans	Interventions
Primary	reduce risks	trauma noise	wear headgear/helmets wear earplugs avoid prolonged exposure
		ototoxic drugs	monitor lab levels discontinue medications
		infectious diseases	vaccination; infection control
Secondary	early detection and referral		screen at 65 yrs and older screening monitor for vertigo and tinnitus
Tertiary	maintenance of function		hearing rehabilitation hearing aids implement coping and communication skills

18. OUTCOME: Client will develop effective methods to communicate needs and will be included in conversation
    INTERVENTIONS: writing requests, visual aids (pictures, diagrams), use of an expert interpreter
19. 3
20. 1, 2, 4, 6
21. a. meticulous cleaning of ear canal, b. warming solution to body temperature
22. complete
23. 2, 3, 4
24. corticosteroids
25. boric acid and alcohol
26. 1, 3, 4

CHAPTER 69
1. See Figure U16-1 in the textbook.
2. See Figure U16-10 in the textbook.
3. stroke
4. 5
5.

Area	Clinical significance
Growth and development	Was neurologic dysfunction present at early age?
	Prenatal exposure to disease
	Full term vs. pre-term
	Did client accomplish major developmental tasks?
Family health history	Presence of genetic risk factors
	Epilepsy
	Huntington's disease
	ALS
	Muscular dystrophy
	HTN/stroke
	Psychiatric disorders
Psychosocial history	Educational background
	Level of performance
	Changes in sleep patterns
	Perceived stressors
	Exposure to toxic substances at work

6. Level of consciousness
7. 1, 2, 3, 4
8. 7s, 3s
9. a. inspection, b. palpation, c. percussion, d. auscultation
10. Raccoon eyes
11. nuchal rigidity

12.

Cranial Nerve	Function	Testing Method
I	smell	ask client to identify aromatic odor (coffee, vanilla)
II	visual acuity	Snellen chart; visual fields
III, IV, VI	eyes; eye movement	test direct/consensual response
		test accommodation
		pupillary light reflex
		check 6 cardinal directions of gaze
V	muscles of mastication	clamp jaws shut, open mouth against resistance
		open mouth widely
		test corneal reflex
VII	facial expression	ask client to frown, smile
		raise eyebrows, tightly close eyes
		show teeth, puff out cheeks
VIII	hearing; bone and air conduction; equilibrium	listen to whispered voice
		tuning forks
		Romberg's test
IX, X	pharynx	open mouth wide and say "Ah"
		test gag reflex
		ask client to cough and speak
XI	sternocleido-mastoid; trapezius muscles	elevate shoulders with/without resistance
		turn head to one side, then other
		resist attempt to pull chin back to midline
		push head forward against resistance
XII	tongue	open mouth wide, stick out tongue; check to see if midline

13. Ask the client to stand quietly with feet together; assess balance and sense of body position.

14.

Type	Method of testing
Stereognosis	place 3 small familiar objects into client's hands; ask client to identify with eyes closed
Graphesthesia	trace different, separate letters and numbers on client's palm; ask client to identify with eyes closed
Extinction phenomenon	simultaneously prick client's skin at same point on two sides of the body at same time; ask client whether they felt one or two pricks
Two-point simulation	simultaneously prick the skin with two pins at varying distances; identify the smallest distance which the client can perceive 2 pricks

15. Babinski
16. False, True, True, False, True
17. blood flow
18. brain death
19. Clients who are confused, combative, or ventilator-dependent may require assistance of the nurse during the procedure.
20. lateral
21. the results are known
22. metal
23. 150
24. a. CSF leakage, b. infection
25. a. assessing area for LP
    b. keep the spinous processes horizontal
    c. keep spine horizontal
    d. separate and increase space between vertebrae
    e. to keep the client's upper shoulder from falling forward, prevent rotation of spine
26. To restore CSF volume and help prevent spinal headache.
27. The agents are iodine-based and would be contraindicated if the client were allergic.
28. Many over-the-counter medications contain ingredients that affect the CNS and can alter functioning. Many herbal remedies, which are advertised as "natural," have active chemical components that alter CNS function too.

CHAPTER 70
1. Structural lesions
2. Metabolic disorders
3. True
4. metabolic
5. contractures
6. a. aphasia, b. apraxia, c. agnosia

7.

Manifestation	Example
Disorder of attention	patient may fear they are "going crazy"
	may appear preoccupied
Fluctuations in cognition	totally irrational one moment; then lucid
	more disoriented at night
	unfamiliar surroundings
	unfamiliar noises
	unfamiliar people
	lack of window in room: disoriented
Loss of memory for recent events	hallmark of metabolic disorders
	quickly lose orientation to time
Perceptual errors	mistaking the nurse for daughter
	hallucinations, illusions, delusions

8. The client cannot actively participate in care/decisions; therefore the family serves as the client in these circumstances.
9. impaction
10. 1, 2, 3, 4, 5
11. doll's eye
12. 1, 2, 3, 4, 5, 6, 7, 8
13. mortality or significant morbidity
14. Glasgow Coma
15. 3
16. Reposition the patient often and tape the eyes closed if needed
17. False, True, True, True, False
18. high Fowler's
19. Turn off tube feedings several hours before the meal to stimulate appetite.
20. Resume the tube feeding. Volumes under 100 ml do not require delaying tube feeding.
21. 1, 2, 3, 4, 6
22.

Task	Responsibility	Can RN Delegate?
Verification of MD order	RN	no
Verification of placement of feeding tube	RN	no
Reconstitution of feeding	RN/licensed	yes*
Preparation of feeding	RN/licensed	yes*
Priming the feeding pump	RN/licensed	yes*
Irrigation of feeding tube	RN	no
Tube site care	RN/licensed	yes*

Monitoring fluid/
nutritional balance   RN   no

*RN is responsible for the care of the patient. If tasks are delegated, the RN retains the responsibility for ensuring proper instructions were given and verifying competence in performing.

23. diazepam
24. Empty the catheter bag to assist with clear assessment of diuretic effect per urine volume obtained.
25. seizure threshold

CHAPTER 71

1. seizure
2. Epilepsy
3. During continued seizure activity, the brain requires increased oxygen and glucose to meet the energy demands. If the seizures continue, as in status epilepticus, the supplies are exhausted and result in anaerobic metabolism.
4.

Area of Brain	Manifestations
Parietal region:	sensory phenomena; numbness or tingling
Occipital region:	bright, flashing lights in field of vision opposite the side of the focus
Posterior temporal area:	difficulty speaking or aphasia
Anterior temporal lobe:	begin with psychic manifestations; "aura"

5. a. 3, b. 4, c. 1, d. 5, e. 2
6. True, False, True, True, False, True
7.

Area of Brain	Manifestations
Frontal lobe	Inappropriate behavior
	Speech disturbance
	Bowel/bladder incontinence
	Gait disturbances
Temporal lobe	Receptive aphasia
	Visual field changes
	Tinnitus
	Headache
Parietal lobe	Sensory deficits
	Right/left disorientation
	Psychomotor seizures
Occipital lobe	Headache
	Homonymous hemianopsia
Cerebellar	Unsteady gait
	Falling/incoordination
	Tremors
	Nystagmus

Brain stem	Vertigo/dizziness
	Vomiting
	Sudden death from cardiac/respiratory failure
Pituitary/hypothalamus	Hormonal dysfunction
	Sleep disturbance
	Temperature fluctuations
	Cushing's syndrome
Ventricle	Obstruction of CSF circulation
	Hydrocephalus
	Rapid rise in ICP
	Postural headache

8. 1
9.

Type	Etiology	Manifestation
Tension	muscle contraction fatigue and stress	tight, band-like posterior neck
Cluster	form of migraine triggered by alcohol	cyclical pattern boring, intense pain constricted pupils
Migraine	vascular headache	vasospasm unilateral throbbing/pulsatile

10. EEG
11. Details about the seizure, its starting point, and progression can aid in diagnosing cause.
12. The nurse should look at the stereotypical movements and paroxysmal nature of seizures. Clients exhibiting pseudoseizures make different movements with each seizure.
13. 1, 2, 4
14. aneurysm
15. blood
16. a. Nuchal rigidity: stiffness of the neck, pain upon movement
    b. Brudzinski's sign: forward neck flexion of a supine client results in flexion of both thighs at the hips and flexion of ankles
    c. Kernig's sign: with client recumbent, thigh flexed at right angle to abdomen, knee flexed 90 degrees; extending the leg causes pain, spasm of hamstring, and resistance to further extension.
17. a. prevent injury during seizures
    b. eliminate factors that precipitate seizures
    c. diagnose and treat cause of seizures
    d. control seizures to allow desired lifestyle
18. 1, 2, 3, 5
19. Complete history and physical assessment with documentation of LOC orientation, neurologic checks, cranial nerve function and limb strength and movement.

20. Immediate notification of observation to physician to evaluate for presence of CSF fluid.
21. b
22. Monitor dosage and side effects carefully due to decreased elimination and increased half-life resulting in higher plasma levels of medications.
23. immediately
24. Alcohol lowers the seizure threshold and is detoxified by the liver. Most anticonvulsant drugs are also metabolized by the liver; this would place an increased strain on the metabolizing functions of the liver.
25. diazepam
26. vasopressin
27. The osmotic diuretic, mannitol, disrupts the barrier allowing greater concentration of the chemotherapy agents.
28. Corticosteroids
29. gastrointestinal motility

CHAPTER 72
1. a. Ischemic: caused by a thrombotic or embolic blockage of blood to the brain
   b. Hemorrhagic: bleeding into the brain tissue; may be due to aneurysm
2. ischemic
3. oxygen
4. Atherosclerosis causes a narrowing of the blood vessel with deposits; turbulent blood flow causes platelets to adhere to the plaque.
5. diabetes
6. hypertension
7. a. hyperlipidemia, b. cigarette smoking, c. heavy alcohol consumption, d. cocaine use, e. obesity
8. 50
9. middle cerebral artery
10. The speech center for most right-handed clients is in the left cerebral hemisphere. Therefore a stroke to the left side of the brain results in loss of speech control and right-sided hemiplegia.
11. With dysarthria, the client understands language but has difficult pronouncing words and may slur them. Aphasia may involve deficits in speaking, reading, and writing.
12. TIAs are brief episodes of neurologic dysfunction, lasts less than 24 hours and recovery is complete. TIAs serve as a warning sign of an impending stroke, the effect of which may be permanent.
13.

Type	Characteristics
Wernicke's	receptive aphasia
	clients can speak but do not understand spoken words
Broca's	expressive aphasic
	clients can understand spoken words but cannot speak clearly
Global	affects both speech comprehension and speech production

14.

Type of Stroke	Warning Manifestations
Ischemic	Transient hemiparesis
	Loss of speech
	Hemisensory loss
Thrombotic	Occurs suddenly, without warning
Hemorrhagic	Occurs rapidly
	Severe occipital headache
	Vertigo/syncope
	Paresthesias
	Transient paralysis
	Epistaxis
	Retinal hemorrhage

15. 1, 2, 4
16. a. level of consciousness, b. pupillary response to light, c. visual fields, d. movement of extremities, e. speech, f. sensation, g. reflexes, h. vital signs
17. a. acoustic aphasia: Clients can hear the sounds of speech but the parts of the brain that give meaning to these sounds is damaged. They do not understand.
    b. visual aphasia: Clients cannot read words but can see them. They do not understand the symbols.
18. 1, 4
19. 2
20. maintaining a patent airway
21. Elevated temperatures require increased metabolic needs, which in turn will cause cerebral edema and increased risk of ischemia.
22. a. prevents joint immobility, contractures and muscle atrophy, b. stimulates circulation, c. helps to reestablish neuromuscular pathways
23. Assist client to lie prone for 15-30 minutes several times a day and place a pillow under the pelvis to hyperextend the hip joints.
24. To rule out hemorrhagic stroke as the cause of acute neurologic changes. Hemorrhage would contraindicate using thrombolytics.
25. 1, 3, 4, 7
26. 24
27. 1.5-2.5

CHAPTER 73

1.

Cause	Example
Biomechanical and destructive	Compression of disks
	Herniation of disks
	Torsion injuries
Destructive origins	Infections, tumors
	Rheumatoid disorders
Degenerative	Osteoporosis
	Spinal stenosis

2. Changes in cartilage and elasticity of the disk cause the disk to prolapse.
3. True, True, False
4. a. Lordosis: excessive backward concavity of lumbar spine; results in swayback and ky-phosis
   b. Spondylothesis: forward slipping of verte-bra; occurs at L4-L5; loss of spinal align-ment
   c. Spondylosis: defect of lamina; vertebral arch slips forward; lumbar area most common
   d. Spinal stenosis: narrowing of spinal canal; produces pressure on entire spinal cord, weakness or paralysis
5. contralateral paralysis
6. Neurofibromas, meningiomas
7. fifth
8. seventh, unilateral paralysis
9.

Type	Manifestation
Motor nerves	muscle weakness
	cramps
	spasms
	loss of balance/coordination
Sensory nerves	tingling
	numbness
	pain: burning, freezing, or electric-like sensations
Autonomic nerves	orthostatic hypotension
	bradycardia
	reduced ability to perspire
	constipation
	bladder dysfunction
	sexual dysfunction

10. carpal tunnel
11. buttocks, back of the thigh to leg/ankle
12. to identify workplace causes for back strain and correct them
13. bone graft donor
14. swelling
15. See Figure 73-12 in the textbook.
16. Surgeons frequently inject local anesthetic into surgical site. Assessment of sensation can be done after the effects have worn off.
17. Document client's occupation and identification of dominant hand. This information is necessary to plan for adjustments in lifestyle and work conditions.
18. Place the client in a lateral position with knees flexed.
19. 1, 2, 4
20. strengthening of back and abdominal muscles through daily exercises
21. logrolling
22. Pillows should not be placed under the popliteal space as this increases risk of DVT
23. eight
24. 1, 2, 3, 5
25. 2
26. opioids
27. The chemical in the hot pepper extract added to the cream is useful in relieving neuropathic pain by blocking pain impulses.
28. The discomfort is an indicator of the need to make adjustments in lifestyle to preserve func-tion. Medicating will mask the need for changes.
29. Tegretol

CHAPTER 74

1.

Type	Characteristics
Alzheimer's disease	progressive decline in 2 or more areas of cognition
	most common form of dementia in people 65+ years of age
	cause is unknown
	presence of neurologic plaques/tangles widely distributed throughout brain
Multi-infarct disease	second most common cause of irreversible dementia
	blood clots block small vessels in brain
	men over 50 years old
	progressive decline in cognition
Lewy body dementia	similar to Alzheimer's
	progresses more rapidly
	abnormal brain cells "Lewy bodies"
Pick's disease	form of dementia, different from Alzheimer's
	"Pick's bodies" within neuron cells
	sharply confined to front parts of brain

2.

Stage	Manifestations
Preclinical	disease begins near hippocampus (essential for short and long-term memory); affected regions begin to shrink
	memory loss begins
	period can last 10-20 years
Mild Alzheimer's	cerebral cortex begins to shrink
	memory disturbances noticed by family or co-workers before client does
	may have poor judgment or problem-solving skills
	may become careless in work habits
	confused where they are/get lost easily
	client may become irritable, agitated
Moderate Alzheimer's	language disturbances: circumlocution
	paraphrasias
	palilaia
	echolalia
	motor disturbances: apraxia
	forgetfulness: safety concerns
	depression and irritability worsens
	delusions/psychosis may appear
	wandering at night is common
	occasional incontinence
Severe Alzheimer's	clients cannot recognize family/friends
	do not communicate in any way
	voluntary movement is minimal
	limbs are rigid
	urinary/fecal incontinence frequent
	high risk for aspiration

3. 50
4. 2
5. 1, 3, 4, 5, 7
6. descending
7. ACh receptors
8. cognition
9. respiratory failure and death from pneumonia
10. Myasthenic crisis: precipitated by infection or sudden withdrawal of anticholinesterase drugs; difficulty swallowing or breathing
    Cholinergic crisis: result of overmedication; abdominal cramps, diarrhea, excessive pulmonary secretions
11. 1, 2, 3, 4, 5
12. a. bradykinesia; b. (cogwheel) rigidity; c. tremor at rest
13. muscle weakness and fatigue that worsens with exercise and improves with rest
14. ptosis
15. improvement

16. a. identification of potential safety hazards (loose rugs, hot tap water, inadequate lighting, unlocked doors); b. teach family members how to safeguard home, c. place identification badge on client in case they become lost, d. place dangerous items out of reach, e. supervise potentially dangerous activities
17. a. stretch spastic muscles at least twice a day through full range of motion, b. employ strengthening exercises that are active movement exercises, c. administer medications to relieve muscle spasms, d. schedule rest periods after activity, e. use ambulation aids such as cane or walker
18. 1
19. 1, 2, 3, 5
20. 1, 2, 3
21. 1, 3, 4, 5
22. They are used to help retain ACh in the neurojunctions in clients with Alzheimer's disease. Clients will experience improvements in thinking abilities and are less likely to demonstrate manifestations of wandering, agitation, or socially inappropriate behavior.
23. Levodopa is a precursor to dopamine, a necessary neurotransmitter, which is deficient in Parkinson's disease.
24. Haloperidol
25. IV corticosteroids (methylprednisolone)

CHAPTER 75

1. 20
2. a. space occupying tumors, b. cerebral infarction, c. obstruction of the outflow of CSF, d. ingested or accumulated toxins, e. impaired blood flow to or from the brain, f. systemic hypertension
3. a. movement of CSF out of the cranium, b. reduction of blood flow to the brain, c. displacement of brain tissue (herniation)
4. a. any alteration in level of consciousness, b. decrease in the Glasgow Coma Scale
5. motor vehicle accidents
6.

Injury	Characteristics
Concussion	no break in the skull
	no visible damage on CT or MRI
Open head injury	penetrates the skull
Closed head injury	blunt trauma
Contusions	more extensive damage
	brain is damaged
Subdural hematoma	collection of blood in the subdural space
	brain or blood vessel laceration

7. males, 16, 30
8. Flexion injuries
9. 1, 2, 3, 4
10. quadriplegia
11. paraplegia
12. 1, 2, 3, 4, 5, 6, 7
13. 3
14. 1, 2, 3, 4, 5, 6
15. basilar skull fracture of the frontal and temporal bones
16. It helps to determine the extent of the injury, client's activity, and LOC before and after the injury.
17. 2
18. dermatomes
19. 1, 2, 3, 4
20. a. intubation to maintain PaO2 between 90-100 mm Hg, b. osmotic diuretics: Mannitol, c. elevation of the head: to promote venous drainage
21. depressed, compound skull
22. 1, 2, 4
23. a. elevate the head of the bed to a sitting position immediately, b. check blood pressure, c. check for possible sources of irritation, d. remove stimulus if possible, e. administer antihypertensives if needed
24. logrolling
25. 2, 3, 4
26. a. proper fitting of wheelchair to meet client's ability
   b. ROM exercises, oral antispasmodic medications
   c. intermittent catheterization, suprapubic catheters
   d. use of suppositories or digital stimulation every day
   e. frequent turning, pressure relieving devices; thorough skin assessment
   f. incentive spirometry, diaphragmatic breathing
   g. non-opioid analgesics, TENS units
   h. peer group counseling sessions, vocational rehabilitation
27. Seizures significantly increase metabolic requirements and cerebral blood flow and volume, increasing ICP.
28. muscle relaxants
29. True, False, True, True
30.

Medication	Indication for Use
Vasoactive agents	support blood pressure
Steroids	reduce inflammation/prevent damage
Thyrotropin releasing hormone	decrease post-traumatic ischemia
H$_2$ receptor blocking agents	reduce risk of gastric/intestinal bleeding

31. Urecholine, Ditropan
32. Neurontin (Gabapentin)
33. etidronate disodium (Didronel)

CHAPTER 76
1. See Figure U17-1 in the textbook.
2. a. very young, b. very old
3. 3
4. a. inhalants, b. contact agents, c. ingested agents, d. injectable agents
5. because there is a consequent reduction in absorption of vitamin B$_{12}$
6. increased hemoglobin levels
7. 1, 2, 3
8. 1
9. Tachycardia is a compensatory mechanism to increase cardiac output due to decreased oxygen carrying capacity associated with anemia.
10. three
11. True, False, True, False, True, True
12. 1
13. a. anemia, b. thrombocytopenia, c. bleeding disorders, d. congenital blood disorders, e. jaundice, f. frequent infections, g. delayed healing, h. cancer, i. autoimmune disease.
14. a. superficial lymph nodes, b. liver, c. spleen
15. a. complete blood count, b. differential white blood count, c. coagulation studies, d. a peripheral blood smear for red blood cell morphology
16. A Coombs' test is used to detect certain antigen-antibody reactions between serum antibodies and RBC antigens, to differentiate between various forms of hemolytic anemia, to determine unusual blood types, and to identify hemolytic disease in newborns.
17. a. platelet count, b. PT, c. PTT, d. bleeding time
18. a. low, b. normal, c. normal, d. low, e. high, f. low, g. high, h. normal, i. high, j. normal, k. high, l. normal, m. normal
19. True, True
20. Donating blood or blood products can affect laboratory values for days or weeks.
21. 1
22. observe for bleeding
23. salicylates
24. a. sulfonamides, b. penicillins
25. NSAIDs
26. a. 7, b. 6, c. 2, d. 5, e. 1, f. 3, g. 4
27. False, True

CHAPTER 77

1. 4
2. 2
3. a. severity of blood loss, b. speed of blood loss, c. chronicity of the anemia, d. other co-morbid conditions
4. a. decreased synthesis of normal hemoglobin, b. defective DNA synthesis, c. reduced availability of erythrocyte precursors
5. blood loss, most commonly from the GI tract
6. globin
7. RBCs, Vitamin B$_{12}$, folic acid
8. 3
9. aplastic
10. Aspergillus
11. pluripotent stem cells
12. joint pain
13. phlebotomy
14. neutrophils
15. bone pain
16. a. intact blood vessels, b. an adequate number of functioning platelets, c. sufficient amounts of 12 clotting factors, d. a well-controlled fibrinolytic system
17. idiopathic thrombocytopenic purpura
18. vitamin K
19. a. infection, b. introduction of tissue coagulation factors into the circulation, c. damage to vascular endothelium, d. stagnant blood flow
20. a. purpura, petechiae, and ecchymoses on the skin, mucous membranes, heart lining and lungs, b. prolonged bleeding from venipuncture, c. severe, uncontrolled hemorrhage, d. excessive bleeding from gums and the nose, e. intracerebral and GI bleeding, f. renal hematuria, g. tachycardia and hypotension, h. dyspnea, hemoptysis, and respiratory congestion
21. males
22. False, True, False, True, True, False, True, True, True, True, True, False, True, True, True, True, True, True, True, True, False, False, True
23. 2
24. 2
25. 4
26. 1–6 decreased, 7 increased
27. 3
28. splenic rupture secondary to trauma, hypersplenism
29. False, True
30. a. iron therapy, b. nutritional therapy, c. surgery, d. splenectomy, e. removal of toxic agents, f. stem cell or bone marrow transplantation, g. corticosteroid therapy, h. immunosuppressive therapy
31. blood transfusion

32. Stop the transfusion and keep the IV open with normal saline; treat any respiratory or circulatory manifestations immediately; notify the physician and blood bank. Obtain blood samples according to policy from a large peripheral vein using a 19-gauge needle.
33. 1
34. Walking places stress on the long bones and thus increases calcium absorption.
35. emotional support due to the frightening nature of the symptoms
36. True, False, False, False, False, True, True, True, True
37. reticulocytes, 5 – 10 days
38. high doses of folate, cobalamin, and pyridoxine
39. an opioid
40. 2
41. allopurinol 100 – 300 mg/daily
42. True, False, True, True, False, False, False
43. 4
44. 3
45. 4

CHAPTER 78

1. 1
2. 1, 2, 4
3. a. inhalation, b. injection, c. ingestion, c. direct contact
4. 2, 3
5. a. 5, b. 1, c. 3, d. 2, e. 4
6. T cells
7. a. immediate/anaphylactic, b. cytolytic/cytotoxic, c. immune complex, d. cell-mediated or delayed
8. 4
9. a. 4, b. 1, c. 3, d. 2
10. 4
11. Arthus
12. 3
13. a. client history, b. clinical manifestations during or after an allergic exposure, c. results of commonly used allergy tests
14. a. food allergies, b. food intolerances
15. 4
16. a. 5, b. 3, c. 1, d. 2
17. a. 6, b. 4, c. 1, d. 3, e. 2, f. 5
18. True, True, False, False, True, True
19. 4
20. 1, 3
21. 3
22. a. stop the transfusion, b. maintain an open IV line, c. assess the client's vital signs, d. notify the physician
23. Obtain an allergy history and document findings in the medical record.

24. 3
25. a. apply a cool compress, a topical steroid or antihistamine, b. administer an oral antihistamine.
26. Clients are asked to wait so that immediate reactions can be treated.
27. client education
28. 3
29. The newer agents do not cross the blood brain barrier and therefore do not cause significant drowsiness.
30. 4
31. a. antihistamines, b. topical corticosteroids, c. antibiotics
32. antihistamine
33. True, True

CHAPTER 79
1. Arthritis
2. 1, 2, 4, 5, 6, 7
3. 2, 3, 4
4. a. swan-neck deformity, b. boutonniere deformity, c. carpal tunnel syndrome
5. C: calcium deposits in the tissues
R: Raynaud's phenomenon
E: esophageal hardening
S: scleroderma of the digits
T: telangiectasis (capillary dilations on face, lips and fingers)
6. WHITE: Vasospasm causes constriction of blood vessels: pallor of fingers
BLUE: Venous congestion and cyanosis: blue coloring
RED: Vasospasm resolves with hyperemia due to vasodilation: red coloring
7. Lyme disease
8. ACR 20
9. 1, 2, 3, 4, 5
10. ulnar nerve entrapment
11. systemic lupus erythmatosus
12. Repetitive actions can produce trauma to the joint and result in bursitis. This information will also aid in measures to prevent further trauma.
13. 1, 2, 3
14. 3
15. a. improve joint motion; passive ROM can assist in preventing contractures
b. preserve or improve the muscle's ability to do work
c. build strength and prevent injury
16. a. making the client comfortable according to what has worked in the past, b. listening to and learning from clients, c. reducing anxiety, d. enlisting family and community support
17. 1, 2, 3, 4

18. 1, 2, 4, 5
19. 1, 2, 3, 4, 5
20. steroids, immunosuppressive agents
21. impaired renal function
22. Nifedipine
23. Penicillamine
24. a. L-tryptophan to increase sleep, b. tricyclic antidepressants to inhibit serotonin uptake, c. NSAIDs/corticosteroids for pain control
25. It decreases the production of rheumatoid factors which cause inflammation, edema, and pain. It also decreases the number of immune complexes which are deposited in the synovium, causing inflammation and pain
26. The inflammation releases lysosomal enzymes which attack the synovial tissue resulting in swelling and eventual loss of joint space.
27. Glucocorticoids, ASA, and NSAIDs
28. Inflammation causes release of macrophages and leukocytes to the area, which normally attack "foreign" tissue. Rheumatoid arthritis is an autoimmune disease that causes immune cells to attack "self" causing destruction.
29. joint swelling, muscle spasms
30. joint fusion, loss of joint space. Rheumatoid nodules are most often temporary.

CHAPTER 80
1. subtype B
2. a. sexual practices, b. exposure to blood, c. perinatal transmission
3. needle stick
4. a, d, c, e, g, b, f
5. 22/mm³
6. A long-term non-progressor is someone who is HIV positive and after many years shows no signs of disease progression. A long-term survivor is someone who has lived for more than 8 years after an AIDS diagnosis.
7. 4 to 12
8. 4
9. a. bacterial, b. fungal, c. protozoal, d. viral
10. 4
11. a. ingestion of contaminated food, b. drinking contaminated water, c. ingesting contaminated drugs or diagnostic agents, d. directly handling contaminated feces, e. sexual activity involving oral-anal contact
12. a. needle sharing, b. environmental exposure, c. heavy alcohol use, d. smoking, e. inadequate nutrition
13. intertrigo
14. coughing

15. False, True, True, True, False, True, False, True, True
16. a. laboratory data (CD4 cell counts), b. clinical presentation
17. 3
18. existing level of knowledge
19. a. severity of symptoms, b. presence of renal or hepatic disease
20. False, True
21. Follow Standard Precautions when handling blood and body fluids and when performing procedures that could lead to exposure to blood and body fluids.
22. a. time of initial HIV-positive diagnosis, b. time of initial AIDS diagnosis, c. changes in treatment, d. development of new manifestations, e. recurrence of problems or relapse, f. terminal illness
23. 1, 4, 5, 6
24. 8 ounces of yogurt made from live cultures
25. a. keep the client in a warm room to avoid shivering, b. apply a sheet and loosely woven blanket, c. avoid fanning bed covers, exposing the skin or rapidly removing clothing
26. This causes defensive vasoconstriction and shivering which may increase the temperature.
27. 3
28. True, True, False, True, False, True
29. a. do not inject drugs, b. use sterilized injection paraphernalia and never share needles and syringes, c. clean injection paraphernalia with full-strength bleach before injecting
30. 4
31. zidovudine (Retrovir, AZT)
32. a. 3, b. 4, c. 5, d. 2, e. 1
33. 95%
34. a. isoniazid, b. rifampin, c. pyrazinamide
35. True, True, True, True, False, False

CHAPTER 81

1. a. 2, b. 4, c. 1, d. 3
2. a. genetic factors, b. exposure to ionizing radiation and chemicals, c. congenital abnormalities, d. primary immunodeficiency and infection
3. acute lymphoblastic leukemia (ALL)
4. acute myeloid leukemia (AML)
5. a. anemia, b. thrombocytopenia, c. leukopenia
6. tumor lysis syndrome
7. 1, 2, 3
8. Allogeneic bone marrow is obtained from a relative or unrelated donor having a closely matched HLA type. Syngeneic bone marrow is donated by an identical twin. Autologous marrow is removed from the intended recipient dur-

ing the remission phase to allow another course of ablative therapy to be given if relapse occurs.
9. 7, 30
10. True, True, True
11. 3
12. bone marrow aspiration
13. 4
14. a. the blood should be human leukocyte antigen (HLA) matched, b. the blood should be cytomegalovirus (CMV) negative
15. 4
16. 3
17. 2
18. True
19. to prevent infection, detect and treat infection early in an effective manner as evidenced by absence of fever, no respiratory difficulty, and neutrophil count greater than 1000/mm³
20. $(1\% + 42\%) \times 1650 = 709.50$
21. No; protective isolation is indicated when the ANC count falls below 500.
22. The nurse should explain that because of the risk of infection the client is on a low-bacteria diet that prohibits raw fresh fruits and vegetables.
23. d. The nurse should question the order for Tylenol because the client should not receive rectal suppositories and the Tylenol may mask the fever.
24. During the acute phase there is an increased risk of introducing blast cells into the CNS.
25. Teach the client that he or she needs a high-carbohydrate diet, that cold foods are tolerated better than hot, spicy foods, and that small, frequent meals may be tolerated more easily.
26. Explain to the client that the hair loss is temporary; however, the hair may have a different texture and color when it returns.
27. They assist the client and family in understanding the disease process and treatment, and in identifying strategies for successful transition from the hospital to home and outpatient care.
28. 1
29. Aspirin decreases platelet aggregation and further contributes to the risk for bleeding.
30. a. adriamycin, b. bleomycin, c. vinblastine, d. dacarbazine. This treatment regimen can be easily delivered with full doses, has fewer side effects, and carries less risk of developing subsequent leukemia.

CHAPTER 82

1. 2
2. Infection

3. within the first 3 months after transplantation
4. after the first 3 months of transplantation
5. 1, 2, 3
6. 1, 2, 3, 4
7. 1, 2, 3, 4
8. Social Security Act
9. 1, 2
10. 4
11. Xenotransplantation
12. 1
13. 1, 2, 3
14. True, True
15. 1, 2, 3
16. 1, 2, 3
17. 1, 2, 3
18. 1, 2, 3
19. 1, 2, 3, 4, 5
20. 1, 2
21. 1, 2, 3, 4, 5

CHAPTER 83
1. 1
2. 1, 2, 3
3. 1
4. 1, 2
5. 2
6. 1, 2, 3
7. 1, 2
8. 1
9. 1, 2, 3
10. 1, 2, 3, 4
11. respiratory failure
12. 1
13. 2

14. 1, 2
15. 1
16. 1
17. 1
18. 1, 2
19. 1, 2
20. 1, 2, 3, 4
21. MAST garment
22. 1, 2, 3
23. 1, 2, 3
24. 1, 2, 3, 4
25. 1, 2
26. 1
27. 1, 2, 3, 4

CHAPTER 84
1. Autotransfusion
2. a. 7, b. 4, c. 2, d. 5, e. 8, f. 6, g. 3, h. 1
3. 1, 2, 3, 4
4. a. 4, b. 2, c. 6, d. 1, e. 5, f. 3, g. 2, h. 8
5. Patient Self Determination Act
6. 1, 2, 3
7. 3
8. 1, 2, 3, 4
9. 1, 2, 3, 4
10. 1
11. 1
12. 2, 3
13. 1, 2, 3
14. 2, 3
15. 2
16. 1, 2, 3, 4
17. 1, 2, 3, 4
18. 2